Stress and Cardiovascular Disease

Paul Hjemdahl • Annika Rosengren
Andrew Steptoe

Editors

Stress and Cardiovascular Disease

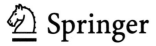 Springer

Editors
Paul Hjemdahl, M.D., Ph.D.
Department of Medicine
Solna; Clinical Pharmacology Unit
Karolinska Institute, Karolinska
University Hospital/Solna, Stockholm
Sweden

Andrew Steptoe, D.Sc.
Department of Epidemiology
and Public Health
University College London
London
UK

Annika Rosengren, M.D., Ph.D.
Institute of Medicine, Sahlgrenska
Academy, Sahlgrenska University
Hospital, Ostra, Gothenburg
Sweden

ISBN 978-1-84882-418-8   e-ISBN 978-1-84882-419-5
DOI 10.1007/978-1-84882-419-5
Springer London Dordrecht Heidelberg New York

British Library Cataloguing in Publication Data
A catalogue record for this book is available from the British Library

Library of Congress Control Number: 2011937320

Printed on acid-free paper

Springer is part of Springer Science+Business Media (www.springer.com)

Preface

Stress is a multifaceted issue which is of considerable interest to physicians and other health care professionals, as well as to their patients and to people in general. The term "stress" is frequently used in different contexts by both professionals and lay people, and means different things to different people. There are many accounts, starting centuries ago, of how acutely stressful situations may precipitate cardiovascular events, especially myocardial infarction and sudden death, and stress is then seen as the culprit by both laymen and professionals. Chronic stress is increasingly being acknowledged as an etiological factor in the development of ischaemic heart disease and other atherosclerotic manifestations, as well as in the development of hypertension and metabolic disturbances which fuel the atherosclerotic process. Research into mechanisms involved in stress-related cardiovascular disease and investigations concerning the role of acute and chronic stress in the causation of cardiovascular disease, and how to manage stress-related problems have attracted much attention. Thus the importance of "stress" for cardiovascular disease is of considerable interest to both researchers and health care professionals with different areas of expertise.

A simple Medline search in 2011 using the term "stress and cardiovascular disease" yields more than 50,000 "hits" with more than 10,000 of them being overviews. Limiting the search to "mental stress and cardiovascular disease" yields 8,500 articles of which more than 1,400 are overviews. Thus there is a wealth of knowledge concerning stress and cardiovascular disease, much of it being valuable information based on high-quality studies. Unfortunately, as in all fields of research, there are also lower-quality studies which may confound interpretation. As editors who collectively have experience from experimental and epidemiological research, as well as in therapeutics, we felt it was timely to summarize the field of research on stress and cardiovascular disease. In doing so, a number of experts on different aspects of stress were invited to contribute, and thereby to focus on what is actually evidence-based in the field.

The book provides up to date information about mechanistic factors, clinical and epidemiological aspects and management issues. The mechanistic part starts out with animal research documenting the capability of inducing coronary heart disease in social stress models, and continues with neuro-hormonal factors, haemostasis and inflammation, as well as recent developments using brain imaging techniques. The clinical and epidemiological section starts out with chapters on the triggering of acute cardiac events and stress cardiomyopathy, and continues with various issues related to chronic stress. Stress at the workplace is dealt with from both epidemiological and practical perspectives. The much discussed, but somewhat elusive, relationship between depression and coronary heart disease is the subject of a thoughtful and critical review. The evolving role of posttraumatic stress and the importance of sleep and recuperation in the context of coronary heart disease are highlighted, as are the contributions of chronic stress to the development of hypertension, and metabolic syndrome and type 2 diabetes. The value of incorporating increased physical activity into stress management programs and individual patient care is addressed in several chapters. The evidence base for psychological treatment of cardiac patients is critically, yet optimistically, addressed in a comprehensive overview and several other chapters. Finally, useful hands-on suggestions on how to deal with stress-related problems in the doctor's office and increase adherence to lifestyle advice are given.

The initiative for this book was taken by Grant Weston at Springer, and we are deeply indebted to him and the development editor Michael Griffin for their support and patience on the sometimes bumpy road towards completion. Most of all, we are very grateful for the high-quality work from all the experienced authors who contributed their knowledge and wisdom in different chapters. It is our hope that this book will contribute to the recognition of "stress" as an important and modifiable risk factor for cardiovascular disease, and that stress and psychosocial factors will be dealt with more seriously than is often the case today in the care of patients who already suffer from such disease. Although research in the area has provided a wealth of knowledge, we also hope that the book will stimulate interest in further studies of stress and cardiovascular disease. There is still much to be uncovered and/or more firmly established concerning the mechanisms involved and how to best manage stress-related problems in the community as well as among patients suffering from cardiovascular disease!

Paul Hjemdahl
Annika Rosengren
Andrew Steptoe

Contents

1 **Introduction to Cardiovascular Disease, Stress and Adaptation** 1
Andrew Steptoe, Annika Rosengren,
and Paul Hjemdahl

Part I   Mechanisms

2 **Social Stress and Cardiovascular Disease in Primates** 17
Carol A. Shively

3 **Cardiovascular and Autonomic Responses to Stress** 31
Paul Hjemdahl and Murray Esler

4 **Sympathetic Neural and Adrenal Medullary Mechanisms in Depression and Panic Disorder** 55
Murray Esler

5 **Hypothalamic–Pituitary–Adrenal Axis and Cardiovascular Disease** 71
Gregory Kaltsas, Anthony S. Zannas,
and George P. Chrousos

6 **Haemostatic Effects of Stress** 89
Paul Hjemdahl and Roland von Känel

7 **Stress, Inflammation, and Coronary Heart Disease** 111
Andrew Steptoe

8 **Brain Imaging of Stress and Cardiovascular Responses** 129
Marcus Gray, Yoko Nagai,
and Hugo D. Critchley

Part II   Acute Stress and Triggering

9   **Psychological Triggers for Plaque Rupture** 151
     Geoffrey H. Tofler, Alexandra O'Farrell,
     and Thomas Buckley

10   **Stress Cardiomyopathy** 169
     Ilan S. Wittstein

Part III   Chronic Stress

11   **Psychosocial Factors at Work:**
     The Epidemiological Perspective 195
     Mika Kivimäki, Archana Singh-Manoux, G. David Batty,
     Marianna Virtanen, Jane E. Ferrie, and Jussi Vahtera

12   **Depression and Cardiovascular Disease Progression:**
     Epidemiology, Mechanisms and Treatment 211
     Petra Hoen, Nina Kupper, and Peter de Jonge

13   **Post-Traumatic Stress Disorder:**
     Emerging Risk Factor and Mechanisms 235
     Roland von Känel and Marie-Louise Gander Ferrari

14   **Sleep, Stress, and Heart Disease** 257
     Torbjörn Åkerstedt and Aleksander Perski

15   **The Causal Role of Chronic Mental Stress**
     in the Pathogenesis of Essential Hypertension 273
     Murray Esler

16   **Metabolic Syndrome and Diabetes** 285
     Annika Rosengren

Part IV   Treatment

17   **Stress Management and Behavior:**
     From Cardiac Patient to Worksite Intervention 299
     Daniela Lucini and Massimo Pagani

18   **Exercise to Reduce Distress and Improve**
     Cardiac Function: Moving on and Finding the Pace 317
     Hugo Saner and Gunilla Burell

Part V   Psychological Management

19   **The Psychological Treatment of Cardiac Patients** 335
     Alena Talbot Ellis and Wolfgang Linden

20 Integrating the Management of Psychosocial and Behavior Risk Factors into Clinical Medical Practice 355
Alan Rozanski

Part VI Conclusions

21 Concluding Remarks 377
Paul Hjemdahl, Annika Rosengren, and Andrew Steptoe

Index 383

Contributions

Torbjörn Åkerstedt Ph.D. Stress Research Institute, Stockholm University, Stockholm, Sweden

G. David Batty M.Sc., Ph.D. Department of Epidemiology and Public Health, University College London, London, UK

Thomas Buckley B.Sc., M.N., Ph.D. Department of Cardiology, Royal North Shore Hospital, Sydney, NSW, Australia
Sydney Nursing School, University of Sydney, Sydney, NSW, Australia

Gunilla Burell Ph.D. Department of Public Health and Caring Sciences, University Hospital of Uppsala, Uppsala, Sweden

George P. Chrousos M.D. First Department of Pediatrics, Aghia Sophia Children's Hospital, Athens, Greece

Hugo D. Critchley M.B.Ch.B., D.Phil., M.R.C.Psych. Department of Psychiatry, Brighton and Sussex Medical School, University of Sussex, Brighton, East Sussex, UK

Alena Talbot Ellis M.A. Department of Psychology, University of British Columbia, Vancouver, BC, Canada

Murray Esler M.B.B.S., Ph.D. Hypertension Thrombosis and Vascular Biology Division, Baker IDI Heart and Diabetes Institute, Melbourne, VIC, Australia

Jane E. Ferrie Ph.D. Department of Epidemiology and Public Health, University College London, London, UK

Marie-Louise Gander Ferrari M.D. Department of General Internal Medicine, Inselspital, Bern University Hospital, Bern, Switzerland
Department of Psychosomatic Medicine, Inselspital, Bern University Hospital, Bern, Switzerland

Marcus Gray Ph.D. Department of Experimental Neuropsychology Research Unit, School of Psychology and Psychiatry, Faculty of Medicine Nursing and Health Sciences, Monash University, Clayton, VIC, Australia

Paul Hjemdahl M.D., Ph.D. Department of Medicine, Solna, Clinical Pharmacology Unit, Karolinska Institute, Karolinska University Hospital/Solna, Stockholm, Sweden

Petra Hoen B.S. Department of Interdisciplinary Center for Psychiatric Epidemiology, University Medical Center Groningen, Groningen, The Netherlands

Peter de Jonge Ph.D. Department of Interdisciplinary Center for Psychiatric Epidemiology, University Medical Center Groningen, Groningen, The Netherlands

Roland von Känel M.D. Department of General Internal Medicine, Inselspital, Bern University Hospital, Bern, Switzerland
Division of Psychosomatic Medicine, Inselspital, Bern University Hospital, Bern, Switzerland

Gregory Kaltsas M.D., F.R.C.P. (Lon.) Department of Pathophysiology, Laiko Hospital, National University of Athens, Athens, Greece

Mika Kivimäki Ph.D. Department of Epidemiology and Public Health, University College London, London, UK

Nina Kupper Ph.D. Department of Medical Psychology, Center of Research on Psychology in Somatic Diseases, Tilburg University, Tilburg, The Netherlands

Wolfgang Linden Ph.D. Department of Psychology, University of British Columbia, Vancouver, BC, Canada

Daniela Lucini M.D., Ph.D. Department of Clinical Science, L. Sacco, University of Milan, Milan, Italy

Yoko Nagai Ph.D. Department of Psychiatry, Brighton and Sussex Medical School, University of Sussex, Brighton, East Sussex, UK
Brighton and Sussex Medical School, Department of Psychology, University of Essex, Brighton, East Sussex, UK

Alexandra O'Farrell B.N. Department of Cardiology, Royal North Shore Hospital, Sydney, NSW, Australia

Massimo Pagani M.D. Department of Clinical Science, L. Sacco, University of Milan, Milan, Italy

Aleksander Perski Ph.D. Stress Research Institute, Stockholm University, Stockholm, Sweden

Annika Rosengren M.D., Ph.D. Institute of Medicine, Sahlgrenska Academy, Sahlgrenska University Hospital, Ostra, Gothenburg, Sweden

Alan Rozanski M.D. Director, Cardiology Fellowship Training Program, Department of Medicine, St. Luke's Roosevelt Hospital Center, Columbia University College of Physicians and Surgeons, New York, NY, USA

Hugo Saner M.D. Cardiovascular Prevention and Rehabilitation, University Hospital Inselspital, Bern, Switzerland

Carol A. Shively Ph.D. Department of Pathology/Comparative Medicine, Wake Forest University School of Medicine, Winston-Salem, NC, USA

Archana Singh-Manoux Ph.D. Centre for Research in Epidemiology & Population Health, Hôpitaux de Paris, Villejuif Cedex, France

Andrew Steptoe D.Sc. Department of Epidemiology and Public Health, University College London, London, UK

Geoffrey H. Tofler M.B.B.S, M.D., F.R.A.C.P., F.A.C.C Department of Prevantative Cardiology, University of Sydney, Sydney, NSW, Australia
Department of Cardiology, Royal North Shore Hospital, Sydney, NSW, Australia

Jussi Vahtera M.D., Ph.D. Department of Public Health, University of Turku and Turku University Hospital, Turku, Finland

Marianna Virtanen Ph.D. Unit of Expertise for Work Organizations, Finnish Institute of Occupational Health, Helsinki, Finland

Ilan S. Wittstein M.D. Department of Medicine/Division of Cardiology, Johns Hopkins University School of Medicine, Baltimore, MD, USA

Anthony S. Zannas M.D., M.Sc. Department of Psychiatry and Behavioral Sciences, Duke University Medical Center, Durham, NC, USA

Chapter 1
Introduction to Cardiovascular Disease, Stress and Adaptation

Andrew Steptoe, Annika Rosengren, and Paul Hjemdahl

Keywords Cardiovascular disease • Stress • Adaptation • Animal research • Naturalistic monitoring • Ambulatory monitoring

Psychological stress is increasingly being recognised as a modifiable cardiovascular risk factor, and is being vigorously investigated in animal studies, human experimental and clinical research, and in population-level epidemiological studies.[1] There is a growing trend for the incorporation of stress management into cardiac rehabilitation programmes and into preventive cardiology. However, stress is multi-faceted and often misunderstood, and requires as much scientific scrutiny as other pathological processes relevant to cardiology. There is thus a need for better understanding of stress and its ramifications by cardiologists and other clinicians caring for cardiac patients, and by those involved in primary prevention. The quality of research into stress management is variable, and care is required in identifying effective evidence-based methods.

The purpose of this multidisciplinary volume is to provide an up-to-date survey of research relating stress with cardiovascular disease, highlighting the clinical implications of physiological and population studies of stress. Our ultimate aim is to aid physicians in their management of stress-related issues in cardiac patients and

A. Steptoe (✉)
Department of Epidemiology and Public Health, University College London, London, UK
e-mail: a.steptoe@ucl.ac.uk

A. Rosengren
Institute of Medicine, Sahlgrenska Academy, Sahlgrenska University Hospital, Ostra, Gothenburg, Sweden
e-mail: annika.rosengren@hjlgu.se

P. Hjemdahl
Department of Medicine, Solna, Clinical Pharmacology Unit, Karolinska Institute, Karolinska University Hospital/Solna, Stockholm, Sweden
e-mail: paul.hjemdahl@ki.se

P. Hjemdahl et al. (eds.), *Stress and Cardiovascular Disease*,
DOI 10.1007/978-1-84882-419-5_1, © Springer-Verlag London Limited 2012

high-risk individuals. Each chapter addresses a particular aspect of this exciting field of basic and clinical research. The chapters illustrate how the study of stress and cardiovascular disease has broadened over the past few decades to involve disciplines such as neuroimaging, epidemiology, psychiatry, sleep medicine and exercise science as well as clinical and experimental research. This chapter sets out the background for studies of stress and adaptation in cardiovascular disease, outlining the nature and extent of the cardiovascular problems under investigation, the conceptualisation of stress, and the methodological approaches used in research.

1.1 Cardiovascular Disease

Atherosclerotic cardiovascular diseases (CVD) include coronary heart disease (CHD), stroke, and peripheral arterial disease. CVDs are the number one cause of death globally: more people die annually from CVD than from any other cause, with an estimated one-third of all global deaths being due to CVD. Four out of five CVD deaths currently occur in low- and middle-income countries. The increase in CVD that took place during the twentieth century is partially explained by a longer life expectancy, but also by economic and human development such as urbanization and industrialization, with concomitant changes in work conditions, transportation, diet and social networks, all of which have a direct impact on risk factors for CVD. CHD is the single most common cause of death in the Westernized world, and the second globally, with stroke being the fifth most common cause of death in the world. CVD results in substantial disability and loss of productivity and contributes in a large part to the escalating costs of health care.

During the last two decades, considerable evidence has accumulated with respect to the association of markers of stress and other psychosocial factors with CVD, chiefly CHD, but also stroke. Compared with other major risk factors, however, psychosocial variables are more difficult to define objectively because several different dimensions are involved. Despite this, several separate constructs within the broad conceptual framework of psychosocial factors are increasingly considered as being causally related to CHD. Dimensions such as stress at work and in family life, life events, low perceived control, lack of social support, socioeconomic status, and depression have been shown to either influence the risk of CHD or affect prognosis in CHD patients, as will be illustrated in several chapters in this book. The INTERHEART study[2] has highlighted the importance of psychosocial factors for CVD in a global perspective.

1.2 Conceptualisation of Stress

Scientific research into stress began with the American physiologist Walter B. Cannon who coined the term 'fight or flight' to describe the integrated biological and behavioural response to threat in his book *Bodily Changes in Pain, Hunger,*

Fear and Rage (1915). Cannon also brought the concept of homeostasis into wider usage, arguing that a series of regulatory systems maintain constancy in physiological processes such as internal temperature, water balance, glucose metabolism and blood pressure, with different pathways responding to reinstate balance after any perturbation. A somewhat different conception of stress was espoused by the Hungarian endocrinologist Hans Selye in the mid-twentieth century. Selye was immensely influential with books such as *The Stress of Life* (1956), though his reputation is now somewhat tainted by the revelations of his involvement with the tobacco industry.[3] Selye described stress as 'the non-specific response of the body to any demand on it', formulating the notion of the general adaptation syndrome. This was described as a three-stage response to exposure to stressful stimuli, beginning with the alarm phase in which there is a massive alteration in regulatory processes affecting blood pressure, glucose, electrolyte balance, blood flow and membrane permeability.[4] The second phase is that of resistance in which the organism mobilises hormonal processes that increase toleration of the challenge. The third phase that of exhaustion, would follow if the stressor continued, with depletion of adaptational processes and increased susceptibility to a range of pathologies.

Selye placed glucocorticoids centre stage in the stress response. But the concept of non-specificity faced many criticisms from researchers identifying different patterns of biological responses with different challenges. An influential review by Munck et al.[5] argued that the role of glucocorticoids was not to activate stress processes, but to act in a protective fashion by regulating overreactions in other systems such as inflammation and carbohydrate metabolism. Modern conceptualisations of biological stress responses are based less strongly on Selye's theories than on the concepts of allostasis and allostatic load championed by Bruce McEwen from the Rockefeller University.[6,7] Allostasis is the ability to achieve stability and the maintenance of homeostasis through change, arising from activities of the autonomic nervous system, the hypothalamic–pituitary–adrenal (HPA) axis, and cardiovascular, immune and metabolic processes. These systems fluctuate in an integrated fashion to enable the organism to respond to the environment and to support behaviours such as eating, sleeping and exercising. Excessive fluctuations can impair regulatory systems, and this is manifest in a progressive failure to maintain levels within normal operating ranges. Allostatic load is the cumulative biological toll of attempting to maintain allostasis in the face of persistent challenge, and affects neuroendocrine systems, autonomic activity, immune function, metabolic processes, brain structure and reproductive function. Although not all features of this model are universally accepted, features such as normal operating ranges, the importance of low-level chronic activation, the damaging effects of underactivity as well as overactivity, and the manifestations of allostatic load as failures of adaptation and impaired recovery, are widely recognised in stress research.

These developments in physiological stress research have been paralleled by progress in the psychological domain. It has long been recognised that the responses to stressful stimuli are not fixed. Take the case of electric shock, the archetypal experimental stressor used in animal research in the twentieth century. Biological responses to shock administration depend not only on duration and intensity, but on

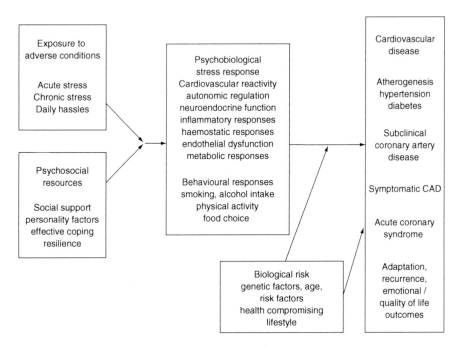

Fig. 1.1 Schematic model of stress and cardiovascular disease

predictability, prior experience, behavioural response requirements, pattern of presentation, the availability of coping strategies and other factors. In humans, the variation in responses to the same stimuli between people, and in the same person at different times is considerable. Even major traumas such as the death of a family member or a natural disaster give rise to a wide spectrum of response intensities.

The fact that the elicitation of a biological stress response is not an inevitable consequence of exposure to a 'stressor' was recognised by Richard Lazarus who formulated the transactional model of stress.[8] This argues that stress responses arise when the demands on the person are not in balance with the adaptive capacity of the person and the resources he or she can bring to bear on the situation. These resources include personality factors, coping strategies, and social factors such as supportive relationships. For example, individuals who are high in hostility tend to be more stress reactive, whereas optimism is associated with diminished inflammatory cytokine responses.[9,10] Lack of social resources is linked with greater acute cortisol reactivity,[11] higher cortisol output over the day,[12] and with lower heart rate variability over the day.[13]

A general conceptualisation of stress and disease is outlined in Fig. 1.1. Biological stress responses arise when the stresses or demands on the individual exceed his or her psychosocial resources. Potential stressors can take several forms, including acute life events, major chronic stressors, and more mundane day-to-day hassles. All three forms are relevant to cardiovascular disease, as is apparent from chapters on acute stress (Tofler et al. Chap. 9, and Wittstein, Chap. 10), and chronic stressors (e.g., Shively, Chap. 2; Esler, Chaps. 4 and 15; Kaltsas et al. Chap. 5; Kivimäki et al. Chap. 11; and Åkerstedt and Perski, Chap. 14). The impact of potential stressors is influenced by their predictability and controllability, and whether habituation takes place with repeated exposure.

The biological stress responses relevant to cardiovascular disease include a complex matrix of haemodynamic, neurohumoral, inflammatory and haemostatic changes that are detailed in Chaps. 3–8. Figure 1.1 also indicates that stress responses do not act in isolation, but against a substrate of genetic, physiological and lifestyle risk factors. It should be emphasised that the purpose of this book is not to argue that stress is the primary cause of cardiovascular disease, or that behavioural methods are the mainstay of cardiovascular prevention and treatment. Rather, these chapters make the case that along with other factors stress-related processes contribute to a range of cardiovascular outcomes, and in some cases may play an important role in disease development. Furthermore, behavioural methods should play a significant role in the care of patients with cardiovascular illnesses.

Understanding the role of stress in cardiovascular disease development and management requires the application of several different scientific methodologies and types of study. No single study or experiment can definitively prove or disprove the impact of stress processes on cardiovascular disease. Rather, the integration of evidence from different sources and types of investigation is required.

1.3   Strategies for Studying Stress in Cardiovascular Disease

1.3.1   Animal Research

Experimental animals must be employed with care in medical research, and utilised under ethically rigorous conditions when the circumstances indicate that there are limited viable alternative methods of investigation. But studies in animals are crucial to understanding the biology of stress and adaptation in cardiovascular disease, the neurochemical systems underlying behaviourally driven physiological adjustments, and the factors contributing to behavioural influences on disease development. Animal research has provided many important insights into the role of stress that could not have been established using other methods. A major advantage of animal studies is that the impact of stress on biological responses and subsequently on objectively determined cardiovascular disease can be examined experimentally within a relatively short period of time. The use of experiments in humans is limited to short-term responses and proxy cardiovascular end points, whereas the complete aetiological process can be documented in animal models. Notable examples include the impact of social stress on coronary artery disease described by Shively (Chap. 2), the animal models of stress in hypertension outlined by Esler (Chap. 15), and the identification of the pathways in the brain regulating neuroendocrine function detailed by Kaltsas et al. (Chap. 5). Animal models are also central to the investigation of behavioural and pharmacological interventions that may ameliorate the impact of stress.

One word of caution about the use of animal models is to avoid the temptation to draw direct parallels between the specific types of stressor that impact on cardiovascular function in animals and humans. The fact, for example, that in some species social disorganisation, or subordinate social status, has a deleterious effect on the cardiovascular system does not mean that the same factors are necessarily relevant to humans. Animal species vary markedly in the effects of the same social factors on physiological systems,[14,15] and human experience depends greatly on psychological and social processes that are difficult to investigate in animals. Animal studies show that stress-related processes can initiate or accelerate cardiovascular pathology, and can provide important insights into relevant pathogenic pathways, but do not show that these mechanisms are necessarily relevant to human disease.

1.3.2 Laboratory Studies in Humans

A second major strategy used in studies of stress and cardiovascular disease involves the measurement of biological responses to experimentally administered stressors in humans. Psychophysiological or mental stress testing involves the measurement of physiological responses to standardised stimuli such as problem-solving tasks or emotionally demanding social interactions. A crucial element is that conditions are perceived as stressful, challenging and involving.[16] When applied carefully, psychophysiological stress testing elicits consistent physiological responses with good test–retest reliability in many biological measures including blood pressure, heart rate, and inflammatory and haemostatic variables.[17,18] The use of psychophysiological stress testing is detailed in this book to understand cardiovascular and autonomic responses by Hjemdahl and Esler (Chap. 3), activation of the hypothalamic–pituitary–adrenal axis by Kaltsas et al. (Chap. 5), haemostatic responses by Hjemdahl and von Känel (Chap. 6), and inflammatory responses by Steptoe (Chap. 7).

Psychophysiological stress testing has several compelling advantages. The first is that responses to psychosocial stimuli can be monitored under environmentally controlled conditions, reducing many of the sources of bias and individual difference that might otherwise be present. Second, direct comparisons of stress responses in different groups can be made, contrasting patients with and without hypertension or coronary heart disease, people at high and low risk of cardiovascular illness, or individuals with and without characteristics such as hostility or panic disorder that may be relevant to cardiovascular risk. Third, experimental designs can be used with randomization to different conditions such as low and high stress controllability,[19] or stress reactivity under standard conditions or in the presence of a supportive friend.[20] Finally, the administration of psychologically stressful stimuli in the laboratory allows responses to be recorded using technically complex methods that would not be possible in other settings. Many of the advances in understanding the biological pathways through which stress impacts on cardiovascular function have emerged because researchers have moved beyond monitoring blood pressure and heart rate to investigate neuroendocrine and immune measures, kidney function, detailed haemodynamic responses, noradrenaline spillover and nerve recordings, vascular endothelial dysfunction and myocardial blood flow. The monitoring of autonomic responses during functional brain imaging has greatly enhanced our understanding of central nervous system processes, as detailed by Gray et al. (Chap. 8).

A typical psychophysiological stress testing session involves instrumentation of the participant, which might be complex if blood is being drawn or regional haemodynamics is being monitored, followed by a period of rest so that baseline levels of physiological function can be established. The participant is then administered standard tasks or stressors for periods that may last anything from a few minutes to several hours depending on the protocol in question. Physiological monitoring may continue throughout the task period and during a varying post-task recovery period. Early research on stress responses focused almost exclusively on the task period itself, but there is increasing interest in the post-task period for two main reasons. First, important differences in responses may emerge following stress that are not apparent during the tasks themselves. For example, it appears that lower socioeconomic status is associated with delayed post-task recovery in cardiovascular and haemostatic variables.[21] This is consistent with the allostatic load concept that emphasises dysregulation of recovery processes as a consequence of sustained stress. Second, some physiological responses are not immediate, but only emerge after several minutes; levels of cortisol in the saliva or blood can take up to 30 min to peak, while inflammatory cytokines such as IL-6 may continue to rise for up to 2 h following stress.[22]

The tasks used in psychophysiological stress testing are not interchangeable, but have distinctive characteristics. Dimensions such as predictability or unpredictability, the level of control and the availability of coping responses are relevant, as is the involvement of social challenges.[23] For example, a meta-analysis of laboratory studies of cortisol responses clearly demonstrated that the largest cortisol increases are observed in response to social-evaluative challenges such as simulated public speaking, rather than during exposure to difficult tasks or aversive stimuli.[24] Some studies involve types of challenge that are specifically designed to tap into certain psychological characteristics, for instance, the use of discussions between married couples about areas of conflict in order to elicit hostile responses.[25] The choice of challenge requires careful consideration, depending on the purpose of the investigation.

Psychophysiological stress testing has been subject to a number of criticisms, including the potential instability of responses, and the relevance of short-term physiological reactions to arbitrary stimuli for long-term cardiovascular health.[26] A recent meta-analysis by Chida and Steptoe[27] of more than 40 longitudinal studies showed that both the magnitude of hemodynamic responses to acute stress and impairment of post-stress recovery predicted future cardiovascular risk, though there was substantial variation between studies. A more challenging criticism is that only relatively short-term biological responses can be recorded, whereas chronic stressors may elicit different response patterns because of habituation, adaptation, and chronic disturbances in autonomic or neuroendocrine regulation. In order to address this issue, laboratory stress testing has been increasingly complemented by naturalistic and ambulatory monitoring methods.

1.3.3 Naturalistic and Ambulatory Monitoring

These studies involve sampling biological variables during everyday life and take several forms, from recordings during stressful tasks such as public speaking, to repeated measures of blood pressure or salivary cortisol over an ordinary day. Naturalistic monitoring in cardiovascular stress research has benefitted considerably from advances in measurement technology, including the development of lightweight ambulatory blood pressure monitors and Holter monitors of the electrocardiogram. These methods are used in cardiovascular stress research to evaluate function in relation to chronic everyday stress, such as studies linking work stress with elevated ambulatory blood pressure and reduced heart rate variability.[28,29] The advantage of these methods is that biological activity is assessed under natural conditions, circumventing some of the problems of ecological validity that are present for laboratory studies. The dynamic covariation between everyday activities, emotions, and biology can also be evaluated. The multiple measures obtained during naturalistic monitoring may provide more stable estimates of cardiovascular risk than are available from clinical measures, since observations are made in many different situations.[30]

There are of course limitations to studies of this kind. The range of biological markers that can be assessed is relatively small in comparison with the more extensive possibilities available in the clinic and the laboratory. Blood pressure, heart rate, heart rate variability, physical activity and salivary cortisol are among the commonest measures, which are relatively easy to record in everyday life. The measurement techniques need to be relatively unobtrusive, so as not to interfere with ongoing activities, and this typically rules out blood sampling. There are factors that influence biological function in everyday life that need to be taken into account in naturalistic studies, including time of day, cigarette smoking, food and caffeine intake, sleep and physical activity. These factors need to be monitored and added to the statistical modelling, so that the independent impact of stress can be examined. Multi-level modelling has become a popular method in the analysis of such data.[31] Another important issue is whether and to what extent participants change their behaviour because they are being monitored in a study. The aim of naturalistic monitoring is to study biology in everyday life, but if behaviour is not typical, this aim is not achieved. For example, there is evidence that physical activity may be reduced during days of ambulatory blood pressure monitoring in comparison with other days, perhaps because participants are uneasy or embarrassed by wearing the equipment.[32]

1.3.4 Observational Epidemiological Studies

Observational studies provide the main evidence base for establishing the contribution of psychosocial factors to the development of cardiovascular disease, and can also be used to identify plausible biological mediators of these associations. Several chapters of this book capitalise on the epidemiological approach, including the contributions from Kivimäki et al. (Chap. 11), Steptoe (Chap. 7), Hoen et al. (Chap. 12), von Känel (Chaps. 6 and 13), Åkerstedt and Perski (Chap. 14), and Rosengren (Chap. 16). Epidemiological studies take several forms, but perhaps the most fruitful in cardiovascular stress research has been the longitudinal observational cohort or population study. Such studies have a number of components: first, the recruitment of a large, preferably representative, population that is screened to ensure they do not already suffer from the end point under investigation (e.g. diabetes, CHD); second, the measurement of exposure to the risk factors being tested (e.g. chronic stress, low social support), along with other factors known to influence the outcome; third, the monitoring of the population over time, measuring the development of CHD, hypertension or diabetes; and finally, multivariate analysis to test whether exposure to the risk factor is associated with the end point after the covariates have been controlled.

The major advantage of observational cohort studies is that they can be sufficiently large to be able to document associations between stress and future clinical cardiovascular outcomes, unlike laboratory or naturalistic monitoring studies. Only with this strategy is it possible to draw conclusions about whether stress experience predicts cardiovascular morbidity and mortality. But there are also limitations, many of which are discussed in later chapters. Longitudinal observational studies take many years before sufficient numbers of cases accrue for meaningful analysis, so it is difficult to answer scientific questions quickly. Other methods such as case–control studies[1] can be completed more rapidly and produce valuable findings[1] but have disadvantages such as the retrospective nature of data collection.[33] In these retrospective studies lack of or poor attention to the quality of measurements of possibly confounding factors may create problems. However, a nested case–control study, within an observational cohort study or a clinical trial, is also a possibility.

The level of detail in measurement in population studies is often lower than in more intensive clinical and laboratory investigations; biological indicators are typically assessed at rest on a single occasion rather than dynamically, and stress measures are often restricted to brief questionnaires. When a study lasts many years, it is difficult to be confident that the stress exposure is stable, since the circumstances for participants may change. Thus, projects that rely only on baseline assessments only may generate misleading results.[34] In addition, there are difficulties in establishing causality. Because a stress factor is associated with future cardiovascular disease does not mean that it is a causal relationship. The association may be dependent on confounding factors that are related both to stress and cardiovascular end points (such as low socio-economic status). Epidemiologists use multivariate statistics to test confounders, but unmeasured or unappreciated covariates of importance may be involved, and it is often difficult to be confident that residual confounding is not present. Strategies for addressing these issues are described in later chapters.

1.3.5 Clinical Research on Stress

Clinical research is crucial to understanding the contribution of stress to cardiovascular disease, as exemplified in several chapters of this book. Clinical research takes many forms, and may include physiological investigations of the type summarised earlier. Interviews with patients and the administration of standardised and validated questionnaires about psychological states are central to, for example, the study of stress as a trigger of cardiac events (Tofler et al. Chap. 9; Wittstein, Chap. 10), and the evaluation of depression and post-traumatic stress disorder in patients with CHD (Hoen et al. Chap. 12; von Känel and Gander, Chap. 13). Standardisation of procedures can be challenging, but is vital to the collection of high-quality systematic evidence.

One of the difficulties in the interpretation of assessments of emotional state in cardiac patients is that some evaluations are necessarily retrospective and may be flawed by recall bias. For example, interviews concerning the social and emotional circumstances surrounding the triggering of acute MI or the development of stress cardiomyopathy require patients to recall the situation prior to the cardiac event. Similarly, studies of depression following acute coronary syndrome often include evaluation of the patient's emotional state before hospital admission. Investigators are well aware that such data need to be interpreted cautiously, since patients' retrospective accounts may be coloured by their subsequent experience.[35] For instance, patients who have survived an acute MI may come to the view that it was caused by stress, so re-evaluate their lives before the illness in that light. Because most acute cardiac events are unpredictable, it is difficult to obtain data from the person beforehand. Studies of the emotional experiences of patients also of course exclude individuals who died during the acute cardiac episode. There has been some research involving interviewing of relatives about the emotional states of victims of sudden cardiac death, but this approach is rare.[36,37]

Another issue in the interpretation of psychological data from patients with cardiovascular disorders is the impact of disease awareness and labelling. For example, a substantial proportion of hypertension is undetected in the population because many people never have their blood pressure measured. Identification of hypertension occurs through a number of pathways including routine screening, but often emerges because people go to their physicians complaining of non-specific symptoms. Individuals identified in this way may not be typical of hypertensives in general. In addition, the label of hypertension may elicit distress and impair quality of life.[38] A recent epidemiological study evaluated psychological distress in people who were found to have elevated blood pressure on clinical examination, individuals who had a physician diagnosis of hypertension, and normotensives.[39] It was found that aware hypertensives had raised distress scores, while unaware hypertensives did not. In a series of analyses of young army recruits, it was found that individuals who were told their blood pressure was elevated showed heightened blood pressure and catecholamine responses to acute stress tests, compared with participants with equally high blood pressures who had not been given a diagnosis.[40,41] These findings indicate that care must be taken in the interpretation of psychological and physiological observations on patients with diagnosed cardiovascular disorders.

1.3.6 Prevention and Treatment Studies

Research on understanding the role of stress in cardiovascular disease is ultimately designed to help prevent future illness and enhance the well-being of patients with current disease. Several chapters describe psychological and behavioural methods including stress management, exercise training, and the integration of psychological approaches into clinical practice (Lucini & Pagani, Chap. 17; Saner & Burell, Chap. 18, Tablot-Ellis & Linden, Chap. 19, and Rozanski, Chap. 20). Randomised controlled trials are fundamental in intervention research, so as to rule out the impact of non-specific factors (unknown or known confounders). Protocols for the development and evaluation of complex interventions have been devised,[42,43] and there are many issues that need to be taken into account. These include the distinction between efficacy trials in which the intervention is tested under tight experimental control, and effectiveness studies that evaluate the generalisability of the intervention and its effectiveness in clinical practice. Both types of trial are important, but the combination is rare in psychological and behavioural interventions in the cardiovascular domain.[44,45] The choice of control or comparison condition is also complicated, with standard care conditions, treatment as usual, or enhanced usual care all being employed.[46]

New guidelines analogous to the CONSORT criteria for medical randomised controlled trials are being developed to encourage improvements in the quality of planning and reporting of psychological treatment research.[47] When documenting pharmaceuticals it is especially important to be stringent in the reporting of clinical trial results due to the financial interests involved. Trials nowadays have to be registered in a database such as ClinicalTrials.gov for the sake of accountability, and the CONSORT statement[48] provides detailed advice on how to report trial results. Nonetheless, publication bias and selective reporting are phenomenona which can distort the generally available information on drug efficacy, as shown by studies comparing published data on antidepressant drugs with data submitted to Government Authorities in Europe[49] and the USA[50] which must have access to all data gathered on the drugs to assure their efficacy and safety. Hopefully, this problem will diminish due to the requirements for transparency by making trial protocols publicly available. These issues are more difficult to evaluate with regard to epidemiological studies. When evaluating the literature regarding stress and its management it is thus a considerable advantage if several studies agree on important findings. The application of these methodologies and precautions to studies in the cardiovascular domain will increase the credibility of behavioural intervention research, leading to better integration of the methods into clinical care.

References

1. Fink G (ed.) *Encyclopedia of Stress*, 4 vols. Oxford: Academic Press; 2007.
2. Rosengren A, Hawken S, Ounpuu S, et al. Association of psychosocial risk factors with risk of acute myocardial infarction in 11119 cases and 13648 controls from 52 countries (the INTERHEART study): case-control study. *Lancet.* 2004;364:953-962.
3. Petticrew MP, Lee K. The "Father of Stress" meets "Big Tobacco": Hans Selye and the tobacco industry. *Am J Public Health.* 2010;101(3):411-418.
4. McCarty R, Pacak K. Alarm phase and general adaptation syndrome. In: Fink G, ed. *Encyclopedia of Stress*, vol. 1. 2nd ed. Oxford: Elsevier; 2007:119-123.
5. Munck A, Guyre PM, Holbrook NJ. Physiological functions of glucocorticoids in stress and their relation to pharmacological actions. *Endocr Rev.* 1984;5:25-44.
6. McEwen BS, Stellar E. Stress and the individual. Mechanisms leading to disease. *Arch Intern Med.* 1993;153:2093-2101.
7. McEwen BS. Protective and damaging effects of stress mediators. *N Engl J Med.* 1998;338:171-179.
8. Lazarus RS. *Psychological Stress and the Coping Process.* New York: McGraw-Hill; 1966.
9. Brydon L, Walker C, Wawrzyniak AJ, et al. Dispositional optimism and stress-induced changes in immunity and negative mood. *Brain Behav Immun.* 2009;23:810-816.
10. Chida Y, Hamer M. Chronic psychosocial factors and acute physiological responses to laboratory-induced stress in healthy populations: a quantitative review of 30 years of investigations. *Psychol Bull.* 2008;134:829-885.
11. Eisenberger NI, Taylor SE, Gable SL, et al. Neural pathways link social support to attenuated neuroendocrine stress responses. *Neuroimage.* 2007;35:1601-1612.
12. Grant N, Hamer M, Steptoe A. Social isolation and stress-related cardiovascular, lipid, and cortisol responses. *Ann Behav Med.* 2009;37:29-37.
13. Horsten M, Ericson M, Perski A, et al. Psychosocial factors and heart rate variability in healthy women. *Psychosom Med.* 1999;61:49-57.
14. Abbott DH, Keverne EB, Bercovitch FB, et al. Are subordinates always stressed? A comparative analysis of rank differences in cortisol levels among primates. *Horm Behav.* 2003;43:67-82.
15. Ely D, Caplea A, Dunphy G, et al. Physiological and neuroendocrine correlates of social position in normotensive and hypertensive rat colonies. *Acta Physiol Scand Suppl.* 1997;640:92-95.
16. Singer MT. Engagement – involvement: a central phenomenon in psychophysiological research. *Psychosom Med.* 1974;36:1-17.
17. Kamarck TW, Lovallo WR. Cardiovascular reactivity to psychological challenge: conceptual and measurement considerations. *Psychosom Med.* 2003;65:9-21.
18. Hamer M, Gibson EL, Vuononvirta R, et al. Inflammatory and hemostatic responses to repeated mental stress: individual stability and habituation over time. *Brain Behav Immun.* 2006;20:456-459.
19. Bohlin G, Eliasson K, Hjemdahl P, et al. Pace variation and control of work pace as related to cardiovascular, neuroendocrine and subjective responses. *Biol Psychol.* 1986;23:247-263.
20. Kamarck TW, Manuck SB, Jennings JR. Social support reduces cardiovascular reactivity to psychological challenge: a laboratory model. *Psychosom Med.* 1990;52:42-58.
21. Steptoe A, Feldman PM, Kunz S, et al. Stress responsivity and socioeconomic status: a mechanism for increased cardiovascular disease risk? *Eur Heart J.* 2002;23:1757-1763.
22. Steptoe A, Poole L. Use of biological measures in behavioral medicine. In: Steptoe A, ed. *Handbook of Behavioral Medicine.* New York: Springer; 2010:619-632.
23. Steptoe A, Vögele C. The methodology of mental stress testing in cardiovascular research. *Circulation.* 1991;83:II14-II24.

24. Segerstrom SC, Miller GE. Psychological stress and the human immune system: a meta-analytic study of 30 years of inquiry. *Psychol Bull.* 2004;130:601-630.
25. Kiecolt-Glaser JK, Loving TJ, Stowell JR, et al. Hostile marital interactions, proinflammatory cytokine production, and wound healing. *Arch Gen Psychiatry.* 2005;62:1377-1384.
26. Parati G, Trazzi S, Ravogli A, et al. Methodological problems in evaluation of cardiovascular effects of stress in humans. *Hypertension.* 1991;17(4 Suppl):III50-III55.
27. Chida Y, Steptoe A. Greater cardiovascular responses to laboratory mental stress are associated with poor subsequent cardiovascular risk status: a meta-analysis of prospective evidence. *Hypertension.* 2010;55:1026-1032.
28. Landsbergis PA, Schnall PL, Pickering TG, et al. Life-course exposure to job strain and ambulatory blood pressure in men. *Am J Epidemiol.* 2003;157:998-1006.
29. Vrijkotte TG, van Doornen LJ, de Geus EJ. Effects of work stress on ambulatory blood pressure, heart rate, and heart rate variability. *Hypertension.* 2000;35:880-886.
30. Conen D, Bamberg F. Noninvasive 24-h ambulatory blood pressure and cardiovascular disease: a systematic review and meta-analysis. *J Hypertens.* 2008;26:1290-1299.
31. Schwartz JE, Stone AA. Strategies for analyzing ecological momentary assessment data. *Health Psychol.* 1998;17:6-16.
32. Costa M, Cropley M, Griffith J, et al. Ambulatory blood pressure monitoring is associated with reduced physical activity during everyday life. *Psychosom Med.* 1999;61:806-811.
33. Elwood M. *Critical Appraisal of Epidemiological Studies and Clinical Trials.* 3rd ed. Oxford: Oxford University Press; 2007.
34. Stringhini S, Sabia S, Shipley M, et al. Association of socioeconomic position with health behaviors and mortality. *JAMA.* 2010;303:1159-1166.
35. Strike PC, Steptoe A. Behavioral and emotional triggers of acute coronary syndromes: a systematic review and critique. *Psychosom Med.* 2005;67:179-186.
36. Rissanen V, Romo M, Siltanen P. Premonitory symptoms and stress factors preceding sudden death from ischaemic heart disease. *Acta Med Scand.* 1978;204:389-396.
37. Greene WA, Goldstein S, Moss AJ. Psychosocial aspects of sudden death. A preliminary report. *Arch Intern Med.* 1972;129:725-731.
38. Pickering TG. Now we are sick: labeling and hypertension. *J Clin Hypertens (Greenwich).* 2006;8:57-60.
39. Hamer M, Batty GD, Stamatakis E, et al. Hypertension awareness and psychological distress. *Hypertension.* 2010;56:547-550.
40. Rostrup M, Kjeldsen SE, Eide IK. Awareness of hypertension increases blood pressure and sympathetic responses to cold pressor test. *Am J Hypertens.* 1990;3(12 Pt 1):912-917.
41. Rostrup M, Mundal HH, Westheim A, et al. Awareness of high blood pressure increases arterial plasma catecholamines, platelet noradrenaline and adrenergic responses to mental stress. *J Hypertens.* 1991;9:159-166.
42. Craig P, Dieppe P, Macintyre S, et al. Developing and evaluating complex interventions: the new Medical Research Council guidance. *BMJ.* 2008;337:a1655.
43. Ogilvie D, Craig P, Griffin S, et al. A translational framework for public health research. *BMC Public Health.* 2009;9:116.
44. Lewin B, Robertson IH, Cay EL, et al. Effects of self-help post-myocardial-infarction rehabilitation on psychological adjustment and use of health services. *Lancet.* 1992;339:1036-1040.
45. Moore RK, Groves DG, Bridson JD, et al. A brief cognitive-behavioral intervention reduces hospital admissions in refractory angina patients. *J Pain Symptom Manage.* 2007;33:310-316.
46. Freedland KE, Carney RM, Lustman PJ. Trial design in behavioral medicine. In: Steptoe A, ed. *Handbook of Behavioral Medicine.* New York: Springer; 2010:925-939.
47. Boutron I, Moher D, Altman DG, et al. Extending the CONSORT statement to randomized trials of nonpharmacologic treatment: explanation and elaboration. *Ann Intern Med.* 2008;148:295-309.

48. Moher D, Hopewell S, Schulz KF, et al. CONSORT 2010 explanation and elaboration: updated guidelines for reporting parallel group randomised trials. *BMJ.* 2010;340:c869.
49. Melander H, Ahlqvist-Rastad J, Meijer G, et al. Evidence b(i)ased medicine – selective reporting from studies sponsored by pharmaceutical industry: review of studies in new drug applications. *BMJ.* 2003;326:1171-1175.
50. Turner EH, Matthews AM, Linardatos E, et al. Selective publication of antidepressant trials and its influence on apparent efficacy. *N Engl J Med.* 2008;358:252-260.

Part I
Mechanisms

Chapter 2
Social Stress and Cardiovascular Disease in Primates

Carol A. Shively

Keywords Social stress • Coronary artery atherosclerosis • Social reorganization • Social isolation • Social strangers • Social status • Cholesterol • Ovarian function • Ovariectomy • Depression • Autonomic nervous system • Sympathetic nervous system • Hypothalamic–pituitary–adrenal axis • Visceral obesity • Inuslin resistance • Hyperglycemia • Dyslipidemia • Proinflammatory cytokines

2.1 Introduction

2.1.1 Coronary Artery Atherosclerosis (CAA) and Coronary Heart Disease (CHD) Risk

Atherosclerosis of the coronary arteries (CAA) and its complications are the principal pathological processes that result in coronary heart disease (CHD). Cynomolgus monkeys (*Macaca fascicularis*) are a well-characterized animal model of susceptibility to diet-induced atherogenesis. Cynomolgus monkeys imported as adults have little or no atherosclerosis. Atherogenesis begins when the monkeys begin to consume diets containing fat and cholesterol. Like human beings, the monkeys become hypercholesterolemic, and develop fatty streaks in the coronary and other arteries, which progress to the formation of atherosclerotic plaque. If the plaques are allowed to progress they will develop necrosis, mineralization, and crystalline clefts of cholesterol, similar to the plaques of human beings. Cynomolgus monkeys will eventually develop clinical manifestations including myocardial

C.A. Shively
Department of Pathology/Comparative Medicine,
Wake Forest University School of Medicine,
Winston-Salem, NC, USA
e-mail: cshively@wfubmc.edu

P. Hjemdahl et al. (eds.), *Stress and Cardiovascular Disease*,
DOI 10.1007/978-1-84882-419-5_2, © Springer-Verlag London Limited 2012

infarction.[1-3] Thus, this species has been used widely for many years as a model of CAA. Unless stated otherwise, in the experiments discussed below imported monkeys were fed a moderately atherogenic diet containing 0.25–0.39 mg cholesterol/cal and 38–43% of calories from primarily saturated fat.

2.1.2 Laboratory Social Stressors

Like human beings, cynomolgus monkeys have an obligate social system; that is, they rely on social relationships to provide for many of the necessities of life. While the benefits of social living are numerous, there are costs which include the strife that comes with social density and proximity. Individuals compete for access to resources which may become critical when resources are scarce. Those that have prioirty of access to resources are dominant. Unfamiliar animals face the social challenge of working out their status relationships. Monkeys exhibit preferences for specific individuals in their groups as evidenced by spending time with them in grooming bouts and passive physical contact. Preferred partners are often allies in disputes over resources. The effects of several types of social stressors on CAA and CAA risk factors have been studied in nonhuman primates. Most of these are reminiscent of social challenges commonly experienced by human beings.

1. *Social reorganization*: Monkeys are housed in small social groups for several weeks to months until the constituents have formed stable social relationships. Then the constituency of the group is changed requiring the reestablishment of dominance relationships and social alliances. Human beings are subject to the stresses of joining new groups when they change schools, jobs, and locations, events that have become commonplace in Western society.

2. *Social strangers*: A related laboratory manipulation involves placing a social stranger in a small group of monkeys for a brief period of time (hours to a few days) as a social challenge. Acute social challenge in the presence of strangers is reminiscent of public-speaking engagements and also similar to aspects of the Trier Social Stress Test used in clinical studies.[4]

3. *Social isolation*: Social isolation, or a lack of social support in human beings is associated with increased cardiovascular disease (CVD) morbidity and mortality.[5,6] Like people, monkeys prefer to be with conspecifics, at least those with which they have friendly relationships. Thus, isolating monkeys from each other in single cages can be used as a laboratory social stressor.

4. *Low social status*: Socioeconomic status in human beings is inversely related to morbidity and mortality of a large number of diseases including CVD and depression, two that will be discussed in depth below.[5,7] Inverse linear relationships between status and disease rates are observable in studies in which the poorest still have the basic necessities including employment, income, and

access to health care such as the Whitehall studies of British civil servants. It is hypothesized that this health gradient results from the increases in the social stress of everyday life due to decreasing resources and control over life that accompany decreasing social status. Social status hierarchies are a central organizing mechamism of virtually all gregarious societies that have been studied including monkey societies. In social groups of macaques, those that are dominant have priority of access to resources, which may become critical during lean times when resources are scarce. Dominants control space and other resources, whereas subordinates have little control over factors which impact the quality of their lives. As reviewed below, health disparities also charcterize low social status in macaques.

2.2 Social Reorganization Stress and Coronary Artery Atherosclerosis in Males

Kaplan and colleagues studied the effects of social reorganization on CAA in adult male cynomolgus monkeys in two experiments. In the first, 30 adult male monkeys were fed a moderately atherogenic diet (0.34 mg cholesterol/cal and 43% of calories from primarily saturated fat) for 22 months and housed in social groups of about five animals each. The constituency of half of the groups was reorganized quarterly the first year and monthly the second year. Social instability resulted in exacerbated CAA, but only in dominant animals. Dominants in unstable social groups had twice the CAA as dominants in stable groups, and twice the CAA as their subordinate counterparts in unstable social groups (Fig. 2.1).[8] The second study used a similar protocol; however, the animals were fed a very low fat and cholesterol diet (0.05 mg cholesterol/cal and nearly devoid of saturated fat). Social instability also resulted in a fivefold increase in CAA in the absence of an atherogenic diet.[9]

Kaplan and colleagues followed up these observations with investigations into the role of autonomic arousal in exacerbation of CAA in response to repeated social reorganization.

To test the hypothesis that sympathetic activation may be an important mechanism through which social factors may promote atherogenesis, all adult male monkeys in a subsequent study were housed in periodically reorganized social groups and fed an atherogenic diet for 26 months. The monkeys in half of the groups also received a β-adrenoreceptor antagonist throughout the study period.[10,11] Untreated dominant monkeys again had twice the amount of coronary atherosclerosis of their subordinate counterparts. However, dominant monkeys treated with the β-adrenoreceptor antagonist developed less than half the coronary atherosclerosis of untreated dominants, and had CAA extent similar to both treated and untreated subordinate animals. Beta-adrenergic blockade did not alter the behaviors or serum lipid concentrations, suggesting that sympathetic activation is a primary mechanism through which social reorganization stress exacerbates CAA.

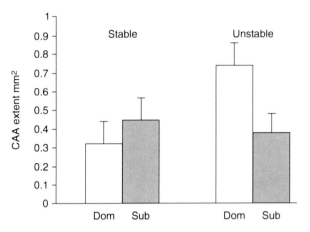

Fig. 2.1 Social instability and coronary artery atherosclerosis (CAA) in males. *Dom* dominant, *Sub* subordinate. Social instability exacerbates coronary artery atherosclerosis, but only in dominant animals ($p = 0.03$) (Adapted from Kaplan et al. (1982)[4])

2.3   Social Subordination Stress, Ovarian Function, and Coronary Artery Atherosclerosis

In the studies discussed below, social status was determined based on the outcomes of agonistic interactions. Simply put, the loser of the interaction is subordinate to the winner. This is also sometimes termed "agonistic dominance." Subordinates receive more aggression, less affiliative social contact in the form of being groomed, are more vigilant, and spend more time alone.[12] Subordinates are also hypercorti-solemic and have higher heart rate responses in an open field test than their domi-nant counterparts.[12] Thus, social subordination in cynomolgus macaques appears stressful both behaviorally and physiologically.

The reproductive system of female mammals is exquisitely sensitive to at least some types of stress. This is most apparent in women with the clinical manifestation of hypothalamic anovulation, but suppression of ovarian function by social factors is well established throughout the mammalian class.[13,14] Female cynomolgus monkeys have menstrual cycles like those of women in length, and cyclic gonado-tropin and ovarian steroid secretion.[15,16] Thus, they are a good model in which to study social stress effects on reproductive function. Subordinate females have impaired ovarian function relative to their dominant counterparts as indicated by low luteal phase peak progesterone concentrations.[17] Since social status is stable over long time periods (years), the ovarian function of subordinate females may be suppressed for long time periods.[18] Females that produce relatively low amounts of progesterone in the luteal phase also produce relatively low amounts of estradiol in the follicular phase. Thus, subordinate females with poor ovarian function are estrogen-deficient.[19]

Although women are protected relative to men, CHD is the leading cause of death in women in the Western world. The female protection from CHD that women enjoy is due to the protective effects of ovarian steroids, particularly estrogen. Female cynomolgus monkeys are also protected relative to males from CAA.[20] Ovariectomy

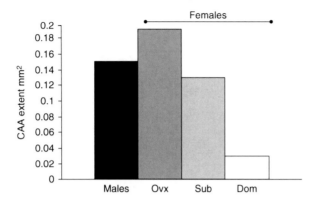

Fig. 2.2 Sex, social status, and coronary artery atherosclerosis (CAA) in females. *Ovx* Ovariectomized females, *Sub* intact subordinate females, *Dom* intact dominant females. Ovariectomy abolishes female protection against CAA ($p<0.02$). CAA is also exacerbated in intact socially subordinate females that have poor ovarian function resulting in no difference between subordinates and ovariectomized females ($p>0.2$) (Adapted from Kaplan et al. (1984) and Adams et al. (1985)[19,21])

results in extensive CAA similar to that observed in males (Fig. 2.2).[19] If estrogen therapy is begun right after ovariectomy, female protection from CAA is restored.[22]

Social subordination in females also results in extensive CAA. A significantly greater proportion of subordinate females develop severe lesions in their coronary arteries than dominant females. CAA extent is associated with the ovarian dysfunction common in subordinate females[19,21,23] (Fig. 2.2). Since subordinates are estrogen-deficient due to ovarian dysfunction, and estrogen protects against CAA, one mechanism through which social subordination stress exacerbates CAA in female monkeys is by suppression of ovarian function.[22,23] It was later observed that women with a history of irregular menses are at increased risk for CHD.[24,25]

2.4 Sex Differences in the Relationship Between Specific Stressors and Coronary Artery Atherosclerosis

From a cardiovascular risk perspective it seems that social instability is a particularly potent social stressor for males resulting in exacerbated CAA, whereas in females social subordination appears to confer the greatest risk for CAA. This may reflect sex differences in sensitivity to particular social stressors. Kaplan and colleagues addressed this possibility in a recent meta-analysis of all relevant studies since 1982 which included 200 females and 219 males from 11 separate investigations. They found that, among males, dominants developed more extensive atherosclerosis than subordinates when housed in recurrently reorganized (unstable) social groups. Dominant males in stable social groups tended to have less atherosclerosis than similarly housed subordinates, but this effect was not significant. In contrast, dominant

Fig. 2.3 Social deprivation and coronary artery atherosclerosis (CAA). *Dom* dominant, *Sub* subordinate. Females housed in single cages had more extensive CAA than those housed in social groups ($p = 0.03$) (Adapted from Shively et al. (1989)[27])

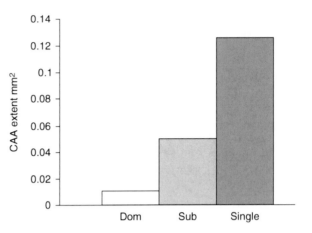

females developed reliably less atherosclerosis than subordinates.[26] Thus, there appear to be sex differences in the biological relevance of specific social stressors.

2.5 Social Isolation Stress and Coronary Artery Atherosclerosis in Females

In the 1980s, studies began to accumulate which suggested that social support might affect CHD. The proper way to quantify this aspect of the social psychological health of human beings was the subject of much discussion. We compared the extent of CAA in female cynomolgus monkeys fed a moderately atherogenic diet for 31 months that were housed either in single cages ($n = 30$) or small social groups of four or five females each ($n = 47$). While socially subordinate females had five times the CAA of dominants, those housed in single cages had more than twice the CAA of social subordinates, and 12 times the CAA extent of social dominants (Fig. 2.3). These differences occurred in the absence of significant differences in plasma lipids.[27] Thus, social deprivation resulted in exacerbated CAA in adult female cynomolgus monkeys. These and the results of subsequent human studies support the conclusion that social isolation or a lack of social support is associated with increased CAA/CHD.[5]

2.6 Social Subordination, Depression, and Coronary Artery Atherosclerosis in Females

There are individual differences in behavioral and physiological responses to social stressors that are relevant to CAA and CHD. For example, compared with dominants, socially subordinate females more frequently exhibit depressive behavior, defined as a slumped or collapsed body posture accompanied by a relative lack of

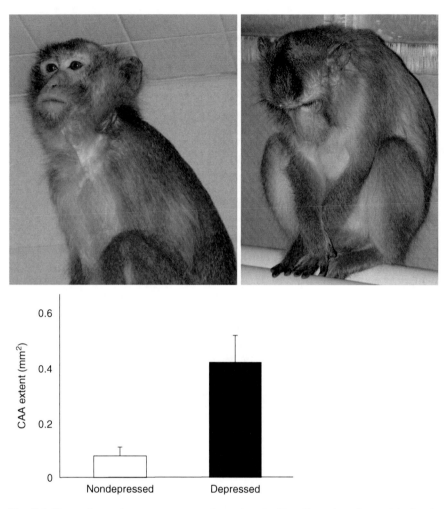

Fig. 2.4 Depression and coronary artery atherosclerosis. *Top*: Examples of an adult female cynomolgus monkey exhibiting behavioral depression, and a nondepressed counterpart; *Bottom*: Depressed monkeys have more coronary artery atherosclerosis than nondepressed females ($p < 0.001$) (Adapted from Shively et al. (2008)[30])

responsiveness to environmental stimuli to which other monkeys are attending, and open eyes.[28] Monkeys that exhibit behavioral depression have many characteristics observed in human depression including perturbed hypothalamic–pituitary–adrenal (HPA) axis function, high heart rates,[29] high insulin-like growth factor, low body weight and body mass index, low activity levels, dyslipidemia, and poor ovarian function. With these number of systems perturbed in depressed female cynomolgus monkeys perhaps it is not surprising that they develop more CAA than their nondepressed counterparts (Fig. 2.4)[30]

While the correlation between CAA and depressive behavior was $r=-0.73$ in this study, the corresponding correlation between social status and CAA was $r=-0.26$. Thus, since more subordinates than dominants exhibit depressive behaivor, depressive behavior seems to identify more precisely which subordinates develop the most extensive CAA.

2.7   Physiological Mechanisms of Social Stress Effects on Atherogenesis and CHD

The two major systems thought to communicate social stress effects to tissues are the autonomic nervous system, and the HPA axis. Perturbations in both appear to affect arterial endothelial function, and the HPA axis is also implicated in platelet aggregation and thrombosis.

Strawn et al.[31] investigated the role of the autonomic system in social-stress-induced endothelial dysfunction in 20 male cynomolgus monkeys fed an atherogenic diet for 10 weeks while housed in single cages. Each monkey was then introduced as a stranger into a four-member social group for 3 days (social stranger challenge). Half the monkeys were treated with a β1-adrenergic blocking agent by subcutaneous implant 2 days before and during group housing. The heart rates of untreated monkeys increased, suggesting a relative increase in sympathetic versus parasympathetic activity, whereas those of the treated monkeys decreased. Endothelial injury as indicated by immunoglobulin G incorporation, endothelial cell replication, and low density lipoprotein concentrations were significantly greater in untreated monkeys than treated monkeys. These results indicate that social disruption is associated with a relative increase in sympathetic nervous system arousal and endothelial dysfunction, and that this effect is mediated via β1-adrenoceptor activation. The observation of endothelial cell injury as indicated by immunoglobulin G incorporation was also observed in male cynomolgus monkeys housed socially for 11 weeks, and then exposed to the 3-day social stranger challenge. This effect was also attenuated by β1-adrenergic blocker treatment.[32]

Mechanisms through which HPA axis secretions may promote CAA or CHD have not been investigated in nonhuman primates. However, in healthy human volunteers subjected to mental stress, stress-related endothelial dysfunction and impairment of baroreceptor sensitivity is prevented by blocking cortisol production with metyrapone. This suggests that cortisol may have a direct or facilitative role on endothelial function and baroreceptor sensitivity, and suggests that stress effects on HPA axis function may contribute to CAA and CHD.[33,34] Fantidis and colleagues[35,36] have demonstrated in pigs that adrenocorticotropin (ACTH), a key peptide in the HPA axis which is released by the pituitary in response to stress, promotes platelet aggregation and thrombosis providing another potential direct effect of the HPA axis on CAA/CHD. The HPA axis may also indirectly affect CAA/CHD risk by promoting visceral obesity, reviewed below, or by inhibiting the gonadal axis contributing to ovarian dysfunction. Since social subordination stress and depression are associated with deleterious effects, and exercise is associated with beneficial effects on HPA axis function in cynomolgus monkeys, it would be useful to investigate HPA mechanisms in social-stress-induced atherogenesis in this model.[12,28,37,38]

2.8   Social Stress, Visceral Fat Deposition, and Cardiovascular Disease

Another mechanistic pathway through which stress may exacerbate CVD is via effects on energy metabolism (Fig. 2.5). Specifically, it appears that stress may affect patterns of fat deposition. In human beings, fat deposited in the viscera is associated with metabolic changes that are known to increase CVD including dylipidemia, hypertension, hyperglycemia, and insulin resistance, as well as a procoagulant and proinflammatory state.[39] Taken together these are referred to as the metabolic syndrome, a powerful predictor of type 2 diabetes mellitus and CVD.[40] In cynomolgus monkeys, central obesity measured anthropometrically, or visceral obesity measured with computed tomography (CT), are associated with similar metabolic changes and exacerbated carotid artery atherosclerosis and CAA.[41-44]

Males that are subjected to repeated social reorganization have more fat deposited in the viscera than those that live in stable social groups.[45] Socially subordinate

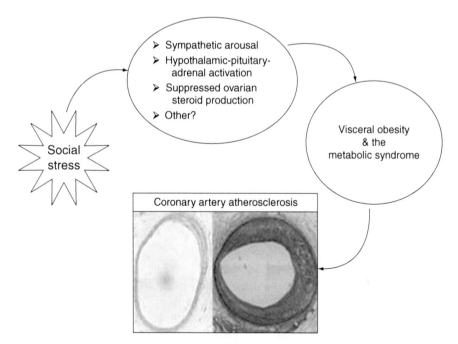

Fig. 2.5 Model of the relationships between social stress, physiological responses to stress, and coronary artery atherosclerosis

females have relatively more fat deposited on the trunk than the periphery.[46] Most recently we studied 41 socially housed females that consumed an atherogenic diet for 32 months. Social behavior and ovarian function were continuously recorded; dexamethasone suppression tests, telemetered overnight heart rate, BMI, visceral (VAT) and subcutaneous abdominal (SAT) adipose tissue were measured with CT before necropsy. Females with high ratios of visceral to subcutaneous abdominal fat (VAT:SAT) were relatively subordinate, socially isolated, received more aggression and less grooming, desensitized to circulating glucocorticoids, had impaired ovarian function, higher heart rates late in the day, and more CAA than low VAT:SAT females. In contrast, the only behavioral or physiological difference observed in females with high-versus-low BMI was that females with high BMI had higher heart rates than low-BMI females. Poor ovarian function in high VAT:SAT females is a novel observation suggesting the need for studies of fat distribution and ovarian function in women. The results of this study were the first to demonstrate a relationship between CAA and visceral obesity, and suggest that social stress may exacerbate CAA in part by increasing the ratio of visceral:subcutaneous fat mass in selected individuals susceptible to diet-induced CAA.[43] These data support the hypothesis that social stress may cause visceral fat deposition and the metabolic syndrome, which, in turn increases CHD.[44]

There are several possible mechanisms through which social stress may promote visceral fat deposition. First, stress may result in sustained glucocorticoid production, which is thought to promote visceral obesity.[47] In the study described above, monkeys with high visceral obesity were relatively insensitive to glucocorticoid negative feedback. Thus, they do not downregulate cortisol production in the face of high cortisol levels, sustaining hypercortisolemia. Another potential mechanism involves sex steroid concentrations. Sex steroids are known to influence fat patterning; thus the suppression of ovarian function resulting in relatively low progesterone and estradiol concentrations may promote visceral obesity.[48] Third, high heart rates are indicative of a shift in autonomic nervous system function in the direction of relatively increased sympathetic arousal. Sympathetic stimulation may also promote the deposition of visceral fat.[43,49,50] Thus, socially stressed monkeys have several characteristics that may promote visceral fat deposition. Further studies are needed to understand the complex and multifactorial temporal relationship among relative social stress, visceral obesity, and CAA.

2.9   Summary

In summary, several types of social stress result in increased CAA and carotid artery atherosclerosis extent in nonhuman primates. The effects of acute social stressors on arterial endothelial function are consistent with the effects of chronic social stress on CAA and CHD risk factors. The effects of some social stressors are sex-specific. Physiological perturbations in response to social stress that appear to promote cardiovascular disease include perturbations in the HPA axis and autonomic nervous system. Both of these appear to promote visceral obesity and the metabolic syndrome which have profound deleterious effects on CVD. There are a number of other important factors that have yet to be studied and for which primate models might be particularly illuminating. These include maternal stress effects on offspring cardiovascular health; relationships between social stress, sleep, metabolic perturbation, and CHD risk; the prothrombotic effects of social stress; and the relationship between social stress effects on eating behavior and CVD risk.

References

1. Armstrong ML, Trillo A, Prichard RW. Naturally occurring and experimnetally induced atherosclerosis in nonhumna primates. In: Kalter SS, ed. *The Use of Nonhuman Primates in Cardiovascular Diseases*. Auistin: University of Texas Press; 1980:58-101.
2. Clarkson TB. Symposium summary. In: Kalter SS, ed. *The Use of Nonhuman Primates in Cardiovascular Diseases*. Austin: University of Texas Press; 1980:452-473.
3. Bond MD, Bullock BC, Bellinger DA, et al. Myocardial infarction in a large colony of nonhuman primates with coronary artery atherosclerosis. *Am J Pathol*. 1980;101:675-692.
4. Kirschbaum C, Pirke KM, Hellhammer DH. The 'Trier Social Stress Test'–a tool for investigating psychobiological stress responses in a laboratory setting. *Neuropsychobiology*. 1993;28 (1–2):76-81.
5. Rozanski A, Blumenthal JA, Kaplan J. Impact of psychological factors on the pathogenesis of cardiovascular disease and implications for therapy. *Circulation*. 1999;99(16):2192-2217.
6. O'Donovan A, Hughes BM. Access to social support in life and in the laboratory: combined impact on cardiovascular reactivity to stress and state anxiety. *J Health Psychol*. 2008;13(8): 1147-1156.
7. Adler NE, Boyce T, Chesney MA, et al. Socioeconomic status and health. The challenge of the gradient. *Am Psychol*. 1994;49(1):15-24.
8. Kaplan JR, Manuck SB, Clarkson TB, Lusso FM, Taub DM. Social status, environment, and atherosclerosis in cynomolgus monkeys. *Arteriosclerosis*. 1982;2(5):359-368.
9. Kaplan JR, Manuck SB, Clarkson TB, Lusso FM, Taub DM, Miller EW. Social stress and atherosclerosis in normocholesterolemic monkeys. *Science*. 1983;220(4598):733-735.
10. Kaplan JR, Manuck SB, Adams MR, et al. Inhibition of coronary atherosclerosis by propranolol in behaviorally predisposed monkeys fed an atherogenic diet. *Circulation*. 1987;76: 1364-1372.
11. Kaplan JR, Manuck SB. The effect of propranolol on social interactions among adult male cynomolgus monkeys (*Macaca fascicularis*) housed in disrupted social groupings. *Psychosom Med*. 1989;51:449-462.
12. Shively CA. Social subordination stress, behavior and central monoaminergic function in female cynomolgus monkeys. *Biol Psychiatry*. 1998;44:882-891.
13. Berga SL, Loucks TL. The diagnosis and treatment of stress-induced anovulation. *Minerva Ginecol*. 2005;57(1):45-54.
14. Shively CA. Reproduction, effects of social stress on. In: Fink G, ed. *Encyclopedia of Stress*. 2nd ed. Oxford: Elsevier; 2007:360-365.
15. Mahoney CJ. A study of the menstrual cycle in *Macaca irus* with special reference to the detection of ovulation. *J Reprod Fertil*. 1970;21:153-163.
16. Wilks JW, Hodgen GD, Ross GT. Endocrine characteristics of ovulatory and anovulatory menstrual cycles in the rhesus monkey. In: Hafez ESE, ed. *Human Ovulation*. Amsterdam: ElsevierMorth-Holland Biomedical Press; 1979:205-218.
17. Kaplan JR, Manuck SB. Ovarian dysfunction, stress, and disease: a primate continuum. *ILAR J*. 2004;45:89-115.

18. Shively CA, Kaplan JR. Stability of social status rankings of female cynomolgus monkeys, of varying reproductive condition, in different social groups. *Am J Primatol.* 1991;23:239-245.
19. Adams MR, Kaplan JR, Clarkson TB, Koritnik DR. Ovariectomy, social status, and athero-sclerosis in cynomolgus monkeys. *Arteriosclerosis.* 1985;5:192-200.
20. Hamm TE Jr, Kaplan JR, Clarkson TB, Bullock BC. Effects of gender and social behavior on the development of coronary artery atherosclerosis in cynomolgus macaques. *Atherosclerosis.* 1983;48:221-233.
21. Kaplan JR, Adams MR, Clarkson TB, Koritnik DR. Psychosocial influences on female 'protection' among cynomolgus macaques. *Atherosclerosis.* 1984;53(3):283-295.
22. Adams MR, Kaplan JR, Manuck SR, et al. Inhibition of coronary artery atherosclerosis by 17-beta estradiol in ovariectomized monkeys. *Arteriosclerosis.* 1990;10:1051-1057.
23. Kaplan JR. Origins and health consequences of stress-induced ovarian dysfunction. *Interdiscip Top Gerontol.* 2008;36:162-185.
24. Solomon CG, Hu FB, Dunaif A, et al. Menstrual cycle irregularity and risk for future cardiovascular disease. *J Clin Endocrinol Metab.* 2002;87:2013-2017.
25. Ahmed B, Bairey Merz CN, Johnson BD, et al. Diabetes mellitus, hypothalamic hypoestrogen-emia, and coronary artery disease in premenopausal women (from the National Heart, Lung, and Blood Institute sponsored WISE study). *Am J Cardiol.* 2008;102:150-154.
26. Kaplan JR, Chen H, Manuck SB. The relationship between social status and atherosclerosis in male and female monkeys as revealed by meta-analysis. *Am J Primatol.* 2009;71(9):732-741.
27. Shively CA, Clarkson TB, Kaplan JR. Social deprivation and coronary artery atherosclerosis in female cynomolgus monkeys. *Atherosclerosis.* 1989;77:69-76.
28. Shively CA, Laber-Laird K, Anton RF. The behavior and physiology of social stress and depression in female cynomolgus monkeys. *Biol Psychiatry.* 1997;41:871-882.
29. Shively CA, Williams JK, Laber-Laird K, Anton RF. Depression and coronary artery athero-sclerosis and reactivity in female cynomolgus monkeys. *Psychosomatic Med.* 2002;64(5): 699-706.
30. Shively CA, Register TC, Adams MR, Golden DL, Willard SL, Clarkson TB. Depressive behavior and coronary artery atherogenesis in adult female cynomolgus monkeys. *Psychosom Med.* 2008;70(6):637-645.
31. Strawn WB, Bondjers G, Kaplan JR, et al. Endothelial dysfunction in response to psychosocial stress in monkeys. *Circ Res.* 1991;68(5):1270-1279.
32. Skantze HB, Kaplan J, Pettersson K, et al. Psychosocial stress causes endothelial injury in cynomolgus monkeys via a1-adrenoceptor activation. *Atherosclerosis.* 1998;136:153-161.
33. Broadley AJ, Korszun A, Abdelaal E, et al. Inhibition of cortisol production with metyrapone prevents mental stress-induced endothelial dysfunction and baroreflex impairment. *J Am Coll Cardiol.* 2005;46:344-350.
34. Broadley AJ, Korszun A, Abdelaal E, et al. Metyrapone improves endothelial dysfunction in patients with treated depression. *J Am Coll Cardiol.* 2006;48(1):170-175.
35. Pozzi AO, Bernardo E, Coronado MT, Punchard MA, González P, Fantidis P. Acute arterial thrombosis in the absence of inflammation: the stress-related anti-inflammatory hormone ACTH participates in platelet-mediated thrombosis. *Atherosclerosis.* 2009;204(1):79-84.
36. Fantidis P. The role of the stress-related anti-inflammatory hormones ACTH and cortisol in atherosclerosis. *Curr Vasc Pharmacol.* 2010;8(4):517-525.
37. Cohen S, Line S, Manuck SB, Heise E, Kaplan JR. Chronic social stress, social dominance and susceptibility to upper respiratory infections in nonhuman primates. *Psychosom Med.* 1997;59:213-221.
38. Williams JK, Kaplan JR, Suparto IH, Fox JL, Manuck SB. Effects of exercise on cardiovascu-lar outcomes in monkeys with risk factors for coronary heart disease. *Arterioscler Thromb Vasc Biol.* 2003;23(5):864-871.
39. Després JP, Lemieux I. Abdominal obesity and metabolic syndrome. *Nature.* 2006;444: 881-887.
40. Després JP. Cardiovascular disease under the influence of excess visceral fat. *Crit Pathw Cardiol.* 2007;6:51-59.

41. Shively CA, Clarkson TB, Miller LC, Weingand KW. Body fat distribution as a risk factor for coronary artery atherosclerosis in female cynomolgus monkeys. *Arteriosclerosis*. 1987; 7:226-231.

42. Shively CA, Kaplan JR, Clarkson TB. Carotid artery atherosclerosis in cholesterol-fed cynomolgus monkeys: the effects of oral contraceptive treatments, social factors and regional adiposity. *Arteriosclerosis*. 1990;10:358-366.

43. Shively CA, Register TC, Clarkson TB. Social stress, visceral obesity, and coronary artery atherosclerosis in female primates. *Obesity (Silver Spring)*. 2009;17(8):1513-1520.

44. Shively CA, Register TC, Clarkson TB. Social stress, visceral obesity, and coronary artery atherosclerosis: product of a primate adaptation. *Am J Primatol*. 2009;71(9):742-751.

45. Jayo JM, Shively CA, Kaplan JR. Effects of exercise and stress on body fat distribution in male cynomolgus monkeys. *Int J Obesity*. 1993;17:597-604.

46. Shively CA, Clarkson TB. Regional obesity and coronary artery atherosclerosis in females: a non-human primate model. *Acta Med Scand Suppl*. 1988;723:71-78.

47. Anagnostis P, Athyros VG, Tziomalos K, Karagiannis A, Mikhailidis DP. Clinical review: the pathogenetic role of cortisol in the metabolic syndrome: a hypothesis. *J Clin Endocrinol Metab*. 2009;94:2692-2701.

48. Mayes JS, Watson GH. Direct effects of sex steroid hormones on adipose tissues and obesity. *Obes Rev*. 2004;5:197-216.

49. Kyrou I, Tsigos C. Stress mechanisms and metabolic complications. *Horm Metab Res*. 2007;39:430-438.

50. Kyrou I, Tsigos C. Chronic stress, visceral obesity and gonadal dysfunction. *Hormones*. 2008;7:287-293.

Chapter 3
Cardiovascular and Autonomic Responses to Stress

Paul Hjemdahl and Murray Esler

Keywords Cardiovascular response • Autonomic responses • Cardiovascular homeostasis • Autonomic nervous system • Sympatho-adrenal system • Catecholamine measurements • Acute mental stress • Chronic mental stress • Peripheral vascular responses • Limb blood flow • Renal blood flow • Pathophysiological considerations

The cardiovascular system typically adapts to acute mental stress by a response pattern called the "defense reaction" which serves to prepare the organism for fight or flight.[1,2] The changes associated with the defense reaction provide short term survival benefit, but they may also provoke acute cardiovascular complications, as discussed in Chap. 9 on the triggering of plaque rupture, and Chap. 10 on stress cardiomyopathy. When elicited repeatedly in individuals living in an urban society with everyday stresses the "defence reaction" may lose its survival value and initiate disease processes such as hypertension and atherosclerosis. Another, less well-studied, response pattern is the "defeat reaction" which has been characterized in animals and may be similar to hopelessness reactions in humans.[3] The deleterious effects of chronic stress and the mechanisms involved have been delineated in a series of interesting primate studies described by Shively in Chap. 2. Chronic stress may be caused by many different factors, as discussed in detail elsewhere in this book, and may involve mechanisms that are quite different from those associated with acute stress.

P. Hjemdahl (✉)
Department of Medicine, Solna, Clinical Pharmacology Unit, Karolinska Institute, Karolinska University Hospital/Solna, Stockholm, Sweden
e-mail: paul.hjemdahl@ki.se

M. Esler
Hypertension Thrombosis and Vascular Biology Division,
Baker IDI Heart and Diabetes Institute, Melbourne, VIC, Australia
e-mail: murray.esler@bakeridi.edu.au

P. Hjemdahl et al. (eds.), *Stress and Cardiovascular Disease*,
DOI 10.1007/978-1-84882-419-5_3, © Springer-Verlag London Limited 2012

Cardiovascular responses to an acute mental challenge are brought about by centrally elicited neuro-hormonal mechanisms that are easily elicited in humans. The key features of the acute "defense reaction" are elevations of blood pressure and cardiac output, and a redistribution of blood flow from inner organs (the splanchnic area and the kidneys) to skeletal muscle while maintaining perfusion of the brain. The "defeat reaction" involves an elevation of blood pressure without an accompanying elevation of heart rate.

The autonomic nervous system with its stimulatory sympathetic (or sympatho-adrenal) system and inhibitory parasympathetic system is of key importance for short-term adaptation to stress and are also involved in chronic stress responses, but then cortisol secretion becomes more important. This chapter will focus mainly on acute stress responses, and describe the differentiated regulation afforded by sympathetic and parasympathetic nerve activity in relation to the possibility of generalized activation by the circulating hormone adrenaline. It will be argued that the classical "stress hormone" adrenaline is a less important mediator of stress responses than nerve activity, but a good indicator of arousal and the perception of stress. Activation of the hypothalamic–pituitary–adrenal (HPA) axis and its conse-quences during chronic stress is discussed in Chap. 5 by Kaltsas et al.

When studying cardiovascular responsiveness to stress, the basality of resting measurements will determine any expression of reactivity to stress. The adequacy of resting conditions may be monitored by, for example, heart rate and plasma adrenaline measurements. Differences in results between studies may simply reflect differences in the attention to the resting measurements. The stress test used should be standardized when comparing stress reactivity between individuals or between groups,[4] and reproducible when studying treatment effects on responses to repeated exposure. Habituation is a potential problem with most stress tests and must be dealt with by choosing good study designs with adequate control conditions. It goes without saying that the amplitude of the stress response is of considerable importance for the possibility to reveal an effect of any intervention.

Many factors, including personality factors, will modulate the perception of stress and the arousal caused by the stressor, as well as the cardiovascular responses elicited by it. A limitation of physiological stress research in the laboratory setting is what relevance responses to a mentally but not emotionally demanding task have compared to responses to real-life stressors. However, detailed physiological measurements in the laboratory form a conceptual basis for the interpretation of responses in real life.

3.1   Cardiovascular Homeostasis

The cardiovascular system is regulated in a complex manner to maintain homeostasis (Fig. 3.1). Neuro-hormonal activity influences blood volume, cardiac output, and blood flow to various organs according to needs for function and survival, and there

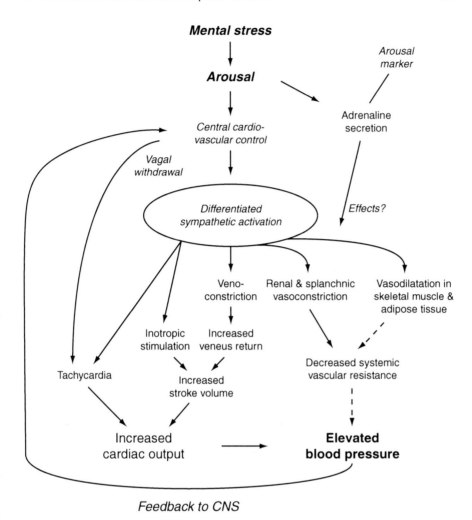

Fig. 3.1 Schematic representation of the cardiovascular response pattern of the defense reaction. The pressor response is mainly cardiac output dependent, and the increase in cardiac output depends mainly on an increase in heart rate. The vascular response is a net reduction of systemic vascular resistance, but responses of individual organs vary considerably. ACTH, cortisol, and adrenaline are markers of the arousal evoked by the stressor (From Hjemdahl[5] with permission from Elsevier)

are compensatory adjustments when the organism is challenged. The fine-tuned cardiovascular system strives to maintain what it perceives as an adequate blood pressure via arterial baroreflexes which serve to dampen short-term changes. If blood pressure rises there is reflexogenic inhibition of the heart and reduced vasoconstrictor nerve activity. Conversely, if the blood pressure decreases there is reflexogenic stimulation of the heart, with increases in heart rate and cardiac output, and a compensatory increase in vasoconstrictor nerve activity which lowers peripheral blood flow (differently in different organs) to maintain central blood pressure and cerebral perfusion. In the long term, baroreflexes may be reset to a new blood pressure level if, for example, a patient with hypertension is treated with a blood pressure lowering drug. There are also receptors which sense venous and cardiac filling pressures, and participate in the regulation of blood volume. If venous pressure decreases reflexogenic and hormonal changes occur, which serve to maintain an adequate filling of the heart during diastole, to conserve salt and water (i.e., to alter renal function), and to maintain blood pressure by adjusting peripheral blood flow. For more detailed information on cardiovascular regulation and the importance of the sympathetic nervous system see, for example, Refs.[1,2,6-9]

The autonomic nervous system and the renin–angiotensin–aldosterone (RAAS) system are keys in cardiovascular adaptation, and the kidney is intimately involved in the regulation of blood pressure according to Guyton's classical theory of cardiovascular homeostasis (see Ref.[1]). Neurogenic mechanisms are important for both short- and long-term levels of blood pressure.[10,11] In addition, autoregulatory mechanisms serve to secure local blood flow and its distribution within an organ. For example, blood flow to the brain is highly autoregulated, and coronary blood flow is governed to a large extent by the metabolic needs of the heart.

Of importance is that the dampening influence of baroreflexes decreases during stress, as centrally elicited pressor mechanisms are less opposed by reflexogenic modulation than blood pressure increases elicited by other maneuvers (Fig. 3.1) (see Refs.[1,2]). As discussed by Julius,[10] there seems to be a blood pressure sensing mechanism which regulates arterial pressure during stress. Interference with one pressor mechanism often leads to another one taking over, resulting in an intact pressor response to the stimulus. Thus, during stress the central nervous system takes greater command over the cardiovascular system to protect the individual.

3.2 Organization and Function of the Autonomic Nervous System

The excitatory sympathetic nervous system (with nerve fibers supplying all organs) and the inhibitory parasympathetic nervous system (from the cardiovascular point of view mainly the cardiac vagal nerves) provide fine-tuned regulation of the cardiovascular system. The adrenal glands secrete the "stress hormone" adrenaline (in US terminology "epinephrine") into the blood stream. The sympathetic neurotransmitter, noradrenaline, may be released in such amounts that spillover into plasma results in levels compatible with a hormonal function also for noradrenaline during intense stress. The parasympathetic neurotransmitter, acetylcholine, is very rapidly cleared at its site of release and thus has no hormonal function. In addition, co-transmission by peptides such as neuropeptide Y (NPY) and calcitonin gene-related peptide (CGRP) stored in the nerves has been identified.[12] Possible roles of co-transmission with peptides and with adrenaline will be briefly commented upon.

3.2.1   The Sympatho-Adrenal System

The sympatho-adrenal system is involved in short-term (phasic) responses to stress via release of noradrenaline and secretion of adrenaline. Sympathetic nerve activity and adrenaline secretion may be simultaneously activated and influence the same (or similar) adrenergic receptors and functions in various organs. However, nerve activity occurs in distinct patterns, and dissociation between the neural and hormonal arms of the sympatho-adrenal system is also seen with certain stimuli. For example, hypoglycemia is a potent and relatively selective stimulus for adrenaline secretion, whereas responses to exercise are mainly neurogenically mediated until the "fuel supply" runs out at exhaustion and adrenaline is recruited to boost metabolism and maintain blood glucose levels.

Noradrenaline is the principal neurotransmitter of sympathetic nerves, although co-transmission by NPY may to some extent contribute to vasoconstrictor responses when sympathetic nerves fire at high frequencies.[13,14] There is variable overflow of NPY-like immunoreactivity from different organs.[15] Mental stress does not appear to activate the sympathetic nerves sufficiently to co-release NPY,[15,16] but strong physical stimuli such as heavy exercise may do so in humans.[15,17]

Adrenaline may, as a circulating hormone, stimulate α- and β-adrenoceptors in all organs. Due to the neuroanatomical distribution of receptor subtypes, the responses to circulating adrenaline will be mainly α_2- and β_2-mediated, whereas neurally released noradrenaline preferentially stimulates α_1- and β_1-adrenoceptors (see Refs.[5,18]). The heart contains both β_1- and β_2-adrenoceptors but responses to cardiac sympathetic stimulation are almost purely β_1-mediated. Comparison of the effects of β_1-selective and nonselective β-blockade on responses to stress thus reveals contributions by adrenaline to cardiovascular responses. Sympathetic nerves may also store and release adrenaline under some circumstances (see below) but adrenaline co-transmission is normally not of importance.

Catecholamines are rapidly cleared from plasma, with half-lives of 1–2 min, but the effect of a sympathetic nerve impulse is much more short-lasting, due to rapid re-uptake of noradrenaline into the nerve and metabolism.[19] Resting levels of noradrenaline in arterial or forearm venous plasma are $\approx$1 nmol/L (169 pg/mL), and threshold levels for hormonal effects are 3–4 nmol/L. Resting adrenaline levels are $\approx$0.2–0.3 nmol/L (30–50 pg/mL) in arterial plasma and half of that in venous plasma due to extraction from arterial plasma in the forearm. During mental challenges there are only mild–moderate elevations of noradrenaline in plasma (depending on the sampling site – see below) but during, for example, intense physical exercise noradrenaline levels may increase to 30–50 nmol/L. Arterial adrenaline levels rarely exceed 1–2 nmol/L; mental stress tests produce only mild elevations (to less than 1 nmol/L), but pronounced hypoglycemia or exhaustive physical exercise can increase adrenaline levels to $\approx$5 nmol/L.[5] Catecholamines in plasma may be measured by different techniques which do not perform equally well in all laboratories; urinary catecholamine measurements are not redundant as they reflect arterial catecholamine levels and thus integrated sympatho-adrenal activity over longer time periods (see Ref.[5]). Urinary catecholamines may be useful for "field" studies, but variations in the renal catecholamine handling (even after normalization for creatinine excretion) make urinary measurements less precise than plasma measurements.

Sympathetic nerve activity may be monitored in humans by:

- Direct recordings of impulse activity in nerves supplying skeletal muscle (MSNA) and skin,[20,21] but not in target organs of perhaps greater interest in the context of mental stress. In animals also cardiac, renal, and splanchnic sympathetic activity can be measured, and inferences from such studies can be made.[1]
- Measurements of noradrenaline levels in plasma and noradrenaline release from various organs.[5,19] Measurements of noradrenaline release and spillover into plasma can be refined by the use of an isotope dilution method involving infusions of radiolabeled noradrenaline.[19] The limitations of conventional measurements of noradrenaline in antecubital venous plasma must be appreciated (see below).
- Analyses of heart rate variability (HRV) which are often thought to reflect cardiac sympathetic activity. However, HRV reflects the balance between sympathetic (stimulatory) and vagal (inhibitory) influences on the heart, and the vagal components of HRV are more easily deduced than the sympathetic components which reduces its specificity regarding cardiac sympathetic activity[8,22-24] (see Fig. 3.2).
- By examining effects of treatment with adrenergic receptor blockers.[5]

These different techniques are all associated with technical difficulties and limitations. They complement each other, since the release of noradrenaline from sympathetic nerves may be influenced by prejunctional regulation (i.e., variable release per nerve impulse), and functional responses may vary due to differences in receptor sensitivity.

Noradrenaline concentrations in plasma do indeed reflect sympathetic nerve activity, but the importance of the sampling site and factors possibly influencing noradrenaline turnover should be appreciated. Since the clearance of noradrenaline from plasma varies both within and between individuals more precise assessments of noradrenaline "spillover" to plasma with the radiotracer infusion technique may be needed to increase precision.[5,19] A clinically relevant example of confounding influences on catecholamine clearance from plasma is the effect of β-blockade. The plasma levels of adrenaline are moderately elevated by β_1-selective blockade and markedly elevated by nonselective β-blockade compared to placebo when adrenaline is infused at fixed doses, presumably due to interference with the hemodynamic effects of adrenaline.[25] Similarly, the clearance of endogenous catecholamines from plasma may be reduced by β-blockade[19] which may confound interpretations of results obtained in β-blocker-treated patients.

3.2.2 Catecholamine Measurements: Importance of Sampling Site

Arterial (or mixed venous) noradrenaline concentrations reflect whole-body noradrenaline release, that is, contributions from sympathetic nerve activity in all organs,

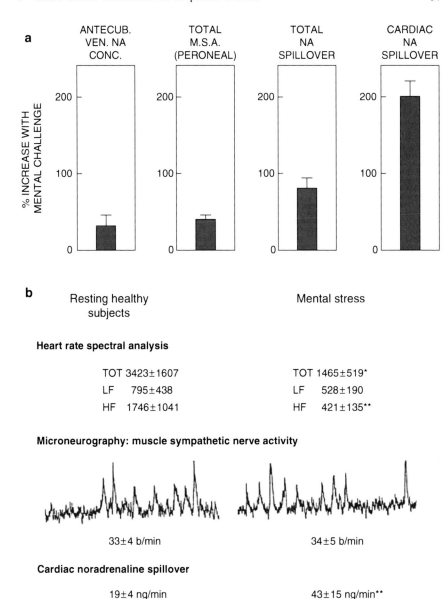

Fig. 3.2 (**a**) Responses of the sympathetic nervous system to mental stress (difficult mental arithmetic) in healthy volunteers. The sympathetic outflow to the skeletal muscle vasculature (MSNA) was little engaged; the failure of antecubital venous plasma noradrenaline concentration to rise reflected this. The response was greatest in the heart, with trebling of cardiac noradrenaline spillover ($P<0.001$), and intermediate for the body as a whole, whole body noradrenaline spillover approximately doubling ($P<0.05$). (**b**) With this same stimulus, in a different group of healthy volunteers, MSNA and cardiac noradrenaline spillover responses are compared to HRV responses. Again, the sympathetic outflow to skeletal muscle was not engaged while there was substantial activation in the cardiac sympathetic outflow ($P<0.01$). Heart rate low-frequency spectral power (*LF*) did not register this cardiac sympathetic activation, contrary to the claims which are sometimes made for this as an index of sympathetic activity in the heart

within a relatively short time frame. The urinary excretion of noradrenaline and adrenaline reflects the arterial plasma levels over longer periods of time,[5,26] whereas noradrenaline released in the kidney upon renal nerve stimulation rapidly appears in renal venous plasma.[27] When assessing regional noradrenaline spillover it is important to measure the extraction of noradrenaline from arterial plasma in the organ studied, preferably using radiolabeled noradrenaline, in order to estimate the contribution of noradrenaline released in the organ.[19] If radiolabeled noradrenaline cannot be infused one can use adrenaline extraction from arterial plasma as a proxy.[5,28]

Half of the noradrenaline in conventionally sampled antecubital venous plasma is derived from the forearm (even though the arterial and venous levels are similar), and changes in sympathetic nerve activity in the forearm and elsewhere during stress may differ substantially.[5,19] Of the noradrenaline in antecubital plasma only 1–2% is derived from the heart and approximately 20% from the kidneys.[19] Thus, "plasma noradrenaline" – as it is measured in most clinical studies – will have little relevance for the evaluation of sympathetic activity in these target organs for stress. Selective measurements of noradrenaline spillover from the heart or the kidney, on the other hand, will provide good reflections of regional sympathetic activity, as will be illustrated below. Failure to recognize the importance of the differentiated patterns in which sympathetic nerves fire, and the need for relevant blood samples for noradrenaline measurements may lead to frustration when results are not as expected, and disbelief in noradrenaline as a sympathetic marker even though it is a good marker when used correctly.

The sympathetic nerves operate in a differentiated fashion with varying levels of activity, and varying responses to stress in different organs and even at different locations in the same organ. For example, simultaneously measured MSNA may even differ between the arm and the leg during mental stress.[29] Thus, the term "sympathetic tone," which indicates uniform nerve activity and uniform neurogenic responses to challenges throughout the body, is not appropriate. If possible, sympathetic activity should be studied selectively in the organ of interest and integrated measures of sympathetic activity should thus be interpreted cautiously with respect to individual organs (see, e.g., Refs.[5,19,30,31]). In particular, antecubital venous plasma noradrenaline measurements should not be overinterpreted since they to a large extent reflect sympathetic nerve activity in the forearm.

3.2.3   Changes in Sympathetic Nerves with Recurrent or Chronic Mental Stress

Patients with panic disorder have been studied as a clinical model of recurrent mental stress responses.[31] Multiple aberrations in sympathetic nerve biology are evident (Fig. 3.3). Single fiber sympathetic nerve recordings commonly, and in the absence of a panic attack, demonstrate multiple firings within a cardiac cycle. Firing salvos of this type are very uncommon in health, but are seen also in patients with depressive illness and essential hypertension, where a relation to chronic mental

Fig. 3.3 Changes occur in sympathetic nerve biology accompanying recurring mental stress responses in patients with panic disorder. These changes take the form of altered sympathetic nerve firing, with firing salvos within a cardiac cycle (**a**), co-release of adrenaline from sympathetic nerves (**b**), and induction of PNMT in sympathetic nerves, and nerve growth factor in subcutaneous veins (NGF is a stress reactant) (**c**). (**b**) Isotope dilution across the heart during an infusion of tritiated adrenaline, indicative of adrenaline release. (**c**) The source of this sympathetic nerve adrenaline cotransmission may be in situ synthesis of adrenaline; on Western blot analysis of proteins extracted from a subcutaneous vein, PNMT was present in two of three patients with panic disorder, but not in three healthy volunteers. The positive control shown is a well overloaded with human cadaver adrenal medulla extract

a

Single fibre sympathetic nerve recording in panic disorder

Control

Panic
disorder

b

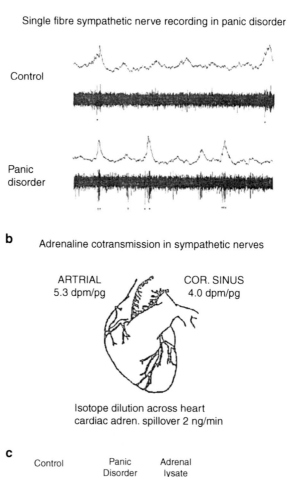

Adrenaline cotransmission in sympathetic nerves

ARTRIAL
5.3 dpm/pg

COR. SINUS
4.0 dpm/pg

Isotope dilution across heart
cardiac adren. spillover 2 ng/min

c

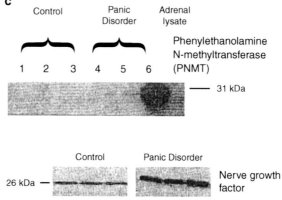

Control   Panic   Adrenal
                 Disorder   lysate

                                            Phenylethanolamine
                                            N-methyltransferase
1   2   3   4   5   6   (PNMT)

————— 31 kDa

Control   Panic Disorder

26 kDa —   Nerve growth
                                             factor

stress has been implicated.[32-34] In sufferers of panic disorder, adrenaline is released as a co-transmitter, originating perhaps from in situ synthesis, or after uptake from plasma during adrenaline surges accompanying a panic attack. Adrenaline co-transmission in sympathetic nerves may also be seen in experimental models of chronic mental stress. Analysis of sympathetic nerve proteins in panic disorder, accessed by a subcutaneous vein biopsy (subcutaneous veins in humans have a dense sympathetic innervation) demonstrates the presence of the adrenaline-synthesizing enzyme, phenylethanolamine N-methyltransferase, PNMT in patients with panic disorder (this is not seen in health), and an increased abundance of nerve growth factor in the vein wall (NGF is a stress reactant).

3.2.4 Cholinergic Mechanisms

The heart is under dual autonomic control. The inhibitory vagal nerve releases acetylcholine (stimulating muscarinic receptors) which is very rapidly inactivated after its release, allowing beat-to-beat control of heart rate. The intrinsic rate of the sinus node is ≈90–100 beats/min, but resting heart rate is usually much lower due to continuous vagal activity. Increased physical fitness reduces resting heart rate by increasing vagal activity. Stress may thus increase heart rate by activating sympathetic nerves and/or by inhibiting the parasympathetic vagal "brake" on the sinus node.[5,18] Heart rate as such is thus not a good indicator of cardiac sympathetic activity, but its variability (HRV) provides clues to the dual autonomic control of the sinus node. When studying HRV, its high frequency variability reflects the beat-to-beat regulation by vagal activity, whereas lower frequency components of HRV include sympathetic influences (see Fig. 3.2, and Chap. 17).

Animal research has demonstrated vasodilator nerves which release acetylcholine in skeletal muscle. Work by Hilton suggested that such vasodilator nerves did not exist in primates, but early studies in humans suggested that it was possible to elicit cholinergic vasodilatation in the forearm with certain stressors (see Ref.[2]). However, the evidence for cholinergic vasodilatation in human skeletal muscle is not solid, and this is most likely not a significant contributor to stress-induced vasodilatation.[35]

3.2.5 Other Mediators and Mechanisms

The renin–angiotensin system may be activated by stress. Renin release from the kidney is under the influence of several factors, one of which is sympathetic nerve activity and β_1-adrenoceptor stimulation; other mechanisms are related to salt concentrations in the macula densa and perfusion pressure in the kidney. Renin catalyzes the formation of angiotensin II, which is a potent vasoconstrictor peptide with several other biological actions, including the enhancement of aldosterone secretion. High sodium intake tends to enhance cardiovascular responses to mental stress (see Ref.[2]), but this is most likely independent of the renin–angiotensin system, which should be down-regulated under such conditions.

Platelets store serotonin, which is released when the cells are activated, and activated platelets also synthesize thromboxane A_2. These substances may stimulate platelets (positive feedback) and cause vasoconstriction, especially when the vascular endothelium is dysfunctional.[36] Stress may activate platelets (see Chap. 6).

Endothelial function is important in local blood flow regulation and endothelial dysfunction promotes the development of athero-thrombotic disease.[37] The principal vasodilators released from the endothelium are nitric oxide (NO) and prostacyclin, and especially NO is involved in flow-mediated dilatation which can be studied in, for example, brachial and coronary arteries as an index of endothelial function in humans.[38,39] The endothelium also releases vasoconstrictors such as endothelin,[38] and endothelium-dependent contracting factor (a prostanoid formed in dysfunctional endothelium).[40]

3.3 Cardiovascular Responses to Acute Stress

Animal experiments have established a typical pattern of cardiovascular responses to acute stress, that is, the defense reaction, which may be elicited by electrical stimulation of certain regions of the brain, and by environmental stimuli in awake animals (see Refs.[1-3]). The "defense reaction" involves sympathetic activation of the heart, kidney, and splanchnic organs, secretion of adrenaline and cortisol, as well as activation of the RAAS system; in animals a surprisingly good correlation between cardiac and renal sympathetic nerve activation has been observed, and the latter also drives the renin release response.[1,41] Vagal withdrawal contributes to increases in heart rate in the "defense reaction," as illustrated in Fig. 3.2. In the "defeat reaction" sympathetic and parasympathetic activation occurs simultaneously to elevate blood pressure without accompanying tachycardia, and the vagal activation also results in gastric hypersecretion and ulcerations.[3,41] Cortisol secretion occurs with both response patterns, but is greater and more important with the defeat reaction pattern and in chronically stressful conditions.

Figure 3.1 illustrates schematically how activation of the "defense reaction" during acute mental stress elevates the blood pressure in humans, based on results from a number of studies (for references, see[2,5,18]). The pressor response is cardiac output dependent, since systemic vascular resistance decreases. In an elegant series of investigations, Brod et al. studied the cardiovascular responses to mental stress, mainly forced mental arithmetics, in normotensive and hypertensive subjects.[42] Figure 3.4 shows that even mild arousal caused by the suggestion of exercise elicited qualitatively similar responses as mental arithmetics. A few examples of our work using the Frankenhaeuser version of Stroop's color word conflict test (CWT), which we found to be both effective and reasonably reproducible (see control group responses in Fig. 3.5), will be mentioned below.

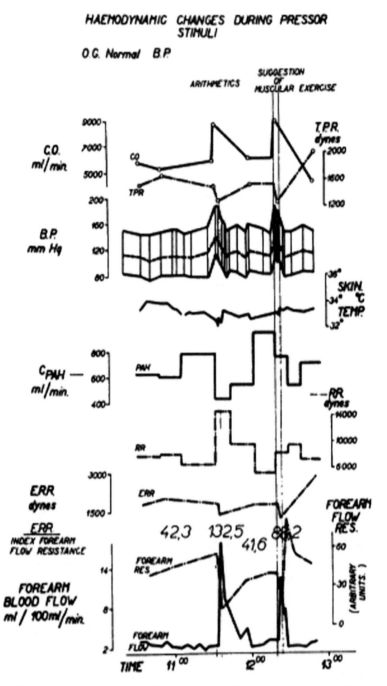

Fig. 3.4 Comparison of systemic and regional hemodynamic responses to mental arithmetic stress and suggestion of heavy muscular exercise in a healthy subject from the studies of Brod et al. Mental stress and the anticipation of physical stress elicited similar cardiovascular responses which resemble the defense reaction. Illustrated are: cardiac output (*C.O.*), systemic vascular resistance (*T.P.R.*), skin temperature, renal blood flow (para-aminohippurate clearance; C_{PAH}), renal vascular resistance (*RR*), extrarenal vascular resistance (*ERR*), and forearm blood flow and vascular resistance (From Brod[42], with permission from the BMJ Publishing Group)

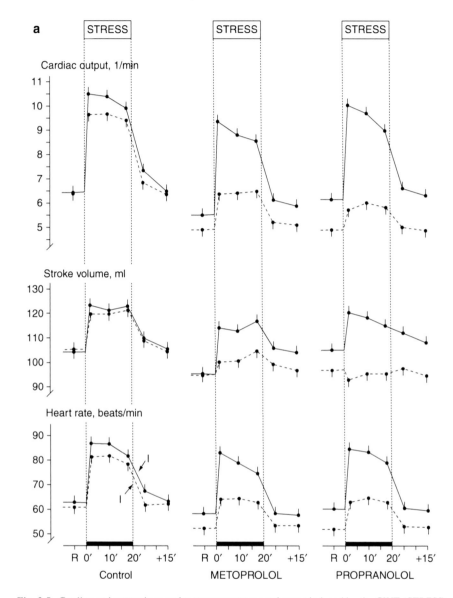

Fig. 3.5 Cardiac and systemic vascular responses to mental stress induced by the CWT (*STRESS*) in healthy male volunteers. There were ten subjects in each group, and CWT was repeated without treatment (*CONTROL*), or after β_1-selective blockade by metoprolol or the nonselective β-blockade by propranolol. (**a**) Cardiac output (thermodilution), stroke volume, and heart rate; (**b**) mean arterial pressure and systemic vascular resistance. The mean arterial pressure response to stress was little affected by the treatments given. The systemic vasodilator response is related to (dependent on?) the cardiac response to stress, as discussed in the text (From Freyschuss et al.[43] With permission from the American Physiological Society)

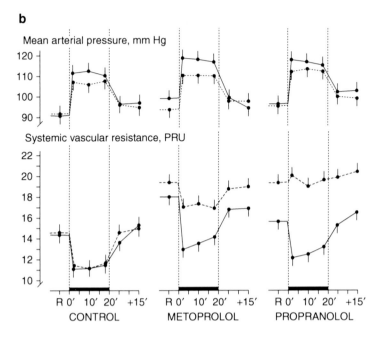

Fig. 3.5 (continued)

3.3.1 Cardiac Responses

Mental stress induced by the CWT increases cardiac output mainly by increasing heart rate, but an increase in stroke volume also contributes (Fig. 3.5 from[43]). Increases in stroke volume are related to increased contractility, and an increase in venous return which supports diastolic filling of the heart. Thus, stress causes veno-constriction and centralization of the blood volume.[44] Studies with pacing have shown that increases in heart rate alone do not efficiently elevate cardiac output – increased contractility and an adequate distension of the heart in diastole are also required for the stress response (see Refs.[2,18,43]). The importance of cardiac sympa-thetic activation during mental stress is reflected by markedly increased cardiac noradrenaline spillover, which occurs simultaneously with a smaller increase in systemic noradrenaline spillover to arterial plasma and no or only minor elevations of antecubital venous plasma noradrenaline (Fig. 3.2).[5,19,24]

The effects of β-blockade by metoprolol (β₁-selective) or propranolol (nonselec-tive) on invasive hemodynamic variables (Fig. 3.5) illustrate the mechanisms involved in the cardiac responses to CWT. The two β-blockers inhibited the heart rate response similarly, indicating β_1-mediated (neurogenic) sympathetic regulation.[43] The partici-pation of vagal mechanisms is reflected in the persisting, although blunted tachycar-dia seen after β-blockade (Fig. 3.5). The stroke volume response was attenuated by metoprolol and abolished by propranolol, suggesting contributions of both neuro-genic (noradrenaline) and hormonal (adrenaline) effects. However, stroke volume is

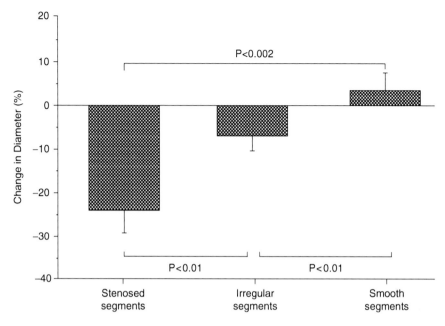

Fig. 3.6 Responses of epicardial coronary arteries to mental arithmetic stress in patients with smooth ($n=25$), irregular ($n=20$), or stenosed ($n=7$) segments on coronary angiography. Heart rate increased by 9 beats/min and mean arterial pressure by 11 mmHg, indicating a relatively mild stimulus. The diameter changes indicate that the coronary vasodilatation in normal segments during stress is converted into vasoconstriction in atherosclerotic segments; this was verified by Doppler flow measurements. Responses to intra-arterial acetylcholine infusions (a stimulus for endothelium-dependent vasodilatation) were correlated with the responses to mental stress (From Yeung et al.[45] With permission from the Massachusetts Medical Society)

dependent on both cardiac contractility and afterload, and the effects of β-blockade on systemic vascular resistance may have influenced the stroke volume response to stress.[43] The cardiac response pattern during adrenaline infusion is quite different (see below), and responses to mental stress are thus mainly neurogenic.

The coronary circulation is to a large extent regulated by cardiac metabolism, and it is difficult to separate β-adrenoceptor-mediated coronary vasodilatation from that induced by increased cardiac metabolism, and flow-mediated vasodilatation. However, α-adrenergic coronary vasoconstriction may occur when the endothelium is dysfunctional, or when cardiac metabolism is inhibited. The vasodilatation which occurs in healthy coronary arteries during stress or intra-arterial acetylcholine infusion may be reverted into vasoconstriction in the presence of atherosclerosis and reduced NO production (Fig. 3.6[45,46]); this may cause ischaemia and increase the risk for arrhythmias and myocardial infarction.

Aging is associated with decreased vagal activity and increased sympathetic activity, as well as a reduction of baroreflex function which leads to greater blood pressure variability.[47-49] Aging also influences adrenal medullary and sympathetic nervous system responses to acute mental stress. When this was explicitly studied with a difficult mental arithmetic test (with rushing and harassment) which caused similar elevations of heart rate in men under 30, and over 60 years,[50] the adrenaline response was much lower in the older men. Conversely the sympathetic response in the heart, based on measurements of cardiac noradrenaline spillover, was substantially higher in the older men, which could possibly be relevant in them to the triggering of cardiac arrhythmias with stress.

3.3.2 Peripheral Vascular Responses

The decrease in systemic vascular resistance during mental stress is related to vasodilatation in skeletal muscle and adipose tissue, which receive a large portion of the cardiac output, whereas there is vasoconstriction in the kidneys, splanchnic organs, and skin.[2,42] Figure 3.4 illustrates how mental stress and mere suggestion of exercise induced marked vasodilatation in the forearm, simultaneously with vasoconstriction in the kidneys and in skin in Brod's experiments[42]; other experiments have shown splanchnic vasoconstriction.

3.3.2.1 Limb Blood Flow

The decrease in systemic vascular resistance illustrated in Fig. 3.5 was intact upon repeated exposure to CWT without treatment, but attenuated by β_1-blockade and abolished by propranolol.[43] These effects of β-blockade may reflect blockade of vascular β-adrenoceptors (of the β_2-subtype), and/or reflexogenic adaptation to the effects of cardiac β-blockade. The increase in mean arterial pressure during CWT was not influenced by β-blockade (Fig. 3.5), in agreement with results from several other studies. If, as discussed by Julius,[10] blood pressure is the primarily regulated variable, attenuation of the increase in cardiac output would result in compensatory (neurogenically mediated?) changes in vascular resistance to achieve the same level of blood pressure during stress with β-blockade as without. Vasodilator responses would then be secondary to, and governed by, the cardiac responses. Further support for this idea was obtained in studies of systemic NO synthesis inhibition by L-NMMA which increased vascular resistance and blood pressure at rest, but did not influence the blood pressure level achieved during CWT.[51]

The studies illustrated in Fig. 3.5 also included measurements of total calf blood flow, and subcutaneous adipose tissue and skeletal muscle blood flow.[52] We found similar degrees of vasodilatation in the adipose tissue, calf skeletal muscle, and the entire calf during CWT. β-Blockade inhibited these local vasodilator responses similarly as for systemic vascular resistance. In other studies we found mild increases in MSNA and noradrenaline spillover from the leg during CWT,[53] in agreement with the results using other stress tests (see Fig. 3.2).[21,29] We found even greater vasodilator responses in the human forearm during CWT (e.g.,[51,54]), and direct comparisons have revealed more pronounced vasodilatation in the arm than in the leg during mental stress.[55] The baroreflex control of skeletal muscle in the arm and leg seems to differ,[7] and simultaneously recorded MSNA increased in the leg but not in the arm during mental stress.[29] We have consistently found no or only minor elevations of antecubital venous plasma noradrenaline during mental stress.[5] Thus, the differing skeletal muscle responses to stress between the upper and lower limbs is an important example of the differentiation of sympathetic nerve activity.

Local inhibition of NO synthesis by intra-arterial infusions of L-NMMA revealed participation of NO and flow-mediated dilatation in the forearm vasodilator response to mental stress.[56] However, the vasodilator response to CWT (a 50% decrease of forearm vascular resistance) was not altered by systemic NO synthesis inhibition.[51] Thus, centrally mediated influences on muscle blood flow may override locally acting influences by, for example, NO released from the endothelium. We found that cholinergic vasodilatation was less likely to be involved in the forearm vasodilator response to stress, in agreement with other data (see Ref.[35]). Interestingly, mental stress seems to cause transient endothelial dysfunction, as assessed by flow-mediated vasodilatation in the forearm.[57]

3.3.2.2 Renal Blood Flow

The kidneys, which receive ≈20% of the cardiac output, are important in the regulation of blood pressure – both in the short term, and in the long term – and appear to be a target for stress effects. Several groups have shown renal vasoconstriction, renin release, and/or altered renal function in response to mental stress.[1,2,11] Examples are shown in Fig. 3.4 of the work of Brod et al.,[42] and in Fig. 3.7 of our work.[58] Of particular interest is that the kidney is very sensitive to stress in hypertension. Thus, Hollenberg and coworkers found that very mild stress induced by a nonverbal IQ test (which did not increase blood pressure) elicited clear-cut renal vasoconstriction among hypertensives, but not among normotensives without a family history of hypertension; those with a family history of hypertension had an intermediate response.[59] Renin release was similarly differentiated among individuals in the Hollenberg study. Thus the kidney is a sensitive target organ for stress, and closely involved in blood pressure regulation.[1,2,11]

We performed a series of investigations of renal vascular responses to different stimuli, based on a renal venous thermodilution technique which allowed rapid measurements of renal blood flow.[60] Figure 3.7 shows that mental stress (CWT) increased renal vascular resistance by 50%, and increased the renal overflow of noradrenaline threefold; renin release also increased.[58] Isometric handgrip exercise was less efficient, especially regarding renin release, despite a similar increase in mean arterial pressure,[60] whereas dynamic exercise was a more potent stimulus.[17] The renal vasoconstrictor response to mental stress was similar to that elicited by dynamic exercise of moderate intensity (≈60% of maximum effort). The importance of renal sympathetic nerve activity in hypertension is discussed in [1,11] and underscored by the blood pressure lowering effect of renal denervation in resistant hypertension (see Chap. 15).

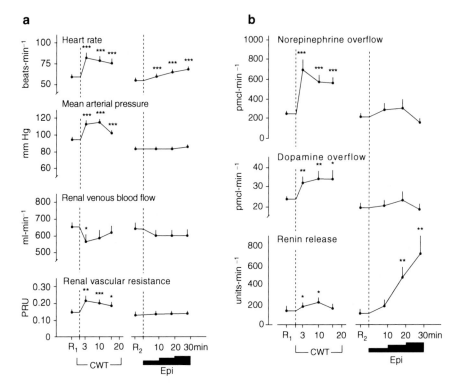

Fig. 3.7 Renal responses to mental stress induced by the CWT and intravenous adrenaline infusion (Epi) elevating arterial plasma adrenaline stepwise from 0.26 ± 0.04 nmol/L at rest to mean values of 0.9, 2.5 and 6.4 nmol/L in 12 healthy volunteers. During CWT the arterial adrenaline levels peaked at 0.7 nmol/L after 3 min. Illustrated are: (**a**) heart rate, mean arterial pressure, renal blood flow, and renal vascular resistance; (**b**) renal noradrenaline and dopamine overflows and renin release from the kidney. Stress elicited clear-cut renal vasoconstriction which was accompanied by a threefold increase in renal noradrenaline overflow (whereas arterial noradrenaline levels increased by only 78%, from 0.78 to 1.34 nmol/L), and an increase in renin release from the kidney. Adrenaline infusion did not influence renal vascular resistance or mean arterial pressure (systolic pressure increased and diastolic pressure decreased dose-dependently). The plasma adrenaline response to CWT could only account for 6% of the heart rate and 21% of the renin release response based on the parallel findings during adrenaline infusion (From Tidgren and Hjemdahl[58], with permission from the American Physiological Society)

3.3.2.3   Is Adrenaline an Important Stress hormone?

When given intravenously, adrenaline increases invasively determined cardiac output mainly by increasing stroke volume.[61] This is perceived as tachycardia (or "the heart is pumping harder"), even though heart rate is little influenced at plasma levels of adrenaline that are encountered during a laboratory stress test (see above). The increase in stroke volume is related to an increase in cardiac contractility, as well as a reduction of afterload due to systemic vasodilatation. Systolic blood pressure rises and diastolic blood pressure decreases, as consequences of increased stroke volume and peripheral vasodilatation, respectively, and mean arterial pressure is maintained even with high doses of adrenaline.[17,61] However, blood pressures increase dose-dependently due to unopposed α-mediated vasoconstriction when adrenaline is infused after β-blockade.[26] During stress, on the other hand, increases in cardiac output are mainly related to increases in heart rate, and diastolic blood pressure increases. As seen in Fig. 3.7 adrenaline infusion did not influence renal blood flow, but increased renin secretion. The plasma levels of adrenaline attained during CWT in these experiments could explain only 6% of the increase in heart rate and 21% of the renin release response during stress.[58] Similarly, direct comparisons of forearm vasodilator responses to CWT and intravenous or intra-arterial adrenaline infusions showed that adrenaline contributed only 10–30% to the marked vasodilatation seen during stress.[54] However, the arterial plasma adrenaline response to stress is correlated to the cardiac noradrenaline overflow response.[5,28] The adrenaline response to mental stress may thus signal a "defense reaction"–like response pattern of sympathetic nerve activity.

The response pattern during mental stress and our plasma concentration-effect studies with adrenaline do not support an important role for adrenaline as mediator of cardiovascular stress responses. The concept that adrenaline is *the* "stress hormone" can thus be questioned from a functional point of view. However, adrenaline responses to stress do reflect the arousal of the individual and the stress perceived, and is therefore a good marker for the stimulus intensity of a stressor and the mainly neurogenic responses elicited.[5]

3.4 Pathophysiological Considerations

The importance of sympathetic mechanisms for the development of stress-related hypertension is discussed in detail in Chap. 4, and the effects of autonomic mechanisms on hemostasis in Chap. 6. Sympathetic overactivity appears to be involved in the metabolic syndrome and obesity,[8,62] in the cardiovascular consequences of sleep apnea,[8] in the target organ damage (cardiac and vascular hypertrophy) seen in long-standing hypertension,[63] and apparently also in the development of atherosclerosis and CHD[9] (see also Chap. 2). Furthermore, sympathetic overactivity signals a worsened prognosis in heart failure.[8]

A high heart rate is indicative of high cardiac sympathetic activity and/or low vagal activity, and is associated with elevated blood pressure, cardiometabolic risk factors, cardiovascular disease, and even longevity.[64] Increased sympathetic activity is of special interest in this context, but reduced cardiac vagal activity may contribute to the risk of suffering sudden death, since the ventricular fibrillation threshold is lowered by both reduced vagal activity and increased cardiac sympathetic activity; ischemia may modify these influences.[64-66] Stress raises heart rate by increasing cardiac sympathetic and decreasing vagal activity, and may thus sensitize the heart to arrhythmogenic stimuli, in addition to causing ischemia[9,67] and increasing the risk for plaque rupture and myocardial infarction in vulnerable individuals (see Chap. 9).

Furthermore, surges in cardiac sympathetic activity can precipitate stress cardiomyopathy in predisposed individuals, as discussed in Chap. 10.

Low HRV has been shown to be associated with increased cardiovascular risk in patients with CHD and other cardiovascular disease, as well as in general populations.[22,23] Few studies have examined the prognostic information in catecholamine assessments. In the Angina Prognosis Study in Stockholm (APSIS)[68] – a single-center study of 809 patients with stable angina pectoris and a mean follow-up of 3.4 years – we studied the prognostic implications of venous plasma catecholamines at rest and after exercise, as well as of urinary catecholamines and HRV. We found no prognostic implications of catecholamines in plasma or urine.[69] However, low HRV as assessed by both time and frequency domain indices of low HRV predicted CV death but not nonfatal MI.[69,70] Patients who suffered CV death had low HRV in all frequency domains, and the LF/HF ratio (which reflects "sympathovagal balance"[23]) did not differ.[69] These findings suggest an increased risk of suffering arrhythmic death in angina patients with low vagal activity rather than increased sympathetic activity. Lack of prognostic information in the various catecholamine measurements may reflect the differentiation of sympathetic activity discussed above.

Mental stress induces transient symptomatic or silent ischemia in one-third to half the patients with CHD; there is limited information on the prognostic implications of such ischemia but the available evidence indeed suggests prognostic importance.[67] Individual stress reactivity, as well as the ability to recover after stress, has been shown to predict the development of hypertension and a worsened cardiovascular risk status (e.g., increased intima-media thickness of the carotid artery).[71] Of interest is that arterial plasma catecholamine responses to mental stress predicted future blood pressure increases among young men.[72] This chapter has not focused on gender differences, but it is pertinent to mention that both HPA-axis and autonomic responses to acute psychosocial stress are lower in premenopausal women than in men of the same age; this difference disappears after menopause and appears to be related to estrogen levels.[73] Heart rate and blood pressure surges may precipitate plaque rupture (Chap. 9), and pro-arrhythmic changes involving autonomic mechanisms. Furthermore, both acute and chronic stress can cause pro-thrombotic changes which appear to involve autonomic mechanisms (see Chap. 6). Treatments to reduce stress (behavioral therapies) and sympathetic overactivity, and to increase vagal activity (especially increasing physical fitness) are thus based on a relatively sound mechanistic base.

References

1. Folkow B. Physiological aspects of primary hypertension. *Physiol Rev.* 1982;62:347-504.
2. Herd JA. Cardiovascular responses to stress. *Physiol Rev.* 1991;71:305-330.
3. Henry JP, Stephens PM, Ely DL. Psychosocial hypertension and the defence and defeat reactions. *J Hypertens.* 1986;4:687-697.
4. Steptoe A, Vögele C. Methodology of mental stress testing in cardiovascular research. *Circulation.* 1991;83:II-14-II-24.

5. Hjemdahl P. Plasma catecholamines – analytical challenges and physiological limitations. *Baillère's Clin Endocrinol Metab*. 1993;7:307-353.
6. Rowell LB. Reflex control of regional circulations in humans. *J Auton Nerv Syst*. 1984;11: 101-114.
7. Shepherd JT, Mancia G. Reflex control of the human cardiovascular system. *Rev Physiol Biochem Pharmacol*. 1986;105:3-99.
8. Malpas SC. Sympathetic nervous system overactivity and its role in the development of cardiovascular disease. *Physiol Rev*. 2010;90:513-557.
9. Rozanski A, Blumenthal JA. Impact of psychological factors on the pathogenesis of cardiovascular disease and implications for therapy. *Circulation*. 1999;99:2192-2217.
10. Julius S. The blood pressure seeking properties of the central nervous system. *J Hypertens*. 1988;6:177-185.
11. DiBona GF, Esler M. Translational medicine: the antihypertensive effect of renal denervation. *Am J Physiol*. 2010;298:R245-R253.
12. Lundberg JM. Pharmacology of cotransmission in the autonomic nervous system: integrative aspects on amines, neuropeptides, adenosine triphosphate, amino acids and nitric oxide. *Pharmacol Rev*. 1996;48:113-178.
13. Pernow J, Kahan T, Hjemdahl P, Lundberg JM. Possible involvement of neuropeptide Y in sympathetic vascular control of canine skeletal muscle. *Acta Physiol Scand*. 1988;132:43-50.
14. Pernow J, Schwieler J, Kahan T, et al. Influence of sympathetic discharge pattern on norepinephrine and neuropeptide Y release. *Am J Physiol*. 1989;257:H866-H872.
15. Morris MJ, Cox HS, Lambert GW, et al. Region-specific neuropeptide Y overflows at rest and during sympathetic activation in humans. *Hypertension*. 1997;29:137.
16. Tidgren B, Theodorsson E, Hjemdahl P. Renal and systemic plasma immunoreactive neuropeptide Y and calcitonin gene-related peptide responses to mental stress and adrenaline in humans. *Clin Physiol*. 1991;11:9-19.
17. Tidgren B, Hjemdahl P, Theodorsson E, Nussberger J. Renal responses to dynamic exercise in man. *J Appl Physiol*. 1991;70:2279-2286.
18. Hjemdahl P. Physiology of the autonomic nervous system as related to cardiovascular function: implications for stress research. In: Byrne DG, Rosenman RH, eds. *Anxiety and the Heart*. New York: Hemisphere Publ Corp; 1991:95-158.
19. Esler M, Jennings G, Lambert G, et al. Overflow of catecholamine neurotransmitters to the circulation: source, fate and functions. *Physiol Rev*. 1990;70:963-985.
20. Wallin BG, Fagius J. Peripheral sympathetic neural activity in conscious humans. *Annu Rev Physiol*. 1988;50:565-576.
21. Joyner MJ, Charkoudian N, Walin BG. Sympathetic nervous system and blood pressure in humans – individualized patterns of regulation and their implications. *Hypertension*. 2010; 56:10-16.
22. Task force of the European Society of Cardiology and the North American Society of Pacing and Electrophysiology. Heart rate variability; standards of measurement, physiological interpretation, and clinical use. *Eur Heart J*. 1996;17:354-381.
23. Lahiri MK, Kannankeril PJ, Goldberger JJ. Assessment of autonomic function in cardiovascular disease. *J Am Coll Cardiol*. 2008;51:1725-1733.
24. Kingwell BA, Thompson JM, Kaye DM, et al. Heart rate spectral analysis, cardiac norepinephrine spillover and muscle sympathetic nerve activity during human sympathetic nervous activation and failure. *Circulation*. 1994;90:234-240.
25. Hjemdahl P, Åkerstedt T, Pollare T, Gillberg M. Influence of beta-adrenoceptor blockade by metoprolol and propranolol on plasma concentrations and effects of noradrenaline and adrenaline during i.v. infusion. *Acta Physiol Scand*. 1983;515(Suppl):45-53.
26. Åkerstedt T, Gillberg M, Hjemdahl P, et al. Comparison of urinary and plasma catecholamine responses to mental stress. *Acta Physiol Scand*. 1983;117:19-26.
27. Kopp U, Bradley T, Hjemdahl P. Renal venous outflow and urinary excretion of norepinephrine, epinephrine and dopamine during graded renal nerve stimulation. *Am J Physiol*. 1983; 244:E52-E60.

28. Hedman A, Hjemdahl P, Nordlander R, Åström H. Effects of mental and physical stress on central haemodynamics and cardiac sympathetic nerve activity during QT interval-sensing rate-responsive and fixed rate ventricular inhibited pacing. *Eur Heart J*. 1990;11:903-915.

29. Anderson EA, Wallin BG, Mark AL. Dissociation of sympathetic nerve activity in arm and leg muscle during mental stress. *Hypertension*. 1987;9(suppl 3):114-119.

30. Folkow B, Di Bona GF, Hjemdahl P, et al. Measurements of plasma norepinephrine concentrations in human primary hypertension – a word of caution on their applicability for assessing neurogenic contributions. *Hypertension*. 1983;5:399-403.

31. Friberg P, Meredith I, Jennings G, et al. Evidence of increased renal noradrenaline spillover rate during sodium restriction in man. *Hypertension*. 1990;16:121-130.

32. Lambert E, Dawood T, Schlaich M, et al. Single-unit sympathetic discharge pattern in pathological conditions associated with elevated cardiovascular risk. *Clin Exp Pharmacol Physiol*. 2008;35:503-507.

33. Esler M, Eikelis N, Schlaich M, et al. Chronic mental stress is a cause of essential hypertension: presence of biological markers of stress. *Clin Exp Pharmacol Physiol*. 2008;35:498-502.

34. Esler M, Eikelis N, Schlaich M, et al. Human sympathetic nerve biology: parallel influences of stress and epigenetics in essential hypertension and panic disorder. *Ann NY Acad Sci*. 2008;1148:338-348.

35. Joyner MJ, Dietz NM. Sympathetic vasodilatation in human muscle. *Acta Physiol Scand*. 2003;177:329-336.

36. Willerson JT, Golino P, Eidt J, et al. Specific platelet mediators and unstable coronary artery lesions: experimental evidence and potential clinical implications. *Circulation*. 1989;80: 198-205.

37. Charakida M, Masi S, Lüscher TF, et al. Assessment of atherosclerosis: the role of flow mediated dilatation. *Eur Heart J*. 2010;31:2854-2861.

38. Deanfield J, Donald A, Ferri C, et al. Endothelial function and dysfunction. Methodological issues for assessments in the different vascular beds: a statement by the Working Group on endothelin and endothelial factors of the European Society of hypertension. *J Hypertens*. 2005;23:7-17.

39. Deanfield JE, Halcox JP, Rabelink JP. Endothelial function and dysfunction: testing and clinical relevance. *Circulation*. 2007;115:1285-1295.

40. Vanhoutte PM, Tang EHC. Endothelial contractions: when a good guy turns bad! *J Physiol*. 2008;586:5295-5304.

41. Folkow B. Physiological aspects of the "defence" and "defeat" reactions. *Acta Physiol Scand*. 1997;640(suppl):34-37.

42. Brod J. Haemodynamic basis of acute pressor reactions and hypertension. *Br Heart J*. 1963; 25:227-245.

43. Freyschuss U, Hjemdahl P, Juhlin-Dannfelt A, Linde B. Cardiovascular and sympathoadrenal responses to mental stress: influence of β-blockade. *Am J Physiol*. 1988;255:H443-H451.

44. Brod J, Cachovan M, Bahlman J, et al. Haemodynamic response to an emotional stress (mental arithmetic) with special reference to the venous side. *Aust N Z J Med*. 1976;6(suppl2):19-25.

45. Yeung AC, Vekshtein VI, Krantz DS, et al. The effect of atherosclerosis on the vasomotor response of coronary arteries to mental stress. *N Engl J Med*. 1991;325:1551-1556.

46. Ludmer PL, Selwyn AP, Shook TL, et al. Paradoxical vasoconstriction induced by acetylcholine in atherosclerotic coronary arteries. *N Engl J Med*. 1986;315:1046-1051.

47. Monahan KD. Effect of aging on baroreflex function in humans. *Am J Physiol*. 2007;293: R3-R12.

48. De Meersman RE, Stein PK. Vagal modulation and aging. *Biol Psychol*. 2007;74:165-173.

49. Kaye DM, Esler MD. Autonomic control of the aging heart. *Neuromol Med*. 2008;10: 179-186.

50. Esler MD, Kaye DM, Thompson JM, et al. Effects of aging on epinephrine secretion, and on regional release of epinephrine from the human heart. *J Clin Endocrinol Metab*. 1995;80: 435-442.

51. Lindqvist M, Melcher A, Hjemdahl P. Hemodynamic and sympatho-adrenal responses to mental stress during nitric oxide synthesis blockade. *Am J Physiol.* 2004;287:H2309-H2315.
52. Linde B, Hjemdahl P, Freyschuss U, Juhlin-Dannfelt A. Adipose tissue and skeletal muscle blood flow during mental stress. *Am J Physiol.* 1989;256:E12-E18.
53. Hjemdahl P, Fagius J, Freyschuss U, et al. Muscle sympathetic nerve activity and norepinephrine release during mental challenge in humans. *Am J Physiol.* 1989;257:E654-E664.
54. Lindqvist M, Kahan T, Melcher A, et al. Forearm vasodilator mechanisms during mental stress – possible roles of epinephrine and ANP. *Am J Physiol.* 1996;270:E393-E399.
55. Rusch NJ, Shepherd JT, Webb RC, Vanhoutte PM. Different behaviour of the resistance vessels of the human calf and forearm during contralateral isometric exercise, mental stress, and abnormal respiratory movements. *Circ Res.* 1981;48:I-118-I-130.
56. Dietz NM, Rivera JM, Eggener SE, et al. Nitric oxide contributes to the rise in forearm blood flow during mental stress in humans. *J Physiol.* 1994;480:361-368.
57. Ghiadoni L, Donald AE, Cropley M, et al. Mental stress induces transient endothelial dysfunction in humans. *Circulation.* 2000;102:2473-2478.
58. Tidgren B, Hjemdahl P. Renal responses to mental stress and epinephrine in man. *Am J Physiol.* 1989;257:F682-F689.
59. Hollenberg NK, Williams GH, Adams DF. Essential hypertension: abnormal renal vascular and endocrine responses to a mild psychological stimulus. *Hypertension.* 1981;2:11-17.
60. Tidgren B, Hjemdahl P. Reflex activation of renal nerves in humans – effects on noradrenaline, dopamine and renin overflow to renal venous plasma. *Acta Physiol Scand.* 1988;134:23-34.
61. Freyschuss U, Hjemdahl P, Juhlin-Dannfelt A, Linde B. Cardiovascular and metabolic responses to low dose adrenaline infusion: an invasive study in humans. *Clin Sci (Lond).* 1986;70:199-206.
62. Mancia G, Bousquet P, Elghozi JL, et al. The sympathetic nervous system and the metabolic syndrome. *J Hypertens.* 2007;25:909-920.
63. Mancia G, Grassi G, Giannattasio C, Seravalle G. Sympathetic activation in the pathogenesis of hypertension and progression of organ damage. *Hypertension.* 1999;34(part 2):724-728.
64. Palatini P, Julius S. Heart rate and cardiovascular risk. *J Hypertens.* 1997;15:3-17.
65. Lown B, Verrier RL. Neural activity and ventricular fibrillation. *N Engl J Med.* 1976;294:1165-1170.
66. Verrier RL, Lown B. Behavioral stress and cardiac arrhythmias. *Annu Rev Physiol.* 1984;46:155-176.
67. Strike PC, Steptoe A. Systematic review of mental stress-induced myocardial ischemia. *Eur Heart J.* 2003;24:690-703.
68. Rehnqvist N, Hjemdahl P, Billing E, et al. Effects of metoprolol versus verapamil in patients with stable angina pectoris - the Angina Prognosis Study In Stockholm (APSIS). *Eur Heart J.* 1996;17:76-81.
69. Forslund L, Björkander I, Ericson M, et al. Prognostic implications of autonomic function in patients with stable angina pectoris – analyses of catecholamines and heart rate variability in the APSIS study. *Heart.* 2002;87:415-422.
70. Björkander I, Forslund L, Kahan T, et al. Differential index – a simple time domain heart rate variability method with prognostic implications in stable angina pectoris. *Cardiology.* 2008;111:126-33.
71. Chida Y, Steptoe A. Greater cardiovascular responses to mental stress are associated with poor subsequent cardiovascular risk status. *Hypertension.* 2010;55:1026-1032.
72. Flaa A, Eide IK, Kjeldsen SE, Rostrup M. Sympathoadrenal stress reactivity is a predictor of future blood pressure. An 18-year follow-up study. *Hypertension.* 2008;52:336-341.
73. Kajantie E, Phillips DIW. The effects of sex and hormonal status on the physiological response to acute psychosocial stress. *Psychoneuroendocrinology.* 2006;31:151-178.

Chapter 4
Sympathetic Neural and Adrenal Medullary Mechanisms in Depression and Panic Disorder

Murray Esler

Keywords Sympathetic nervous system • Adrenal medullary mechanisms • Depression • Panic disorder • Psychoneurocardiology • Adrenaline secretion • Sympathetic pathophysiology

The pathway towards the current recognition[1-3] that mental stress and psychiatric illness is a cause of cardiovascular disease has been long, halting and at times vigorously defended by opposing forces of the medical status quo. For many years this claimed relation of acute mental stress to heart attacks was largely based on individual anecdotes, such as the celebrated case of the famous eighteenth-century English surgeon, John Hunter, who wrote that he was at the mercy of any scoundrel who aggravated him, then proved the point by dying suddenly in the middle of a stormy meeting of the board of his hospital. More recently, systematic evidence has been gathered at times of disasters, including war, terrorist attacks on civilians and earthquakes, which strongly supports the proposition of a mental stress–heart attack link.[4] The issues surrounding triggering of heart attacks are dealt with in-depth in Chap. 8.

4.1 Psychoneurocardiology

The mind–heart disease duality, 'psychogenic cardiovascular disease', takes many forms (Table 4.1). Heart disease attributable to depressive illness and to panic disorder are important examples (see also Chaps. 3 and 18; depression, and psychological treatment). A common concept in the field is the presumed importance of neural

M. Esler
Hypertension Thrombosis and Vascular Biology Division,
Baker IDI Heart and Diabetes Institute, Melbourne, VIC, Australia
e-mail: murray.esler@bakeridi.edu.au

P. Hjemdahl et al. (eds.), *Stress and Cardiovascular Disease*,
DOI 10.1007/978-1-84882-419-5_4, © Springer-Verlag London Limited 2012

Table 4.1 Psychogenic cardiovascular disease [1,3]

Acute mental stress, as a 'trigger' for myocardial infarction, Takotsubo cardiomyopathy and sudden death
Major depressive illness and panic disorder, as primary causes of myocardial infarction and cardiac arrhythmias
Accompanying schizophrenia
Attributable to psychotropic drugs
Chronic mental stress, as a cause of coronary heart disease, essential hypertension

mechanisms involving the sympathetic nervous system, captured in the rubric 'psychoneurocardiology'. A causal relation of episodically or chronically activated cardiac sympathetic tone to adverse cardiac events has been demonstrated in several medical contexts (see below). Perhaps surprisingly, with stress-related cardiovascular disease it is not cortisol which is the prime mover, unlike in some other medical settings. The specific neural and adrenal medullary mediating mechanisms of cardiac risk in patients with depressive illness and panic disorder, drawn primarily from multiple studies by my research group over the past three decades, is the theme of this chapter.

4.1.1   Methods

Current concepts of the participation of the sympathetic nervous system in various forms of psychogenic cardiovascular disease were dependent on the development and application of methods for studying regional sympathetic activity in the sympathetic outflows to different organs. These techniques are clinical microneurography, which measures postganglionic sympathetic fibre firing rates in the nerves passing to the skeletal muscle vasculature,[5,6] and the isotope dilution technique for measurement of the overflow of the sympathetic neurotransmitter to plasma, regional noradrenaline spillover measurements[7,8] (Fig. 4.1). With microneurography, multi-fibre recordings of 'bursts' of nerve activity which are synchronous with the heart beat,[5] and more recently single-fibre traces[6,9] are generated. Neurotransmitter release can be studied clinically using radiotracer-derived measurements of the appearance rate of noradrenaline in plasma from individual organs.[7,8,10,11] Microneurographic methods do not give access to sympathetic nerves of internal organs, a limitation which is overcome by using regional noradrenaline spillover measurements. The same isotope dilution principle can be applied to measure the secretion rate of adrenaline. Intravenous infusion of tritiated adrenaline, with arterial blood sampling allows measurement of the whole-body appearance rate of adrenaline in plasma, equivalent to adrenal medullary adrenaline secretion.[11]

4.1.2   Ancillary Measurements of Sympathetic Nerve Biology

Tracer kinetics methodology allows investigation of additional aspects of sympathetic nervous system functioning. Analysis of the uptake and intraneuronal

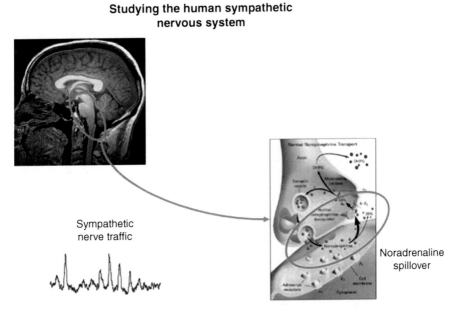

Testing is best done by recording postganglionic nerve traffic (clinical microneurography) and measuring release of the transmitter from sympathetic nerves to plasma (noradrenaline "spillover")

Fig. 4.1 Optimal methodology for studying the human sympathetic nervous system, sympathetic nerve recording with clinical microneurography, and measurement of the release of noradrenaline to plasma, 'noradrenaline spillover', utilising the technique of isotope dilution. These methods can be applied to quantify regional sympathetic activity, in sympathetic efferent fibres passing to skin and the skeletal muscle vasculature with microneurography, and in internal organs including the heart, with regional noradrenaline spillover measurements

processing of infused tritiated noradrenaline allows quantification of neuronal reuptake of noradrenaline,[8,10,12] which is the process which terminates the neural signal, by returning the transmitter to the sympathetic nerve varicosity after its release. Application of regional isotope dilution methodology with infused tritiated adrenaline allows testing for adrenaline co-transmission by sympathetic nerves, which may be seen in pathological conditions but not in healthy subjects.[11,13-15] Impairment of neuronal noradrenaline re-uptake and sympathetic nerve adrenaline co-transmission, in fact, have both been documented in panic disorder.[11,13-15]

4.2 Panic Disorder

Panic disorder sufferers often fear that they have heart disease, because of the nature of their symptoms, but in the past have been reassured that this is not the case. In my own experience with the clinical management of panic disorder sufferers, I began to encounter case material which suggested otherwise. Documented during panic attacks were variously triggered cardiac arrhythmias (atrial fibrillation, ventricular fibrillation), recurrent emergency room attendances with angina and electrocardiographic changes of ischaemia, coronary artery spasm in panic attacks occurring during coronary angiography, and myocardial infarction associated with coronary spasm and thrombosis[14,16] (Fig. 4.2).

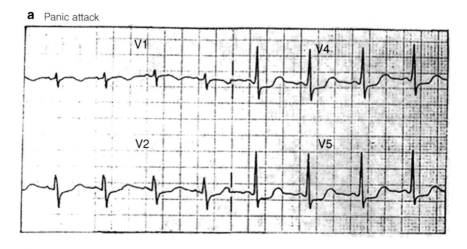

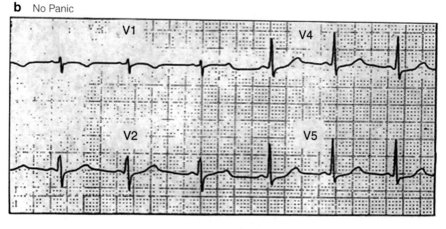

Fig. 4.2 Clinical case material, in two panic disorder patients in whom cardiac complications occurred during a panic attack. (**a**) *Panic attack.* This 36-year-old woman had multiple emergency room attendances with anginal chest pain during panic attacks. The electrocardiograph on each occasion showed ST segment depression, indicative of myocardial ischaemia. There was a good response to medical management, of the type described in the text. A coronary angiogram was not performed. (**b**) *No panic attack.* Development of atrial fibrillation in a 48-year-old female almost coincident with the onset of a panic attack occurring during a period of research monitoring. The atrial fibrillation reverted spontaneously after 6 min, (**c**) *Cardiac risk in panic disorder.* This 49-year-old woman on many occasions had anginal pain during panic attacks. During coronary angiography a panic attack occurred, associated with coronary artery spasm in the left anterior descending coronary artery. This was reversed with infused glyceryl trinitrate. There was no underlying coronary artery atherosclerosis

Coronary spasm during panic attack

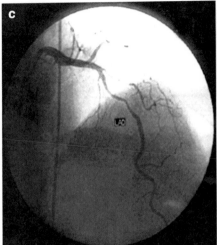 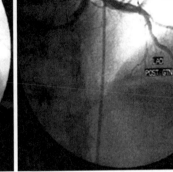

| Spasm in left anterior descending coronary artery | Significant resolution following glyceryl trinitrate |

Fig. 4.2 (continued)

Epidemiological studies affirm the clinical observations that there is an increased risk of myocardial infarction and sudden death in patients with panic disorder.[17-19] This increased cardiac risk applies not only to men who are of such an age that unrecognized underlying coronary artery disease may be present, but also exists in pre-menopausal women who in general have low coronary risk. What might be the mechanisms of this increased cardiac risk in patients with panic disorder? Could patients with panic disorder, perhaps, provide an instructive 'clinical model' for identifying possible mechanisms underlying the general aspects of the stress–heart disease link? This expectation has been fulfilled, with extensive investigation in panic disorder sufferers, pinpointing a primary importance for pathophysiology involving the sympathetic nervous system.[13-16]

4.2.1 The Sympathetic Nervous System and Adrenaline Secretion at Rest

On first appearances, the sympathetic nervous system functions normally in patients with panic disorder at rest, in the absence of a panic attack. Multi-unit sympathetic nerve firing rates and whole-body and cardiac noradrenaline spillover values are within normal limits, as is the secretion of adrenaline by the adrenal medulla.[13-15] Other abnormalities, however, are demonstrable, in the impairment of neuronal noradrenaline re-uptake and sympathetic nerve adrenaline co-transmission mentioned above, and in the anomalous firing pattern of single sympathetic nerve fibres.

4.2.2 Single Fibre Sympathetic Nerve Recordings

Multi-fibre recordings of the sympathetic outflow to the skeletal muscle vasculature are normal in untreated, resting patients with panic disorder. The more instructive analysis of single sympathetic nerve firing patterns indicates, however, that this 'normality' is an illusion. Salvos of multiple single-fibre sympathetic nerve firing are present within a cardiac cycle, in the absence of a panic attack.[20] This is not seen in health. Salvos of single-fibre firings appear to be a 'signature' of stress exposure.[20-23]

4.2.3 Adrenaline Co-transmission in Sympathetic Nerves

Adrenaline is released from the sympathetic nerves of the heart, as an accessory neurotransmitter, in patients with panic disorder (Fig. 4.3). This adrenaline in sympathetic nerves of panic disorder sufferers is presumably taken up from plasma

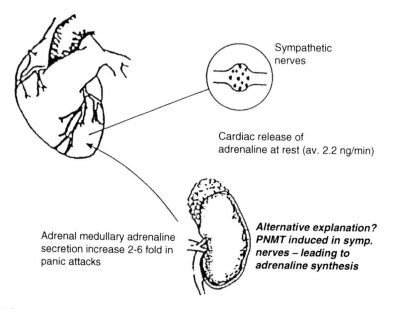

Sympathetic nerves

Cardiac release of adrenaline at rest (av. 2.2 ng/min)

Adrenal medullary adrenaline secretion increase 2-6 fold in panic attacks

Alternative explanation? PNMT induced in symp. nerves – leading to adrenaline synthesis

Fig. 4.3 In patients with panic disorder, adrenaline is a co-transmitter in the sympathetic nerves of the heart, on a 'good day', remote from any panic attacks. Adrenaline release is equivalent to approximately 10% of the concurrent rate of sympathetic nerve release of noradrenaline. The origin of the neurally co-released adrenaline is uncertain, perhaps from loading of sympathetic vesicles by uptake of adrenaline from plasma during the surges of adrenal medullary secretion accompanying panic attacks, or from de novo synthesis in sympathetic nerves, by the enzyme phenylethanolamine methyltransferase (PNMT). PNMT is normally absent from sympathetic nerves, but present in sympathetic nerves of panic disorder patients[15,22]

during panic attacks, or synthesised *in situ* by the adrenaline-synthesising enzyme, phenylethanolamine methytransferase (PNMT), which has been shown in experimental animals to be induced by mental stress[24] and is present in sympathetic nerves in panic disorder.[21]

4.2.4   Reduction in Neuronal Noradrenaline Re-uptake by Sympathetic Nerves

Each pulse of the sympathetic neural signal is terminated in tissues primarily by re-uptake of the released noradrenaline into the sympathetic varicosity via the noradrenaline transporter (NET). The processes of neuronal re-uptake of noradrenaline can be quantified during the course of an infusion of tritiated noradrenaline in humans by measurement of the transcardiac extraction of tritiated noradrenaline from plasma, and analysis of the intraneuronal metabolism of the tracer in the sympathetic nerves of the heart[12,13,25] (Fig. 4.4).

In untreated patients with panic disorder the neuronal re-uptake of noradrenaline is impaired. Such an abnormality would be expected to magnify sympathetically mediated responses, particularly in the heart where noradrenaline inactivation is so dependent on neuronal re-uptake[8,12,26] (Fig. 4.4). No loss of function mutations of coding regions of the NET gene in panic disorder patients, which could explain this,

Does faulty noradrenaline reuptake increase cardiac risk in panic disorder?

NET impairment magnifies sympathetic nervous activation in panic attacks

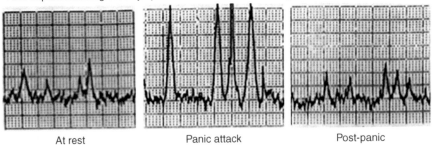

| At rest | Panic attack | Post-panic |

This applies especially in the heart, where approximately 95% of released noradrenaline is recaptured by sympathetic nerves

Fig. 4.4 The figure depicts a massive increase in multi-unit sympathetic nerve activity in the outflow to the skeletal muscle vasculature occurring during a panic attack. Patients with panic disorder have an impairment in the neuronal re-uptake of noradrenaline by sympathetic nerves. If an increase in sympathetic outflow of this magnitude also occurs to the heart, which cannot be measured but is probable, the cardiac neural signal would be markedly intensified, given that in the heart, neuronal re-uptake is of such importance in transmitter disposition.[12,26] This could precipitate a cardiac arrhythmia, of atrial fibrillation, as shown in Fig. 4.2, or of a ventricular tachyarrhythmia

have been found, but epigenetic silencing of the NET gene has been demonstrated.[27] The abundance in sympathetic nerves of the gene product, the transporter protein, sampled from a subcutaneous vein biopsy which can be used as a source of sympathetic nerve proteins, is reduced in patients with panic disorder.[15,21]

4.2.5 Sympathetic Nerve Firing and Secretion of Epinephrine During a Panic Attack

When recorded directly by microneurography, the size of sympathetic bursts increases remarkably during a panic attack, without any increase in firing rate[11] (Fig. 4.4), presumably by recruitment of additional firing fibres. Surprisingly, this response is qualitatively different from that seen during laboratory mental stress with stimuli such as difficult mental arithmetic, where muscle sympathetic nerve activity increases little if at all. Single-fibre measurements have not been made to this point, during mental stress in general or in panic patients. Adrenal medullary secretion of adrenaline increases two- to sixfold.[11] With the pronounced activation of the cardiac sympathetic outflow occurring during a panic attack, the sympathetic nerve co-transmitter, neuropeptide Y (NPY), is co-released from the cardiac sympathetic nerves and appears in measurable quantities in coronary sinus venous blood.[14] This is an intriguing finding, given the capacity of NPY to cause coronary artery spasm.[28]

4.2.6 Panic Disorder: Clinical Correlates and Conclusions

Panic disorder provides a special case further illustrating that mental stress responses can be a cause of triggered adverse heart events such as myocardial infarction and sudden death. In recent years, additional systematic evidence has been gathered at times of disasters, including war, and terrorist attacks on civilians and earthquakes, which also strongly supports the proposition of an acute mental stress–heart attack link. Do these observations have a generality, applicable to the population at large? The answer is that no doubt they do. In individual personal life, 'emotional earthquakes' do occur. Heart attacks have been well documented to be triggered by news of catastrophes involving family members, armed robbery, assaults, and even during gripping sporting events.[1,3,29]

4.3 Depressive Illness

There is strong evidence that patients with major depressive disorder are at increased risk of developing coronary heart disease.[30-32] This elevated risk is independent of classical risk factors such as smoking, obesity, hypercholesterolaemia, diabetes and hypertension. The association is present in males and females, across different age groups and in subjects living in different countries. The risk of coronary heart disease is increased 1.5–2-fold in those with minor/subsyndromic depression and 3–4.5-fold in subjects with major depression and thus appears to be proportional to the severity of the depression. The mechanisms involved are complex (see Chap. 3 on depression and Chap. 18 on psychological treatment). One factor, no doubt, is the loss of volition experienced by patients with depressive illness, which can reduce their adherence to preventive health medical advice, and to the taking of prescribed medication. I will focus here on the possibility of a sympathetic neural component in the cardiac consequences of depression.

4.3.1 The Sympathetic Nervous System and Adrenaline Secretion at Rest

Elevated rates of spillover of noradrenaline to plasma, indicative of chronic sympathetic activation, have long been known in patients with depressive illness,[33] but this abnormality is not straightforward. Whole-body and cardiac noradrenaline spillover rates are extraordinarily high in approximately 35% of patients (to a level seen in cardiac failure), but normal or even low in the remainder[10] (Fig. 4.5). The rate of transmitter release is not manifestly related to clinical characteristics, such as severity of the depression.[10]

Multi-unit sympathetic nerve firing in the outflow to the skeletal muscle vasculature has variously been reported as elevated[35] or normal.[10] Single-fibre sympathetic nerve recording in the clinical neurogram, even in depressed patients with normal multi-unit records, demonstrates an abnormality identical to that seen in panic disorder, with salvos of multiple single-fibre sympathetic nerve firings within a cardiac cycle.[22] Whether the sympathetic nerves to the heart demonstrate this abnormality cannot be tested. As for panic disorder, neuronal re-uptake of noradrenaline is impaired in depressive illness, although the mechanism is unknown.[10] Adrenaline secretion is normal.

4.4 Depressive Illness, Panic Disorder: Contrasting Sympathetic Pathophysiology

Depressive illness and panic disorder often coexist in individual patients. In the studies described above, patient recruitment was such as to minimize this comorbidity. This is crucial for the sympathetic neurobiology of the two conditions to be meaningfully compared (Table 4.2). Points of similarity are the characteristic multiple grouped firings of single sympathetic fibres (firing salvos), and defective re-uptake of noradrenaline by sympathetic nerves in both. But there are many differences. First, the obvious one, is the absence of paradoxical surges of sympathetic activity in depressive illness. Other contrasts are the very high noradrenaline release rates in one third of patients with depressive illness, and in them, the absence of sympathetic

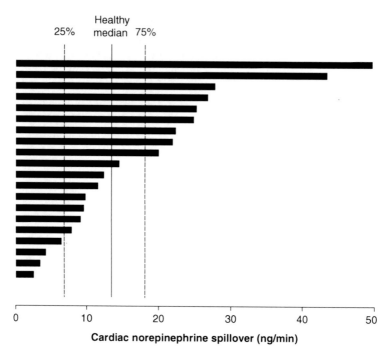

Fig. 4.5 In approximately one third of patients with depressive illness, the sympathetic nervous system is markedly activated.[10] With measurements of whole-body spillover to plasma, the distribution of values is bimodal, with both very high and low-to-normal values.[10] Sympathetic activation is also seen in some patients in the outflow to the heart, based on cardiac noradrenaline spillover measurements, as illustrated in the figure. Individual values for spillover of noradrenaline from the heart are shown in 20 patients with untreated major depressive illness, compared with values in a reference population of healthy men and women. In other clinical contexts, most notably cardiac failure, chronic cardiac sympathetic activity increases risk of death, and in patients with heart failure is beneficially antagonized with beta-adrenergic blocking drugs.[34] Perhaps, anti-adrenergic drug therapy similarly might be helpful in depressive illness, particularly in drug resistant patients in whom remission of the depression cannot be readily achieved. The difficulty here is that the one third of depressed patients with high cardiac sympathetic activity, presumably the ones at highest cardiac risk, cannot be identified on clinical grounds

nerve adrenaline co-transmission (Table 4.2). Well established, but of uncertain significance in relation to disturbances in sympathetic nervous system function, is the increased brain neuronal turnover of serotonin in both disorders.[36,37]

4.5 Mechanism of Cardiac Risk in Depressive Illness and Panic Disorder

A causal relation of episodically or chronically activated cardiac sympathetic tone to adverse cardiac events does seem to generally apply, having been demonstrated elsewhere in patients unexpectedly developing ventricular tachyarrhythmias,[38] in

Table 4.2 Similarities and contrasts in the neural pathophysiology of panic disorder and depressive illness

	Panic disorder	Depressive illness
Multi-unit sympathetic nerve firing rate	Normal	Increased/normal (?)
Single-fibre sympathetic nerve firing	Multiple firings (salvos)	Multiple firings
Total and card. noradren spillover (resting)	Normal	Very high in one third
Symp. nerve noradrenaline reuptake	Impaired	Impaired
Symp. nerve adrenaline co-transmission	Present	Absent
Brain neuronal serotonin turnover	Increased	Increased

Depressive illness and panic disorder commonly coexist in individual patients. If research patient recruitment is such as to minimize this co-morbidity, crucial for the sympathetic neurobiology of the two conditions to be meaningfully compared, there are points of both similarity and contrast. The commonality is in the pattern of single-fibre sympathetic nerve firing, with salvos of firing within a cardiac cycle in both[20,21], in impairment in sympathetic nerve re-uptake of the transmitter[13-15], and in increased brain neuronal turnover of serotonin, measured directly with internal jugular venous sampling[35,36]. Interpretation of the origins of these links does remain problematic

patients with cardiac failure,[39,40] in the inherited long QT syndrome[41] and in end-stage renal disease.[42] The role of sympathetic activation in stress cardiomyopathy is discussed elsewhere in this book (Chap. 9). Might there be specific neural or adrenal medullary mediating mechanisms of cardiac risk in patients with depressive illness and panic disorder?

4.5.1 Panic Disorder

Mediation of heart risk does seem to be explicit during panic attacks, with mechanisms similar or identical to those well characterized during the triggering of adverse cardiac events with acute mental stress in other contexts. In my practice of cardiology I have encountered heart attacks triggered by armed robbery, assaults, and even a racehorse winning by a 'nose'. The report of heart attacks during the 2006 FIFA World Cup of Soccer.[29] is a by now celebrated example of this phenomenon.

The mechanisms proposed[1] for triggering of heart attacks by acute mental stress are:

1. Activation of the sympathetic nervous system, preferentially involving the sympathetic outflow to the heart,[43] which can cause lethal cardiac arrhythmias in the presence of coronary artery narrowing and myocardial ischaemia.
2. Augmented adrenaline secretion by the adrenal medulla, which can activate platelets, predisposing to thrombosis, and reduce serum potassium concentrations, by as much as 0.5–1.0 mmol/L, potentiating the development of disorders of cardiac rhythm.
3. Blood pressure surges accompanying acute mental stress, which can fissure coronary artery atherosclerotic plaques, providing a focus for this thrombosis, and subsequently leading to myocardial infarction.

Panic disorder provides a special case, with additional predisposing features, in which the massive level of sympathetic activation which occurs during a panic attack is no doubt augmented by the single-fibre firing pattern of salvos within a cardiac cycle (thought to cause inordinately high rates of noradrenaline release), and by faulty neuronal re-uptake of noradrenaline (which causes persistence of noradrenaline within the synapse). Adrenaline sympathetic nerve co-transmission additionally is presumably arrhythmogenic. At the very high rates of sympathetic nerve firing in a panic attack, the documented release of neuropeptide Y may possibly be the mediator of coronary artery spasm.[28] This interpretation attributes the increased cardiac risk of panic disorder specifically to the panic attack phenomena, not to the quiescent changes in sympathetic nerve biology (faulty noradrenaline re-uptake, sympathetic nerve adrenaline co-transmission).

4.5.2   Depressive Illness

The neural mechanisms of heart risk in patients with depressive illness presumably differ categorically from those operative in panic disorder. The striking abnormality in depressive illness is a remarkable, chronic activation of the cardiac sympathetic outflow in approximately one third of patients, to a level seen in patients with heart failure. In patients with cardiac failure, this level of sympathetic activity can be lethal,[39] and is beneficially targeted with beta-adrenergic blocking drugs.[34] There is no direct evidence to-date that the depressed patients with very high cardiac sympathetic activity are those particularly at risk, but this is a plausible assumption.

The question might be put: 'In patients with depressive illness, if sympathetic nervous activation increases cardiac risk, why does the sympathetic activation not also elevate blood pressure?' In patients with depressive illness there is no increase in hypertension prevalence,[44] which is perhaps surprising given that there is unequivocal evidence that chronic sympathetic nervous activation is one important mechanism by which the pressure elevation characterizing essential hypertension is generated.[8,25,45] Explicit evidence for this has recently been provided in the anti-hypertensive effect of catheter-based radiofrequency ablation of the renal sympathetic nerves in patients with severe, difficult to control essential hypertension.[46] Perhaps the anomalously normal blood pressure in depression derives from the pattern of sympathetic activation present. Sympathetic nervous system activation in the physiological responses of health and in disease is commonly not global, involving all outflows, but differentiated, with activation of outflows to some organs accompanying no change or sympathetic inhibition in other outflows.[8] Renal sympathetic activation, it seems from clinical observations and the experience with renal denervation in experimental hypertension,[46] is crucial in the pathogenesis of hypertension. Perhaps the sympathetic activation of depressive illness spares the renal sympathetic outflow. This has not yet been tested.

4.5.3   Implications for Therapy

4.5.3.1   Panic Disorder

It is probable that only a small minority of patients with panic disorder, those who have crushing, anginal chest pain during an attack (presumably attributable to coronary artery spasm), are at particular risk for myocardial infarction or the development of cardiac arrhythmias. Conventional cardiac stress tests which are dependent on the demonstration of myocardial ischaemia during increased cardiac work, a sign of persistent coronary artery stenosis, are not diagnostically helpful in patients with panic disorder. A better understanding of the mechanism of coronary artery spasm in panic disorder would facilitate therapeutic intervention. At present I treat patients with panic disorder and clinical evidence of coronary spasm (anginal pain) with conventional measures, selective serotonin re-uptake blocking drugs and cognitive behaviour therapy, aimed at preventing or minimising their panic attacks, plus a dihydropyridine calcium-channel blocker to non-specifically oppose coronary artery spasm, and low-dose aspirin as prophylaxis against coronary thrombosis during spasm.[16] Neuropeptide Y antagonists are not yet available for clinical use. Drugs which act within the central nervous system to inhibit sympathetic outlow, such as the imidazoline agents moxonidine and rilmenidine, might be beneficial but have not yet been trialled.

4.5.3.2   Depressive Illness

In a range of clinical contexts other than depressive illness, ongoing stimulation of the cardiac sympathetic outflow has been demonstrated to contribute to myocardial infarction, ventricular arrhythmias and sudden death.[38-42] Activation of the sympathetic outflow to the heart in patients with cardiac failure is successfully antagonized pharmacologically with beta-adrenergic blocking drugs.[34] Should the chronic sympathetic activation in patients with depressive illness similarly be targeted beta-adrenergic blockers, or alternatively, centrally acting sympathetic inhibitors of the imidazoline class? This might be particularly recommended in patients with treatment-resistant depressive illness, who are at continuing cardiac risk. But there is a difficulty here; only one third of depressed patients have the high cardiac sympathetic activity abnormality,[10] and these cannot readily be identified on clinical grounds. Furthermore, such treatment might influence their mental state.

References

1. Rozanski A, Blumenthal JA, Kaplan J. Impact of psychological factors on the pathogenesis of cardiovascular disease and implications for therapy. *Circulation*. 1999;99:2192-2217.
2. Bunker SJ, Colquhoun DM, Esler MD, et al. "Stress" and coronary heart disease: psychosocial risk factors. National Heart Foundation of Australia position statement update. *Med J Aust*. 2003;178:272-276.

3. Esler M, Schwarz R, Alvarenga M. Mental stress is a cause of cardiovascular diseases: from skepticism to certainty. *Stress Health.* 2008;24:175-180.

4. Leor J, Poole WK, Kloner RA. Sudden cardiac death triggered by an earthquake. *N Engl J Med.* 1996;334:413-419.

5. Hagbarth K-E, Vallbo AB. Pulse and respiratory grouping of sympathetic impulses in human muscle nerves. *Acta Physiol Scand.* 1968;74:96-106.

6. Lambert E, Straznicky N, Schlaich MP, et al. Differing patterns of sympathoexcitation in normal weight and obesity-related hypertension. *Hypertension.* 2007;50:862-868.

7. Esler M, Jennings G, Korner P, et al. Measurement of total and organ-specific norepinephrine kinetics in humans. *Am J Physiol.* 1984;247:E21-E28. Endocrinol Metab 10.

8. Esler M, Jennings G, Lambert G, et al. Overflow of catecholamine neurotransmitters to the circulation: source, fate and functions. *Physiol Rev.* 1990;70:963-985.

9. Macefield V, Wallin BG, Vallbo AB. The discharge behaviour of single vasoconstrictor motoneurones in human muscle nerves. *J Physiol.* 1994;481:799-809.

10. Barton DA, Dawood T, Lambert EA, et al. Sympathetic activity in major depressive disorder: identifying those at increased cardiac risk? *J Hypertens.* 2007;25:2117-2124.

11. Wilkinson DJC, Thompson JM, Lambert GW, et al. Sympathetic activity in patients with panic disorder at rest, under laboratory mental stress and during panic attacks. *Arch Gen Psychiatry.* 1998;55:511-520.

12. Eisenhofer G, Friberg P, Rundqvist B, et al. Cardiac sympathetic nerve function in congestive heart failure. *Circulation.* 1996;93:1667-1676.

13. Alvarenga ME, Richards JC, Lambert G, et al. Psychophysiological mechanisms in panic disorder: a correlative analysis of noradrenaline spillover, neuronal noradrenaline reuptake, power spectral analysis of heart rate variability and psychological variables. *Psychosom Med.* 2006;68:8-12.

14. Esler M, Alvarenga M, Lambert G, et al. Cardiac sympathetic nerve biology and brain monoamine turnover in panic disorder. *Ann N Y Acad Sci.* 2004;1018:505-514.

15. Esler M, Eikelis N, Schlaich M, et al. Human sympathetic nerve biology: parallel influences of stress and epigenetics in essential hypertension and panic disorder. *Ann N Y Acad Sci.* 2008; 1148:338-348.

16. Mansour VM, Wilkinson DJC, Jennings GL, et al. Panic disorder: coronary spasm as a basis for cardiac risk? *Med J Aust.* 1998;168:390-392.

17. Kawachi I, Colditz GA, Ascherio A, et al. Prospective study of phobic anxiety and risk of coronary heart disease in men. *Circulation.* 1994;89:1992-1997.

18. Kawachi I, Sparrow D, Vokanas PS, et al. Symptoms of anxiety and coronary heart disease. The Normative Aging Study. *Circulation.* 1994;90:2225-2229.

19. Albert CM, Chae CU, Rexrode KM, et al. Phobic anxiety and risk of coronary heart disease and sudden cardiac death among women. *Circulation.* 2005;111:480-487.

20. Lambert E, Hotchkin E, Alvarenga M, et al. Single-unit analysis of sympathetic nervous discharges in patients with panic disorder. *J Physiol.* 2006;570:637-643.

21. Lambert E, Dawood T, Schlaich M, et al. Single-unit sympathetic discharge pattern in pathological conditions associated with elevated cardiovascular risk. *Clin Exp Pharmacol Physiol.* 2008;35:503-507.

22. Esler M, Eikelis N, Schlaich M, et al. Chronic mental stress is a cause of essential hypertension: presence of biological markers of stress. *Clin Exp Pharmacol Physiol.* 2008;35:498-502.

23. Lambert E, Dawood T, Straznicky N, et al. Association between the sympathetic firing pattern and anxiety level in patients with the metabolic syndrome and elevated blood pressure. *J Hypertens.* 2010;28(3):543-550.

24. Micutkova L, Krepsova K, Sabban E, et al. Modulation of catecholamine-synthesizing enzymes in the rat heart by repeated immobilization stress. *Ann N Y Acad Sci.* 2004;1018:424-429.

25. Rumantir MS, Kaye DM, Jennings GL, et al. Phenotypic evidence of faulty neuronal noradrenaline reuptake in essential hypertension. *Hypertension.* 2000;36:824-829.

26. Esler M, Wallin G, Dorward P, et al. Effects of desipramine on sympathetic nerve firing and norepinephrine spillover to plasma in man. *Am J Physiol.* 1991;260:R817-R823.

27. Esler M, Alvarenga M, Pier C, et al. The neuronal noradrenaline transporter, anxiety and cardiovascular disease. *J Psychopharmacol*. 2006;20(suppl):60-66.
28. Hass M. Neuropeptide Y: a cardiac sympathetic cotransmitter? In: Goldstein DS, McCarthy R, eds. *Catecholamines: Bridging Basic Science with Clinical Medicine*. New York: Academic; 1998:129-132.
29. Wilbert-Lampen U, Leistner D, Greven S, et al. Cardiovascular events during World Cup soccer. *N Engl J Med*. 2008;358:475-483.
30. Frasure-Smith N, Lesperance F, Talajiic M. Depression following myocardial infarction: impact on 6-month survival. *JAMA*. 1993;270:1819-1861.
31. Anda R, Williamson D, Jones D, et al. Depressed affect, hopelessness, and the risk of ischemic heart disease in a cohort of U.S. adults. *Epidemiology*. 1993;4:285-294.
32. Musselman DL, Evans DL, Nemeroff CB. The relationship of depression to cardiovascular disease. *Arch Gen Psychiatry*. 1998;55:580-592.
33. Esler M, Turbott J, Schwarz R, et al. The peripheral kinetics of norepinephrine in depressive illness. *Arch Gen Psychiatry*. 1982;9:295-300.
34. Dickstein K, Cohen-Solal A, Filippatos G, et al. ESC guidelines for the diagnosis and treatment of acute and chronic heart failure. *Eur Heart J*. 2008;29:2388-2442.
35. Scalco AZ, Rondon MUPB, Trombetta IC, et al. Muscle sympathetic nervous activity in depressed patients before and after treatment with sertraline. *J Hypertens*. 2009;27:2429-2436.
36. Esler M, Lambert E, Alvarenga M, et al. Increased brain serotonin turnover in panic disorder patients in the absence of a panic attack: reduction by a selective serotonin reuptake inhibitor. *Stress*. 2007;10:295-304.
37. Barton DA, Esler MD, Dawood T, et al. Elevated brain serotonin turnover in patients with depression: effect of genotype and therapy. *Arch Gen Psychiatry*. 2008;65:1-9.
38. Meredith IT, Broughton A, Jennings GL, et al. Evidence for a selective increase in resting cardiac sympathetic activity in some patients suffering sustained out of hospital ventricular arrhythmias. *N Engl J Med*. 1991;325:618-624.
39. Kaye DM, Lefkovits J, Jennings GL, et al. Adverse consequences of high sympathetic nervous activity in the failing human heart. *J Am Coll Cardiol*. 1995;26:1257-1263.
40. Brunner-La Rocca HP, Esler MD, Jennings GL, et al. Effect of cardiac sympathetic nervous activity on mode of death in congestive heart failure. *Eur Heart J*. 2001;22:1136-1143.
41. Zipes DP. The long QT interval syndrome. A Rosetta stone for sympathetic related ventricular tachyarrhythmias. *Circulation*. 1991;84:1414-1419.
42. Zoccali C, Mallamaci F, Parlongo S, et al. Plasma norepinephrine predicts survival and incident cardiovascular events in patients with end-stage renal disease. *Circulation*. 2002;105:1354-1359.
43. Esler M, Jennings G, Lambert G. Measurement of overall and cardiac norepinephrine release into plasma during cognitive challenge. *Psychoneuroendocrinology*. 1989;14:477-481.
44. Esler M. Depressive illness, the sympathetic nervous system and cardiac risk. *J Hypertens*. 2009;27:2349-2350.
45. Grassi G, Colombo M, Seravalle G, et al. Dissociation between muscle and skin sympathetic nerve activity in essential hypertension, obesity, and congestive heart failure. *Hypertension*. 1998;31:64-67.
46. Krum H, Schlaich MP, Whitbourn R, et al. Catheter-based renal sympathetic denervation for resistant hypertension: a multicentre safety and proof-of-principle cohort study. *Lancet*. 2009;373:1275-1281.

Chapter 5
Hypothalamic–Pituitary–Adrenal Axis and Cardiovascular Disease

Gregory Kaltsas, Anthony S. Zannas, and George P. Chrousos

Keywords Hypothalamic–Pituitary–Adrenal axis • Cardiovascular disease • Stress system • Stress response • Glucocorticoid circulation • Glucocorticoid metabolism • Glucocorticoid receptor (GR) • Effects on the immune system • Stress and cardiovascular risk factors

5.1 Introduction

Complex biological systems constantly maintain a dynamic equilibrium (homeostasis) that is necessary for survival. This equilibrium is achieved through interactions with the environment, and adaptation to the ever-changing internal and external milieu. Throughout evolution, the *stress system* has remained a relatively well-preserved biological machinery that has served this function efficiently; designed to respond to internal or external challenges (stressors), and to reestablish homeostasis by various physiological and behavioral adaptive responses to stress which have been necessary for the survival of our ancestors in adverse environments. Nonetheless, in modern, "safe" societies, stress very often becomes a maladaptive response to perceived, rather than real, stimuli that threaten homeostasis. Excess severity or duration of the stress response, as well as defective or

G. Kaltsas
Department of Pathophysiology, Laiko Hospital, National University of Athens, Athens, Greece

A.S. Zannas
Department of Psychiatry and Behavioral Sciences, Duke University Medical Center, Durham, NC, USA

G.P. Chrousos (✉)
First Department of Pediatrics, Aghia Sophia Children's Hospital, Athens, Greece
e-mail: chrousge@med.uoa.gr

P. Hjemdahl et al. (eds.), *Stress and Cardiovascular Disease*,
DOI 10.1007/978-1-84882-419-5_5, © Springer-Verlag London Limited 2012

inadequate responses, can lead to several acute and chronic stress-related disorders. Of note, chronic stress can affect the hypothalamic–pituitary–adrenal (HPA) axis and lead to overt or subtle hypercortisolism, a pathophysiological effect that can significantly contribute either directly or indirectly to major risk factors for cardiovascular (CV) morbidity and mortality. In addition, the way that each individual perceives alterations to glucocorticoid exposure at the cellular level can also account for some of these effects.

5.2 Overview of the Stress System and the Stress Response

The integrated stress response occurs as a result of biological, physical, or psychological stimuli that threaten homeostasis (stressors), and involves neuroendocrine, autonomic, behavioral, and immune components. The stress system coordinates these adaptive responses, and is mainly comprised of the hypothalamic- corticotropin releasing hormone (CRH/PVN) and locus ceruleus–norepinephrine (LC/NE) systems, and their peripheral effectors, the pituitary–adrenal axis and the limbs of the autonomic nervous system.[1] These branches functionally relate to each other, and interact with other central systems involved in the stress response (Fig. 5.1). The HPA axis and the sympathoadrenal system represent the primary effectors, via which the brain influences all organs during exposure to threatening stimuli. Each level of the stress system is tightly regulated by various neural and hormonal inputs from both the central nervous system (CNS) and the periphery.

The stress response referred to by Selye as "the general adaptation syndrome,"[2] was considered to be relatively nonspecific, and diverse stressors were thought to exert similar responses. However, experimental studies that involved brain lesions, pharmacological interventions, and early gene expression have shown that several brain regions are differentially activated by physical and psychological stressors. Physical (systemic) stressors (such as hemorrhage, inflammation, and other major threatening events) activate the brain stem and circumventricular areas that project to the paraventricular nucleus (PVN) of the hypothalamus, while psychological stressors (such as social defeat, rejection, and mental illnesses) activate limbic structures that project to the hypothalamus and other regions of the CNS.[3] The limbic system is necessary for the evaluative process that precedes the response to any psychological stressor; stimuli in the social environment which are evaluated as threatening, either real or perceived, activate the stress system. Additionally, each peripheral effector of the stress system may be activated specifically, or to a different extent, by different stressors.[4]

There is also a high level of plasticity in the regulation of the HPA axis, as chronic stress can lead to marked alterations in the control of the HPA axis.[5] For example, in chronically stressed rats as compared to rats not exposed to any stress, it has been shown that an acute stressor leads to reduced HPA axis activation if the applied stimulus is similar to the chronic stimulus (homotypic stress), while the activation of the HPA axis is markedly facilitated if the applied stressor is novel and different from the chronic stimulus (heterotypic stress).[6] This plasticity may result from the

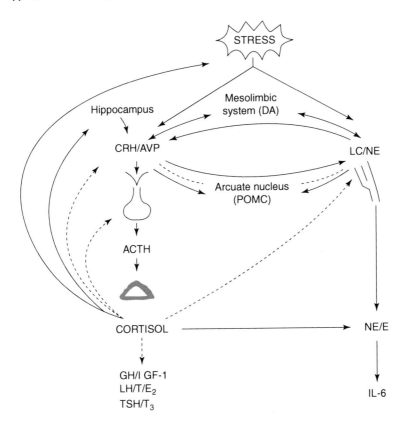

Fig. 5.1 Schematic depiction of the central and peripheral components of the stress system and their complex interactions. The CRH/AVP and the LC/NE reciprocally connect and activate each other, and also interact with multiple areas of the brain, including the mesolimbic system, the amygdala, the hippocampus, and the arcuate nucleus of the hypothalamus. Multiple feedback loops regulate the HPA axis, while activation of the HPA axis leads to suppression of several endocrine systems, including growth, reproductive, and thyroid hormones. *Solid lines* indicate stimulation; *dashed lines* indicate inhibition

convergence of diverse neuronal projections to the hypothalamic PVN, emphasizing that multiple neural circuits and their complex interconnections can affect the stress response and, consequently, the results of stress on bodily organs.

5.3 HPA Axis and Coordination of the Stress Response

The HPA axis (Fig. 5.1) commences with the release of CRH into the hypophysial portal blood, which drives the synthesis and secretion of adrenocorticotropin hormone (ACTH). ACTH in turn is released into the systemic circulation and stimulates the synthesis and secretion of corticosteroids by the adrenal cortex.[1,7] Cortisol, which is the major corticosteroid in humans, is the final effector of the HPA axis and responsible for a wide range of homeostatic activities of the body. Multiple negative feedback loops regulate the basal activity of the HPA axis and the termination of stress responses, thus maintaining homeostasis and achieving adaptation.

CRH is a 41 amino acid neuropeptide that is produced and secreted by nerve terminals in the hypothalamus.[8] From this site, CRH diffuses into the hypophysial-portal circulation and stimulates synthesis of the precursor of ACTH, proopiomel-anocortin (POMC). A proportion of the CRH-synthesizing neurons also produces and secretes arginine-vasopressin (AVP), which acts synergistically with CRH to potentiate ACTH secretion.[9] The secretion of both CRH and AVP follows an ultra-dian rhythm, with two to three secretory pulses per hour,[10] and a circadian pattern, with peak levels in the early morning and trough levels in the evening hours. This circadian pattern drives the diurnal activity of the HPA axis, and is regulated by the negative feedback cotnrol exerted by cortisol. CRH secretion is stimulated by sero-tonin, norepinephrine, and acetylcholine. The potencies of the feedback stimuli may be determined by the state of activation of the CRH neuron.

CRH is also produced in multiple sites in the CNS outside the PVN, and stress stimulates CRH release from both hypothalamic and extrahypothalamic sites.[6,11] CRH-producing neurons are found in the central nucleus of the amygdala, bed nucleus of the stria terminalis, parabrachial nuclei, and the dorsal motor nucleus of the vagus. Corticosteroids significantly affect the expression of CRH in several of these brain areas; CRH expression in the PVN is decreased as a result of negative feedback, whereas CRH expression is increased in the amygdala and bed nucleus, suggesting that corticosteroids differentially regulate CRH at different sites of the brain.

CRH receptors that mediate CRH actions are expressed in several areas of the brain outside the pituitary including the amygdala, the central arousal sympathetic system (LC/NE), several brainstem nuclei, the cerebellar cortex, and areas of the spinal cord.[12,13] CRH receptors located in the locus ceruleus are responsible for the stimulatory effect of CRH on norepinephrine (NE) release from the LC/NE system. NE also activates the amygdala, the brain structure that is responsible for fear-related behaviors and emotional memories of aversive stimuli.[14]

Furthermore, reciprocal interactions exist between the stress system and the meso-cortical/mesolimbic system, the arcuate nucleus-opioid system, and the hippocampus (Fig. 5.1). Both the CRH/AVP and LC/NE systems activate (acutely and transiently) the mesolimbic and mesocortical dopaminergic reward systems.[15] Finally, the stress system acutely activates the hippocampus, an organ that has a major role in intermediate-term memory, whereas it receives tonic, inhibitory input from the hippocampus.[16]

In conclusion, the complex central CRH system appears to play a pivotal role in the stimulation of the neuroendocrine, autonomic, and behavioral components of stress, as well as in the integration and coordination of the overall stress response.[17] Of note is that CRH through its action in the CNS can result in increased arousal, without an accompanying significant increase in ACTH and catecholamines.[18] Selective adminis-tration of CRH into the brains of rodents and primates precipitated several coordinated responses characteristic of stress, whereas oral administration of a CRH receptor antagonist significantly attenuated the behavioral, neuroendocrine, and autonomic manifestations of stress in primates.[19] Finally, CRH type 1 receptor knockout mice exhibit a markedly decreased ability to mount an effective stress response.[20]

5.4 Glucocorticoid Mode of Action and Effects on Bodily Organs, Particularly the Cardiovascular System

GCs are major components of the stress system that affect many different systems. They act to initiate and maintain metabolic, autonomic, psychological, and cardiovascular components of responses to daily stressors. Permissive actions of GCs facilitate the vascular and metabolic effects of other stress hormones, such as catecholamines, glucagon, and angiotensin II.[21] GCs also attenuate inflammation, cellular proliferation, and tissue repair processes aiming at maintaining the inflammatory response at specific tissue level and avoiding a generalized inflammatory response. In addition these compounds prepare the organism for prolonged nutritional deprivation by facilitating proteolysis and insulin resistance (IR) at the muscular level.[22] Due to their multiple action on different tissues they can induce a great number of genes upon binding to specific GC receptors (GRs), and exert both beneficial (suppression of inflammation and cell proliferation) and/or harmful effects (increased blood pressure and insulin resistance) to the CV system, depending on the level of tissue exposure to GCs and the duration of exposure (Table 5.1).

5.4.1 Glucocorticoid Circulation and Metabolism

The plasma half-life of free, biologically active cortisol in plasma is 60–90 min, and is determined by the extent of binding to specific plasma proteins (mainly corticosteroid binding protein, CBP) and by the rate of metabolic inactivation.[23] Only free cortisol is biologically active; it is under tight ACTH regulation and exerts its activity by binding to the GR.[24] GCs are metabolized in the liver whereas cortisol is also converted extensively by the enzyme 11β-hydroxysteroid dehydrogenase (11β-HSD type 2) to the biologically inactive cortisone.[24] This inactivation is particularly important in the kidneys as it protects the mineralocorticoid receptor from occupancy by cortisol, and this prevents cortisol from causing a mineralocorticoid excess state[25] (Fig. 5.2). Conversely, 11β-HSD type 1 converts inactive cortisone into cortisol.

Currently, there are several means of assessing cortisol secretion in basal and stressful situations and thus estimating the adequacy of the HPA axis in these states. Although salivary and plasma cortisol are easy to measure, multiple serial assays are necessary to show hypercortisolism, except in cases of severe and protracted stress where a single measurement may be sufficient.

5.4.2 The Glucocorticoid Receptor (GR)

At the cellular level, the great majority of GC effects are mediated by the GR[25] which is a nuclear receptor that has at least two alternative splice variants leading to two different isoforms[26] (Fig. 5.3). The GR α isoform binds cortisol, DNA, and other transcription factors, thereby modifying the transcriptional activity of target genes. GR β can form heterodimers with GR α and interfere with the function of

Table 5.1 Genes that are regulated by glucocorticoids or glucocorticoid receptors

Site of action	Induced genes	Repressed genes
Immune system	IκB (NFκB inhibitor)	Interleukins
	Haptoglobin	TNF-α
	TCR z	IFN-γ
	p21, p27 and p57	E selectin
	Lipocortin	ICAM-1
		Cyclooxygenase 2
		iNOS
Metabolic	PPAR-γ	Tryptophan hydroxylase
	Tyrosine aminotransferase	Metalloprotease
	Glutamine synthase	
	Glycogen-6-phosphatase	
	PEPCK	
	Leptin	
	γ-Fibrinogen	
	Cholesterol 7α hydroxylase	
	C/EBP/β	
Bone	Androgen receptor	Osteocalcin
	Calcitonin receptor	Collagenase
	Alkaline phosphatase	
	IGF-BP-6	
Channels and transporters	Epithelium sodium channel (ENaC) α, β, γ	
	Serum and glucocorticoid–induced kinase (SGK)	
	Aquaporin	
Endocrine	βFGF	GR
	VIP	PRL
	Endothelin	POMC/CRH
	RXR	PTHP
	GHRH receptor	Vasopressin
	Natriuretic peptide receptors	
Growth and development	Surfactant protein A, B, C	Fibronectin
		A-Fetoprotein
		NGF
		Erythropoetin
		G1 cyclins
		Cyclin-dependant kinases

bFGF basic fibroblast growth factor, *C/EBP/β* CAAT-enchancer binding protein-beta, *GR* glucocorticoid receptor, *GHRH* growth hormone-releasing hormone, *ICAM* intercellular adhesion molecule, *IFN* interferon, *IGF-BP* insulin growth factor-binding protein, *IkB* inhibitory kappa B, *iNOS* inducible nitric oxide synthase, *NFkB* nuclear factor kB, *NGF* nerve growth factor, *PEPCK* phosphoenolpyruvate carboxykinase, *POMC* propiomelanocortin, *PPAR* peroxisome proliferator – activated receptor, *PTHrP* parathyroid hormone–related protein, *RXR* retinoid X receptor, *SGK* serum and glucocorticoid-induced kinase, *TCR* T-cell receptor, *TNF-α* tumor necrosis factor-alpha, *VIP* vasoactive intestinal peptide

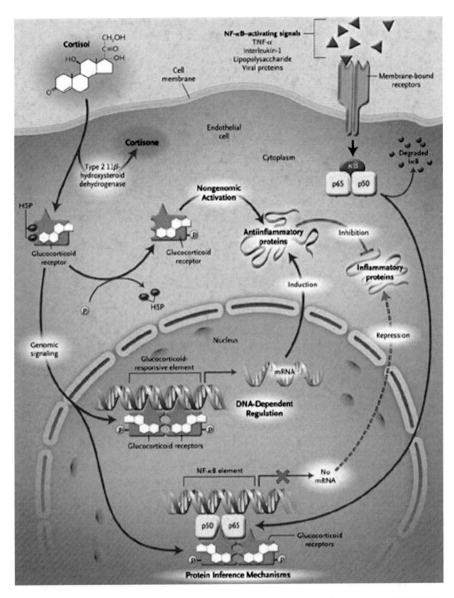

Fig. 5.2 Enzymatic glucocorticoid shuttling. 11β–Hydroxysteroid dehydrogenase (11β-HSD): 11β-HSD catalyzes the interconversion of active cortisol and cortisone. There are two isoenzymes, which are the products of distinct genes. 11β-HSD2 is a nicotinamide adenine dinucleotide (NAD-dependent dehydrogenase that exclusively catalyzes the inactivation of physiological glucocorticoids (Adapted from Rhen and Cidlowski[24])

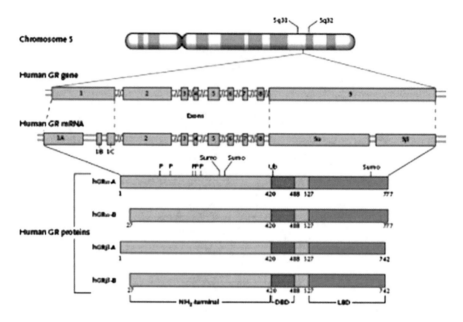

Fig. 5.3 Genomic organization and localization of the glucocorticoid receptor (Adapted from Rhen and Cidlowski[24])

this protein. The relative levels of GR α and β influence cell sensitivity to GCs with higher levels of GR β leading to GC resistance.[27]

5.4.3 GR-Mediated Transcriptional Regulation and Activation

Many effects of GCs are achieved by inhibition rather than activation of target genes[28] (Table 5.2). This is especially true for the anti-inflammatory/immunosuppressive effects of GCs that involve suppressed transcription of immune genes. Another mechanism of action is GC signaling through membrane-associated receptors and second messengers (so-called non-genomic pathways).[25] The most significant example is that of GC-induced fast feedback inhibition of ACTH release; this effect occurs within minutes of GC administration and its rapidity of action suggests that it is not mediated by RNA and protein synthesis.

5.4.4 Biological Effects of Glucocorticoids

Although GCs were originally named because of their effect on glucose metabolism, they are currently defined as steroids that exert their effects after binding to specific

Table 5.2 The principal action of glucocorticoids in humans, highlighting some of the consequences of glucocorticoid excess

System/organ	Effect
Brain/CNS	Depression
	Psychosis
Eye	Glaucoma
Endocrine system	Reduction of LH, FSH release
	Reduction of TSH release
	Reduction of GH secretion
	Increase of appetite
Gastrointestinal tract	Increase in acid secretion (peptic ulceration)
Carbohydrate/lipid metabolism	Increased hepatic glycogen deposition
	Increased peripheral insulin secretion
	Increased gluconeogenesis
	Increased fatty acid production
	Overall diabetogenic effect
	Promotion of visceral obesity
Cardiovascular/renal	Salt and water retention
	Hypertension
Skin/muscle/renal	Protein catabolism/collagen breakdown
	Thinning of the skin
	Muscular atrophy
Bone	Reduction of bone formation
	Reduction of bone mass and development of osteoporosis
Growth and development	Reduction of linear growth
Immune system	Anti-inflammatory action
	Immunosuppression

CNS central nervous system, *GI* gastrointestinal, *FSH* follicle-stimulating hormone, *GH* growth hormone, *LH* luteinizing hormone, *TSH* thyroid-stimulating hormone

GRs, which mediate their actions.[25,28] These receptors are expressed in virtually all tissues and therefore GCs exert a broad spectrum of biological effects almost throughout the body (Table 5.2). It has been estimated that approximately 20% of the human genome is affected by GCs, being either down- or up-regulated by them[29] (Table 5.1, Fig. 5.4). GCs in general inhibit DNA synthesis and in many tissues they also inhibit RNA and protein synthesis, while they accelerate protein catabolism. These actions provide substrate for intermediary metabolism. Accelerated metabolism accounts for the deleterious effects of GCs in several tissues.[28]

5.4.5 *Specific Glucocorticoid Effects on Intermediary Metabolism and the Cardiovascular (CV) System*

GCs increase blood glucose concentrations through their actions on glycogen, protein, and lipid metabolism (Table 5.2). These effects are minimal in the fed state

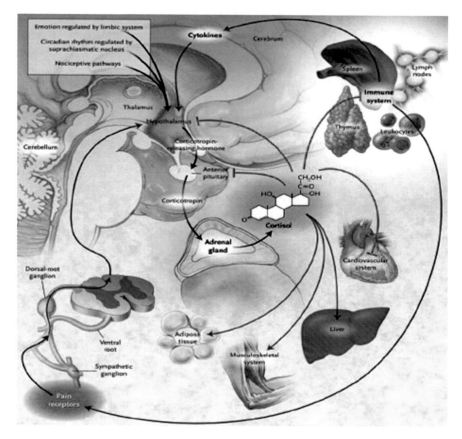

Fig. 5.4 Neuroendocrine control and diversity of action of glucocorticoids (Adapted from Rhen and Cidlowski[24])

but during fasting GCs facilitate the maintenance of adequate glucose concentrations. In the liver, GCs stimulate glycogen deposition and activate hepatic glucose production through the activation of key enzymes involved in gluconeogenesis.[30] In muscle and fat, GCs inhibit glucose uptake and utilization, whereas in adipose tissue they induce lipolysis resulting in the release of free fatty acids into the circulation.[31] GCs also have permissive effects in the actions of other hormones, including catecholamines and glucagon. The net effect of GCs on intermediary metabolism is to cause insulin resistance (IR) and an increase in blood glucose concentration at the expense of muscle and lipid catabolism (Table 5.3). GCs also stimulate adipocyte differentiation and the development of visceral obesity in states of excessive GC production; this may be explained by the increased expression of GR and the type 1 isoenzyme of 11β-HSD in omental compared to subcutaneous adipose tissue.[32]

Table 5.3 Changes associated with glucocorticoid-induced insulin resistance (IR)

Lifestyle	Sedentary behavior
Lipoproteins	Increased apo B, apo C-III
	Decreased Apo A-1
	Small dense LDL and HDL
Pro-thrombotic	Increased fibrinogen, plasma activator inhibitor 1, viscosity
Inflammatory markers	Increased WBC, IL-6, TNF-α, CRP, resistin
	Decreased adiponectin
Vascular	Microalbuminuria
	Increased asymmetric dimethylarginine
Other	Increased uric acid, homocysteine
	Polycyctic ovary syndrome
	Nonalcoholic steatohepatitis
	Obstructive sleep apnea

WBC white blood cell count

GCs may increase cardiac output, and they also increase peripheral vascular tone by augmenting the effects of vasoconstrictors such as catecholamines and angiotensin II, while reducing nitric oxide mediated endothelial vasodilatation.[33] Thus, shock that is refractory to vasoconstrictors may develop when GC deficient individuals are subjected to stress. In the kidney, cortisol can act on the distal nephron, if not converted to the metabolically inert cortisone, causing sodium preservation and potassium loss[34] (Fig. 5.2).

5.4.6 Other GC Endocrine Effects That Can Affect Metabolism

GCs exert permissive effects in growth and development by accelerating the development of several tissues in fetal life, probably through interaction with various growth factors.[28] However, elevated GC levels suppress pituitary growth hormone (GH) secretion and induce resistance to the action of GH and insulin growth factor (IGF) one.[29] GCs suppress the thyroid axis, probably through a direct action on thyroid stimulating hormone (TSH) secretion; in addition, they inhibit 5′ deiodinase activity that mediates the conversion of thyroxine to active triiodothyronine. During inflammatory stress, proinflammatory cytokines, such as TNF-alpha, IL-1, and IL-6, also activate CRH secretion and inhibit 5′-deiodinase activity resulting in decreased T3 and increased rT3 levels.[28,31] Glucocorticoids also act centrally at the hypothalamic level to inhibit the pulsatile secretion of gonadotropin releasing hormone (GnRH) by GnRH neurons and thus luteinizing (LH) and follicle-stimulating hormone (FSH) release; GCs also render target tissues of gonadal steroids resistant to these hormones.[31] These inhibitory effects on the major anabolic hormones and the potential preferential tissue-specific expression of 11β-HSD may account for the development of abdominal obesity in states of excessive GC secretion[31] (Fig. 5.4).

5.4.7   Effects on the Immune System

GCs influence the traffic of circulating leukocytes and inhibit many functions of leukocytes and immune accessory cells. They suppress the immune activation of these cells, inhibit the production of proinflammatory cytokines and other mediators of inflammation, and cause proinflammatory cytokine resistance. During stress IL-6 levels increase substantially and play a major role in the overall control of inflammation by further stimulating GC secretion and by suppressing the secretion of other inflammatory cytokines such as TNF-a and IL-1.[29] Through interaction with the ANS, IL-6 may inhibit IL-12 and stimulate IL-10 secretion, causing suppression of innate and cellular immunity, and stimulation of humoral immunity.[29] This translates clinically into stress-related immunosuppression of mainly innate and cellular immunity[25] (Fig. 5.4).

5.5   Stress and Cardiovascular Risk Factors

The metabolic syndrome is a common metabolic disorder that as a concept has existed the last 70 years following the description of a number of metabolic disturbances, all known risk factors for CV disease (CVD).[35] Its pathophysiology seems to be largely attributable to IR and the presence of a low-grade proinflammatory state.[35] The constellation of metabolic abnormalities includes glucose intolerance (type 2 diabetes, impaired glucose tolerance, impaired fasting glucose), IR, abdominal obesity, dyslipidemia, and hypertension, all documented risk factors of CVD.[36] The chapter by Rosengren in this book discusses the metabolic syndrome and its definitions in detail. It is not surprising that GCs may play an important role in the development of this syndrome as alterations in GC secretion affect insulin secretion/action and lead to a phenotype similar to that of the metabolic syndrome encountered in overt and subclinical Cushing's syndrome (CS). Indeed, the most accepted and unifying hypothesis to describe the pathophysiology of the metabolic syndrome is IR. Insulin resistance has traditionally been defined with a glucocentric view, when a defect in insulin action results in fasting hyperinsulinemia to maintain euglycemia; however, commonly postprandial hyperinsulinemia exists before fasting hyperinsulinemia. GCs induce mainly hepatic IR and can initiate a number of adverse changes explaining the high morbidity and mortality from CVD in patients with CS (Table 4.3). In addition, along with alterations of the HPA axis induced by stress there is also activation of the sympathetic and renin–angiotensin–aldosterone systems that can affect the CV system.[35]

5.6 Effects of Excess Glucocorticoid on Specific Cardiovascular Risk Factors

Body composition: Fat cells are metabolically active, and secrete hormones, cytokines, and metabolites that adversely affect blood pressure, plasma lipoproteins, coagulation, and insulin resistance.[37] Any metabolic change that is associated with obesity, particularly its visceral component, may increase CV risk. In the presence of insulin, GCs promote the terminal differentiation of pre-adipocytes and fibroblast-like stromal vascular precursor cells into mature adipocytes.[38] GCs and insulin act synergistically to increase the activity of 11β-HSD type I in adipocytes, especially in visceral fat depots, augmenting abdominal obesity.[34,38] Desensitization of adipocytes to the lipolytic effects of catecholamines may also contribute to visceral adiposity.[39] Increased visceral adiposity and decreased muscle mass are features of aging in humans, and may be related to increased GC activity along with decreased growth hormone and IGF-1 activity and gonadal steroids.[39] Visceral obesity may be apparent in depressed patients and is then probably related to chronic hypercortisolemia and GC-mediated tissue effects.[33]

Plasma lipoprotein and carbohydrate metabolism: GC excess leading to visceral obesity is associated with low high-density lipoprotein (HDL) cholesterol, high triglyceride (TG) levels and small and dense (atherogenic) low-density lipoprotein (LDL) cholesterol particles.[33] Glucocorticoids also have obesity-independent effects on blood lipids leading to increased LDL-C and TG and reduced HDL-C probably mediated by hyperinsulinemia and IR.[33] As mentioned above, GCs can also cause muscle and hepatic IR and precipitate hyperglycemia. In the liver, GCs oppose the actions of insulin and activate gluconeogenesis by increasing acetyl coenzyme-A levels, whereas increases in citrate lead to inhibition of glycolysis.[33]

Endothelial function, oxidative stress, and vascular tone: Endothelial dysfunction precedes atherosclerosis and is associated with impaired nitric oxide (NO) production, perturbed interactions between platelets, leukocytes, and the vessel wall, and alterations in pro- and anti-thrombotic factors.[40] Endothelial dysfunction is precipitated by hyperglycemia, hypertension, and dyslipidemia, all of which are well-known effects of chronic GC exposure.[40,41] GCs may also impair cholinergic vasodilation mediated in part by reduced activity of inducible nitric oxide synthase (iNOS), or increased oxidative stress.[33,41] GCs may also stimulate the release of the potent vasoconstrictor endothelin-1, an effect that may be partially counter-regulated by a compensatory decrease in endothelin-1 receptors.[33] GCs also increase vascular tone by endothelin-independent mechanisms, that is, by enhancing sympathetic activation, by increased hepatic and adipocyte production of angiotensinogen leading to more angiotensin II being formed, and by reducing vasodilatory prostaglandin E2 synthesis in endothelial and vascular smooth muscle cells.[42]

Inflammation and tissue repair: Atherosclerosis is, in part, an inflammatory disease of the subendothelium.[43] Although acute GC administration may induce a substantial decrease of inflammatory mediators leading to atherosclerosis, sustained and prolonged GC exposure potentiates cytokine-induced CRP increases.[33] The hepatic synthesis of CRP is largely under the regulation of the proinflammatory cytokine IL-6 which has been shown to predict total and CV-mortality over a 5-year follow-up, the association being independent of the presence of other traditional risk factors.[21] IL-6 appears to be the dominant cytokine as it regulates the release and activity of IL-1 and TNFα directly.[21]

Cytokines appear to activate the HPA axis, particularly as IL-6 directly stimulates the hypothalamus to secrete CRH.[28,31] It has been suggested that IL-6 is the "tissue CRH" because of its stimulation of GC secretion especially in chronic stress situations.[44] In addition, IL-6 seems to exert direct effects on insulin secretion and action, release of adhesion molecules by the endothelium and an overall procoagulant effect.[21] Furthermore, stress elevates circulating IL-6 levels, probably through catecholamine-induced IL-6 release from adipose tissue, while inhibiting that from immune cells.[21,33] It is thought that stress-induced increases in IL-6 stimulate the HPA axis, resulting in hypercortisolemia and causing central obesity, IR, and hyperlipidemia; the increased visceral adipose tissue mass further increases IL-6 release and forms the basis for a vicious circle.[21] There is increasing evidence that IR and excess adipose tissue are not only associated with abundance of proinflammatory cytokines but also a relative deficiency of anti-inflammatory cytokines. Such cytokines, mainly adiponectin, are also produced by the adipose tissue and may enhance insulin sensitivity and inhibit many steps of the inflammatory process.[35]

Emotional dysregulation: Stress-induced alterations in GCs, cytokine, and catecholamine secretion are frequently associated with an emotional phenotype similar to adult melancholic depression that leads to perpetuation of the same mechanisms and further dysregulation of the stress response.[29] This form of emotional status is commonly found in patients with the metabolic syndrome and may itself be linked to increased morbidity and mortality from CVD.

5.7 Conclusions

The stress system coordinates the adaptive response of the organism to stressors and plays an important role in the maintenance of basal and stress-related homeostasis. Activation of the stress system leads to behavioral and peripheral changes that improve the ability of the organism to adapt and increase its chances for survival through cortisol and catecholamine hypersecretion. Inadequate and more prolonged responses to stressors may result in a variety of endocrine, metabolic, autoimmune, and psychiatric disorders all of which are associated with increased morbidity and mortality from cardiovascular diseases (Fig. 5.5). Stress-induced hypercortisolism and central obesity are associated with varying degrees and patterns of the metabolic syndrome, and represent common phenomena of major epidemiologic significance. It is of utmost importance to unravel these largely interrelated phenomena as

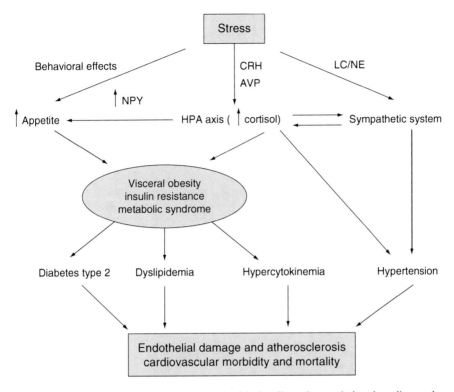

Fig. 5.5 Pathophysiological mechanisms involved in insulin-resistance-induced cardiovascular disease

appropriate changes in lifestyle and possibly pharmacological intervention may help prevent and treat the sequelae of stress and visceral obesity and thus cardiovascular disease. Currently there is an ongoing debate whether such patients should be offered early pharmacological intervention. Lifestyle modification is causal therapy, and can be at least as efficacious – patients should be encouraged to implement lifestyle changes.

References

1. Chrousos GP, Gold PW. The concepts of stress and stress system disorders: overview of physical and behavioral homeostasis. *JAMA*. 1992;267:1244-1252.
2. Selye H. A syndrome produced by diverse nocuous agents. *Nature*. 1936;138:32-36.
3. Herman JP, Cullinan WE. Neurocircuitry of stress: central control of the hypothalamo-pituitaryadrenocortical axis. *Trends Neurosci*. 1997;20(2):78-84.
4. Kvetnasky R, Pacak K, Sabban EL, et al. Stressor specificity of peripheral catecholaminergic activation. *Adv Pharmacol*. 1998;42:556-560.
5. Bhatnagar S, Dallman M. Neuroanatomical basis for facilitation of hypothalamic-pituitary-adrenal responses to a novel stressor after chronic stress. *Neuroscience*. 1998;84(4):1025-1039.

6. Dallman MF, Bhatnagar S, Viau V. Hypothalamic-pituitary-adrenal axis. In: Fink G, ed. *Encyclopedia of Stress*. 1st ed. London: Academic; 2007:421-427.

7. Chrousos GP. Regulation and dysregulation of the hypothalamic-pituitary-adrenal axis. The corticotrophin releasing hormone perspective. *Endocrinol Metab Clin North Am*. 1992;21: 833-858.

8. Antoni FA. Hypothalamic control of adrenocorticotropin secretion: advances since the discovery of 41-residue corticotrophin-releasing factor. *Endocr Rev*. 1986;7(4):351-378.

9. Lamberts SWJ, Verleun T, Oosterom R, et al. Corticotropin releasing factor and vasopressin exert a synergistic effect on adrenocorticotropin release in man. *J Clin Endocrinol Metab*. 1984;58:298-303.

10. Engler O, Pham T, Fullenon MJ, et al. Studies of the secretion of corticotropin releasing factor and arginine-vasopressin into hypophyseal portal circulation of the conscious sheep. *Neuroendocrinology*. 1989;49:367-381.

11. Palkovits M, Young WS, Kovacs K, Toth ZS, Makara GB. Alterations in corticotropin-releasing hormone gene expression of central amygdaloid neurons following long-term paraventricular lesions and adrenalectomy. *Neuroscience*. 1998;85(1):135-147.

12. Wong ML, Licinio J, Pasternak KI, Gold PW. Localization of corticotropin-releasing hormone (CRH) receptor mRNA in adult rat brain by in sity hybridization histochemistry. *Endocrinology*. 1994;135:2275-2278.

13. Potter E, Sutton S, Donaldson C, et al. Distribution of corticotrophin-releasing factor receptor mRNA expression in the rat brain and pituitary. *Proc Natl Acad Sci USA*. 1994;91(19): 8777-8781.

14. Gray TS. Amygdala: role in autonomic and neuroendocrine responses to stress. In: McCubbin A, Kaufmann PG, Nemeroff CB, eds. *Stress, Neuropeptides and Systemic Disease*. New York: Academic; 1989:37-53.

15. Roth RH, Tam SY, Ida Y, Yang J, Deutsch AY. Stress and the mesocorticolimbic dopamine systems. *Ann N Y Acad Sci*. 1988;537:138-147.

16. Mcewen BS. Physiology and neurobiology of stress and adaptation: central role of the brain. *Physiol Rev*. 2007;87:873-904.

17. Dunn AJ, Berridge CW. Physiological and behavioural responses to corticotropin-releasing factor: is CRF a mediator of anxiety or stress responses? *Brain Res Rev*. 1990;15:71-100.

18. Shibasaki T, Imaki T, Hotta M, et al. Psychological stress increases arousal through brain corticotrophin-releasing hormone without significant increase in adrenocorticotropin and catecholamine secretion. *Brain Res*. 1993;618:71-75.

19. Habib KE, Weld KP, Rice KC, et al. Oral administration of a corticotropin-releasing hormone receptor antagonist significantly attenuates behavioral, neuroendocrine, and autonomic responses to stress in primates. *Proc Natl Acad Sci USA*. 2000;97:6079-6084.

20. Smith GW, Aubry JM, Dellu F, et al. Corticotropin releasing factor receptor 1-deficient mice display decreased anxiety, impaired stress response, and aberrant neuroendocrine development. *Neuron*. 1998;20:1093-1102.

21. Yudkin JS, Kumari M, Humphries SE, Mohamed-Ali V. Inflammation, obesity, stress and coronary heart disease: is interleukin-6 the link? *Atherosclerosis*. 2000;148:209-214.

22. Bailey JL, Wang X, Price SR. The balance between glucocorticoids and insulin regulates muscle proteolysis via ubiquitin-proteasome pathway. *Miner Electrol Metab*. 1999;25:220-223.

23. Breuner CW, Orchinik M. Plasma binding proteins as mediators of corticosteroid action in vertebrates. *J Endocrinol*. 2002;175(1):99-112.

24. Rhen T, Cidlowski JA. Antiinflammatory action of glucocorticoids – new mechanisms for old drugs. *N Engl J Med*. 2005;353(16):1711-1723.

25. Bamberger CM, Schulte HM, Chrousos GP. Molecular determinants of glucocorticoid receptor function and tissue sensitivity to glucocorticoids. *Endocr Rev*. 1996;17(3):245-261.

26. Lu NZ, Cidlowski JA. The origin and functions of multiple human glucocorticoid receptor isoforms. *Ann N Y Acad Sci*. 2004;1024:102-123.

27. Pujols L, Mullol J, Perez M, et al. Expression of the human glucocorticoid receptor alpha and beta isoforms in human respiratory epithelial cells and their regulation by dexamethasone. *Am J Resp Cell Mol.* 2001;24(1):49-57.
28. Chrousos GP. Stressors, stress, and neuroendocrine integration of the adaptive response. The 1997 Hans Selye Memorial Lecture. *Ann N Y Acad Sci.* 1998;851:311-335.
29. Chamandari E, Tsigos C, Chrousos G. Endocrinology of the stress response. *Annu Rev Physiol.* 2005;67:259-284.
30. Magnuson MA, Quinn PG, Granner DK. Multihormonal regulation of phosphoenolpyruvate carboxykinase-chloramphenicol acetyltransferase fusion genes. Insulin's effects oppose those of cAMP and dexamethasone. *J Biol Chem.* 1987;262(31):14917-14920.
31. Tsigos C, Chrousos GP. Hypothalamic-pituitary-adrenal axis, neuroendocrine factors and stress. *J Psychosom Res.* 2002;53(4):865-871.
32. Bujalska IJ, Kumar S, Stewart PM. Does central obesity reflect "Cushing's disease of the omentum"? *Lancet.* 1997;349(9060):1210-1213.
33. Girod JP, Brotman DJ. Does altered glucocorticoid homeostasis increase cardiovascular risk? *Cardiovasc Res.* 2004;64:217-226.
34. Stewart PM, Krozowski ZS. 11 beta-Hydroxysteroid dehydrogenase. *Vitam Horm.* 1999;57: 249-324.
35. Eckel RH, Grundy SM, Zimmet PZ. The metabolic syndrome. *Lancet.* 2005;365:1415-1428.
36. Lakka HM, Laaksonen DE, Lakka TA, et al. The metabolic syndrome and total and cardiovascular disease mortality in middle aged men. *JAMA.* 2002;288:2709-2716.
37. Trayhum P, Beattie JH. Physiological role of adipose tissue: white adipose tissue as an endocrine and secretory organ. *Proc Nutr Soc.* 2001;60:329-339.
38. Hauner H, Schmid P, Pfeifer EF. Glucocorticoids and insulin promote the differentiation of human adipocyte precursor cells into fat cells. *J Clin Endocrinol Metab.* 1987;64:832-835.
39. Ramsay TG. Fat cells. *Endocrinol Metab Clin N Am.* 1996;25:847-870.
40. Abrams J. Role of endothelial dysfunction in coronary artery disease. *Am J Cardiol.* 1997;79: 2-9.
41. Mangos GJ, Walker BR, Kelly JJ, et al. Cortisol inhibits cholinergic vasodilation in the human forearm. *Am J Hypertens.* 2000;13:1155-1160.
42. Ullian ME. The role of corticosteroids in the regulation of vascular tone. *Cardiovasc Res.* 1999; 41:55-64.
43. Ross R. Atherosclerosis – an inflammatory disease. *N Engl J Med.* 1999;340:115-126.
44. Venihaki M, Dikkes P, Carrigan A, Karalis KP. Corticotropin-releasing hormone regulates IL-6 expression during inflammation. *J Clin Invest.* 2001;108:1159-1166.

Chapter 6
Haemostatic Effects of Stress

Paul Hjemdahl and Roland von Känel

Keywords Haemostatic effects • Pro-thrombotic mechanisms • Anti-thrombotic mechanisms • Platelets • Blood coagulation • Fibrinolysis • Methodology • Biomarkers • Vital exhaustion

6.1 Introduction

The three major components of haemostasis – platelet activation, blood coagulation and fibrinolysis – are finely tuned to maintain flowing blood in the normal blood vessel, and yet stop bleeding and repair wounds when vessels are damaged. When the system is perturbed, arterial thrombosis may cause myocardial infarction (MI), stroke and other acute ischaemic events. Acute coronary events are often caused by atherosclerotic plaque rupture triggered by haemodynamic factors that increase wall stress and inflammatory weakening of the fibrous cap that covers the plaque.[1] Plaque rupture exposes a highly thrombogenic surface, but arterial thrombosis may also occur without plaque rupture if the endothelium is dysfunctional (as, e.g. in poorly controlled diabetes). In the long term, activated platelets and coagulation seem to contribute to accelerated atherosclerosis,[2-4] and there is an interesting interplay between platelets, coagulation and inflammation (Fig. 6.1). Thus, the effects of

P. Hjemdahl (✉)
Department of Medicine, Solna, Clinical Pharmacology Unit,
Karolinska Institute, Karolinska University Hospital/Solna, Stockholm, Sweden
e-mail: paul.hjemdahl@ki.se

R. von Känel
Department of General Internal Medicine, Inselspital, Bern University Hospital,
Bern, Switzerland

Division of Psychosomatic Medicine, Inselspital, Bern University Hospital,
Bern, Switzerland
e-mail: roland.vonkaenel@insel.ch

P. Hjemdahl et al. (eds.), *Stress and Cardiovascular Disease*,
DOI 10.1007/978-1-84882-419-5_6, © Springer-Verlag London Limited 2012

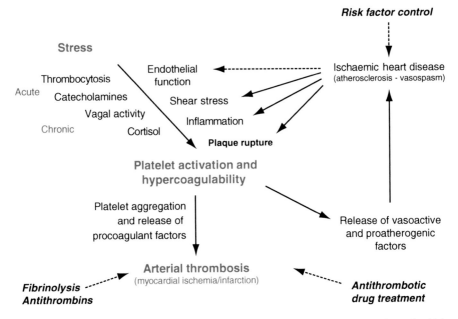

Fig. 6.1 A schematic illustration of pathways and (patho)physiological processes through which stress may promote arterial thrombosis

acute and chronic stress on haemostasis may contribute to an individual's risk of suffering an acute cardiovascular (CV) event, as well as to the slow progression of atherosclerotic disease.

6.2 Pro- and Anti-thrombotic Mechanisms

Primary haemostasis is largely dependent on platelet activation and aggregation, followed by activation of the coagulation system and the formation of thrombin (FII) which cleaves fibrinogen to form fibrin strands that deposit and cross-link to stabilize the thrombus. Anti-thrombotic mechanisms include the release of endogenous anti-platelet and fibrinolytic substances, as detailed below.

6.2.1 Platelets

Resting platelets are discoid, small anuclear cells which are formed from megakaryocytes, and normally circulate 7–10 days. Platelets have a complex intracellular 'machinery' with calcium-dependent contractile elements, several intracellular signalling pathways that respond to different stimuli, and storage granules with

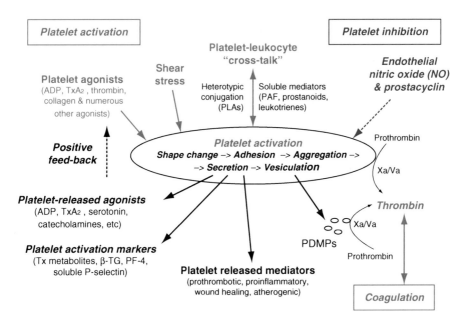

Fig. 6.2 A schematic representation of phenomena leading to platelet activation and inhibition

large amounts of bioactive (e.g. pro-thrombotic, angiogenic, pro-inflammatory and pro-atherogenic) substances that are released upon activation. Strongly activated platelets express a pro-thrombinase complex that catalyses thrombin formation, and releases microparticles which are highly pro-coagulant. Platelets also interact with leukocytes via 'cross-talk' that involves both direct cell–cell contact (conjugation or aggregation) and soluble mediators. For details, see.[5]

A simplified scheme of platelet activation is shown in Fig. 6.2. Activated platelets undergo shape change with the formation of pseudopodia, and spread on surfaces to which they attach. Von Willebrand factor (VWF) released from the endothelium (and from platelets) mediates platelet binding via their GPIb receptors. Platelets can be activated by many agonists, some of which are released from the platelets themselves – for example, thromboxane (Tx) A_2, ATP/ADP, catecholamines and serotonin – and thus provide positive feedback to reinforce platelet aggregation, but also physically, by shear stress. Collagen (which is exposed upon vessel injury and activates GPVI receptors) and thrombin (which activates PAR-1 receptors) are 'strong' platelet agonists, whereas catecholamines and serotonin are 'weak' agonists which mainly act in concert with other stimuli. When platelets are activated, their surface GPIIb/IIIa receptors undergo conformational changes to enable fibrinogen binding and aggregation. Upon activation, the platelets express P-selectin and CD40 which interact with PSGL-1 and CD40L, respectively, in the cross-talk with inflammatory cells. Activated platelets also secrete the endogenous anti-fibrinolytic agent, plasminogen activator inhibitor (PAI)-1, along with other granule contents.

Coagulation and Fibrinolysis Pathways

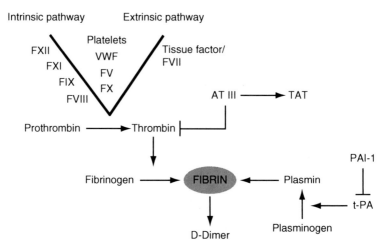

Fig. 6.3 Coagulation and fibrinolysis pathways. The sign '⊥' indicates inhibition of thrombin by anti-thrombin III (*AT III*) in a thrombin–anti-thrombin (*TAT*) complex and of tissue-type plasminogen activator (*t-PA*) by type I plasminogen activator inhibitor (*PAI-1*) in a t-PA/PAI-1 complex. Coagulation steps also involve platelets and the von Willebrand factor (*VWF*). Fibrinolysis steps are detailed in the text. FVIII, VWF, and t-PA are released by endothelial cells into the circulation during acute stress

The normal endothelium releases platelet-stabilizing nitric oxide (NO) and prostacyclin, and a dysfunctional endothelium shifts the haemostatic balance in a pro-thrombotic direction and increases cardiovascular risk.[6] Similarly, COX-2 inhibition attenuates prostacyclin production, and increases the risk of suffering MI.[7]

6.2.2   Blood Coagulation and Fibrinolysis

Activation of haemostasis comprises a sequential interaction between enzymes and inhibitors of the coagulation and fibrinolysis cascades, of platelets, and of the VWF. Figure 6.3 shows the two main pathways of blood coagulation. The intrinsic pathway is initiated by clotting factor XII (FXII), whereas the extrinsic pathway is triggered when tissue factor becomes exposed to the blood at sites of tissue damage, for example, on material in a ruptured atherosclerotic plaque. Tissue factor instantly binds to circulating activated FVII. Both pathways activate cascades of clotting factors that converge in a common activator complex which converts pro-thrombin to thrombin (FII), and results in the conversion of fibrinogen to fibrin.[8] Thus, thrombin formation is the final common pathway of coagulation. Thrombin also influences vascular function and inflammation, which may contribute to athero-thrombotic disease.[9]

Termination of clot formation involves several anticoagulant steps, for example, the binding of anti-thrombin III to thrombin. This neutralizes thrombin, a potent activator of several clotting factors and platelets, in a thrombin/anti-thrombin III (TAT) complex. Fibrinolysis is initiated by tissue-type plasminogen activator (t-PA) which converts plasminogen into fibrin-cleaving plasmin. The breakdown of cross-linked fibrin chains yields soluble fibrin fragments such as D-dimer. PAI-1 is the main inhibitor of t-PA, and neutralizes t-PA in a t-PA/PAI-1-complex.

6.3 Methodology and Biomarkers

Thrombosis and tissue repair are highly localized processes which can be studied in detail with animal models and in vitro techniques to pinpoint mechanisms and mediators of interest. Human stress studies are based on the paradigm that more (re)active circulating platelets and/or pro-thrombotic alterations of markers for blood coagulation and/or fibrinolysis in sampled blood will increase the propensity towards thrombus formation. A brief description of methods and some of the caveats is given below.

6.3.1 Platelet Function

There is no gold standard measure of 'platelet activity' due to the complexity of platelet function (see Fig. 6.2).[5] Furthermore, platelets readily react to artificial surfaces, and sampling and sample manipulation, as well as anticoagulants used, and this may cause artefacts. For example, most studies are performed in citrated blood (with low extracellular calcium), which artificially inflates the Tx dependence of platelet aggregation. Anticoagulation with hirudin preserves calcium levels. The most common platelet function markers and assays for assessments of platelet (re)activity[10,11] are summarized in Table 6.1.

Agonist-induced platelet aggregation may be studied in platelet-rich plasma (PRP) or in whole blood. Light transmittance aggregometry (LTA) in PRP is often thought of as 'gold standard'. LTA requires skilled operators, and there is considerable variability between laboratories. Platelet aggregability in whole blood has traditionally been measured using impedance aggregometry requiring laboratory skills. Several whole blood techniques have been adapted for point-of-care use (Table 6.1), but they also demand good training to yield dependable results. Studies in PRP selectively target platelet function, but contamination by other blood cells and by microparticles and/or loss of large and reactive platelets while preparing PRP may influence results. Studies in whole blood assess platelet function in their natural milieu, with minimal sample handling and allowing interaction with other blood cells.

Table 6.1 Laboratory measures of platelet activation and a hypercoagulable state in connection with mental and/or physical stress

Coagulation	Platelets	Fibrinolysis
Fibrinogen ↑	Platelet counts ↑	PAI-1 activity ↑
	Platelet size distribution ↑	
Von Willebrand factor ↑	Platelet shape change and adhesion ↑	PAI-1 antigen ↑
Antithrombin III ↓	Platelet aggregation in PRP (LTA) ↑	t-PA antigen ↑
		(t-PA/PAI-1 complex)
Thrombin–antithrombin III (TAT) complex ↑	Platelet aggregation in whole blood ↑	t-PA activity ↓
	Impedance aggregometry (Multiplate®)	
	VerifyNow®	
	PFA-100®	
	Cone-and-Plate(let) Analyzer (IMPACT®)	
	PlateletWorks® (with cell counter)	
D-dimer ↑	Whole blood flow cytometry:	
	Platelet fibrinogen binding ↑	
	Activated GPIIb/IIIa expression ↑	
	Platelet P-selectin expression ↑	
	Platelet–leukocyte aggregation ↑	
	PDMP formation ↑	
	Platelet pro-coagulant activity ↑	
Clotting factor XII ↑	Platelet secretion markers in plasma:	
	ß-Thromboglobulin ↑	
	Platelet factor 4 ↑	
	Soluble P-selectin ↑	
Clotting factor VII ↑	Platelet-dependent Tx formation ↑	
	(Serum TxB2)	
Clotting factor VIII ↑	Systemic Tx formation ↑	
	(Urinary 11-dehydro-TxB2)	

Qualitative changes that would indicate a pro-thrombotic to stress are indicated by *arrows* (↑ =increased level, ↓ =decreased level). For platelet aggregation studies in whole blood several techniques which have been developed for point-of-care (clinical) use are listed. Table 6.2 summarizes findings with acute and chronic stress
PRP platelet-rich plasma, *LTA* light transmittance aggregometry, *PDMP* platelet-derived microparticles, *Tx* thromboxane

Flow cytometry is a powerful tool for studies of platelets and other blood cells.[5,10] Flow cytometry can 'gate' various cell populations in unmanipulated whole blood, and may be used to reveal many aspects of platelet function (Table 6.1). The importance of sample handling is illustrated by artefacts introduced when measuring platelet–leukocyte aggregates (PLAs) after commonly used sample preparation procedures.[12,13] Circulating platelet–monocyte aggregates may be a useful marker for platelet activation in vivo.[5]

Platelet secretion can be assessed by markers in plasma (Table 6.1), but care must be taken to minimise artefactual release during sampling and sample handling.[14] This is also important when measuring other plasma constituents that are stored in large amounts in platelets, such as VWF, PAI-1 and fibrinogen.

Tx production can be assessed by measurements of serum TxB_2 (platelet-derived Tx formation in clotting blood) and/or stable Tx metabolites, especially 11-dehydro-TxB_2, in urine. The latter includes $\geq 20\%$ non-platelet-derived Tx in untreated individuals.[15] Intake of COX-1 inhibitors, especially aspirin, must be controlled since this influences results.

6.3.2 Blood Coagulation and Fibrinolysis

Assessment of haemostasis factors in human citrate plasma is typically done by immunoassays or coagulometric methods using factor-deficient standard human plasma and reagents.[16,17] Clotting factors, VWF, and fibrinolytic enzymes are either measured by immunological (i.e. antigen level; e.g. FVIII:Ag) or functional (i.e. molecule activity; e.g. FVIII:C) methods.[8] TAT and D-dimer combine several coagulation steps leading to thrombin and fibrin formation, respectively, and are good hypercoagulability markers. Unlike individual clotting and fibrinolytic factors, D-dimer reflects activation of the entire haemostatic system, particularly fibrin turnover, that is, fibrin formation by the coagulation system and fibrin degradation by the fibrinolytic system.

Sodium citrate plasma is mandatory when assessing the activity levels of coagulation factors, whereas EDTA plasma can also be used to measure antigen levels. A specific anticoagulant, CTAD-PPACK, may prevent artificial coagulation activation by specifically inhibiting thrombin and is useful when assessing the coagulation activation markers TAT and fibrinopeptide A.[18] Antigen levels of t-PA and PAI-1 are assessed in citrated plasma. For determinations of t-PA and PAI-1 activity, a specific platelet stabilizing buffer (with theophylline, adenosine, and dipyridamole) has to be added to the sodium citrate.

In healthy individuals, coagulation factors in plasma (i.e. fibrinogen, VWF:Ag, FVII:C, FVIII:C, FXII:C, D-dimer) increase by about 10% in response to stress. This appears to be reproducible, as stress-induced changes in these factors did not differ across three testings with 1-week intervals.[16] During acute psychosocial stress, plasma is shifted to the extravascular space resulting in concentration of non-diffusible blood constituents.[19] This so-called stress-haemoconcentration is of particular concern for molecules such as coagulation factors which are too big to move passively through vascular pores to the extravascular space.[20] Studies applying arithmetic adjustment of coagulation factor levels for haemoconcentration suggest that increases with acute stress reflect both haemoconcentration and genuine activation of coagulation, particularly of FVIII.[21] However, haemoconcentration accounts for much of the VWF:Ag and soluble ICAM-1 responses to stress.[22] Thus, the influence of stress-haemoconcentration should be taken into account when large molecules are assessed, especially when responses are small.

6.4 Haemostasis During Sympatho-Adrenal Activation and Stress in Humans

There is a rather large literature on haemostasis and stress which has been summarized in overviews, but not subjected to meta-analyses due to methodological diversity.[8,23-27] Overall, there is support for mild activation of platelets and the coagulation system, as well as increased fibrinolysis during sympatho-adrenal activation and acute stress.

6.4.1 Effects of Sympatho-Adrenal Activation

6.4.1.1 Platelets

The micromolar concentrations needed for adrenaline alone to activate platelets in vitro are 3–4 orders of magnitude higher than those found in plasma (0.1–5 nmol/L) even during intense physical stress[23]; noradrenaline levels are about tenfold higher (see Chap. 3 by Hjemdahl and Esler). Platelets may be activated via α_2-adrenoceptors that are stimulated by both catecholamines, and inhibited via β_2-adrenoceptors which are selectively targeted by adrenaline. Studies with catecholamine infusions and adrenoceptor-blocking agents have shown catecholamine-mediated platelet activation.[23-27] Of interest, different platelet function tests may yield apparently conflicting results even in the same study. With filtragometry ex vivo (reflecting platelet aggregability in vivo) we found platelet activation whereas LTA showed reduced platelet sensitivity to ADP-stimulation after adrenaline infusion; the preparation of PRP for LTA may have resulted in a selective loss of large, reactive platelets that had been 'sensitized' in vivo before sampling.[23,28] The less one has to manipulate samples the better when studying platelet responses to stress.

A series of studies using filtragometry consistently showed platelet activation during i.v. infusions of adrenaline[28-31] or noradrenaline[32] in healthy volunteers with thresholds for platelet activation around 4 nM in plasma for both catecholamines. These levels are not reached during laboratory mental stress tasks, but might be reached in an individual during real-life situations perceived as highly stressful or threatening. The platelet-activating effect of adrenaline infusion was confirmed by flow cytometric studies.[33] During physical exercise, noradrenaline is a more likely activator of platelets than adrenaline,[32,34] as suggested also by studies using other techniques.[35] Our studies showed that α-adrenoceptor blockade counteracted responses to adrenaline infusion without influencing resting platelet activity,[29] and studies with ß-blockade showed that platelet activation by adrenaline in vivo is not modulated by β_2-adrenoceptor stimulation.[31] Thus, both noradrenaline and adrenaline may activate platelets in vivo via α_2-adrenoceptor stimulation during intense stress, but their role in milder forms of stress is questionable. Overviews[23-27] show some variability of results depending on the methodology used but support this contention overall.

6.4.1.2 Blood Coagulation and Fibrinolysis

The sympatho-adrenal system may regulate haemostatic activity at times of acute stress.[25] Catecholamines stimulate vascular endothelial β_2-adrenoceptors resulting in release of preformed FVIII, VWF, and t-PA from endothelial storage pools into the circulation.[24] This takes place within a few minutes and the elevation of tPA activity and reduction of PAI-1 activity during adrenaline infusion show dose-dependencies within the physiological range.[36] Adrenaline infusion to high physiological levels elevate VWF:Ag levels via β-adrenergic mechanisms in humans.[24] Isoprenaline infusion increased plasma VWF more in hypertensive individuals than in normotensive controls.[37]

Adrenaline infusion elevates TAT in healthy young men suggesting that catecholamines stimulate thrombin generation in vivo.[24,27] The sensitivity of β_2-adrenoceptors in lymphocytes was positively associated with acute stress-induced thrombin formation as measured by plasma TAT levels,[38] and there was a positive relationship between noradrenaline and D-dimer changes from rest to immediately post-stress.[39] However, the mechanisms involved have not been dissected.

6.4.2 Vagal Activity and the Hypothalamic–Pituitary–Adrenal (HPA) Axis

Activation of the HPA axis and decreased parasympathetic activity might be more important for hypercoagulability with chronic stress than with acute stress. In factory workers we found relationships between the overnight urinary excretion of cortisol and catecholamines on one hand, and morning plasma levels of PAI-1 antigen, fibrinogen, and D-dimer on the other.[40] Plasma cortisol levels correlated directly with fibrinogen and VWF levels in women with stable CHD[41] and with fibrinogen in middle-aged men and women.[42] Decreased vagal function, as reflected by reduced high-frequency (HF) heart rate variability (HRV) and a slower heart rate recovery after exercise, has been associated with hypercoagulability. HF-HRV was inversely associated with PAI-1 antigen levels in healthy individuals[43] and with fibrinogen and activated FVII in women with stable CHD[44] after controlling for a range of co-variates. In healthy factory workers, night-time HF-HRV was inversely related to plasma fibrinogen levels.[45] In healthy men, heart rate recovery after exercise was inversely related to plasma fibrinogen and PAI-1 activity independently of co-variates, including cardio-respiratory fitness.[46]

6.5 Effects of Acute Stress

6.5.1 Platelet Activation

Signs of platelet activation have been found with different stressors using several platelet function tests.[23,25-27] We found elevated platelet counts and signs of mild (barely significant) platelet activation during mental stress (a Stroop colour–word conflict test; see Chap. 8 for cardiovascular responses to this test) using filtragometry[23,28] and flow cytometry.[47] Responses were greater in patients with stable angina than in matched controls.[48] Grignani et al. found that acute stress provoked greater ADP- and collagen-stimulated platelet aggregation in men who had had myocardial infarction than in age-matched healthy controls.[49] Using flow cytometry, small but significant increases in unstimulated platelet P-selectin expression were found after mental stress in CHD patients,[50] whereas Aschbacher et al. found substantial increases among elderly subjects.[51] Steptoe et al. found increased platelet–leukocyte aggregation following mental stress, with greater responses among individuals with high cardiovascular reactivity[52] and more protracted responses in patients with CHD.[53] Other measures, including platelet secretion products in plasma and platelet counts, tend to increase after mental stress.[27] Thus, platelet activation during mental stress is mild in most situations but seems to be greater in CHD patients. There may be more marked platelet activation upon exposure to more challenging or threatening situations than those that can be created in the laboratory.

Physical exercise elicits much larger responses than mental stress,[34,47,48] and platelet activation during high-intensity exercise has been a rather consistent finding.[23,27,54] This is of interest, since exercise may trigger myocardial infarction (see Chap. 9 by Tofler). In our hands, several signs of platelet activation are seen with intense exercise (see, e.g.[34]). Patients with stable angina and matched controls had similar platelet activation during exercise, but responses were intensity-dependent and the patients achieved lower work loads, suggesting platelet hyper-reactivity with CHD.[48] Using the PFA-100, Aurigemma et al. found signs of platelet activation by exercise in CHD patients but not in healthy controls.[55] Moderate exercise may, however, suppress platelet activation[27,56] and exercise training reduces the platelet responsiveness to exercise.[57,58] Interestingly, warm-up exercise attenuates platelet–leukocyte interactions during exercise.[59] Thus, intense exercise activates platelets, especially in sedentary subjects and patients with CHD, whereas lower-intensity exercise and increased fitness appear to be beneficial regarding platelet activation.

Possible mechanisms behind stress-induced platelet activation were studied with exercise testing, since the responses to laboratory mental stress were so small. We found little or no attenuation of platelet activation during exercise when blocking Tx formation by aspirin[34,48] even though Tx formation is enhanced by exercise.[60] Neither ADP receptor blockade by clopidogrel[60,61] nor thrombin inhibition[62] attenuated the platelet activation during exercise. β_1-blockade attenuates haemodynamic responses to exercise, but did not influence the platelet activation response in patients with stable angina.[63] Studies with nonselective β-blockade have yielded equivocal results.[23] The thrombocytosis elicited by stress may introduce newly formed and generally more reactive platelets into the circulation. Of interest from the clinical point of view is that commonly used anti-platelet treatment did not attenuate stress-induced platelet activation. Improving fitness, on the other hand, reduces platelet (re)activity[58] and is thus important in the treatment of CHD patients.

Table 6.2 Reliable changes in haemostasis factors with acute and chronic stress or negative affect

	Acute stress	Chronic stress or negative affect
Fibrinogen	↑	↑
FXII	↑	
FVII	↑	↑
FVIII	↑	
VWF	↑	↑
Platelet activity	↑	↑
TAT	↑	
D-dimer	↑	↑
PAI-1	—	↑
t-PA antigen		↑
t-PA activity	↑	↓

Qualitative changes (↑ = increased level, ↓ = decreased level, — = no change) that have been observed in several studies using one or several of the parameters listed in Table 6.1 are indicated."

6.5.2   *Coagulation and Fibrinolysis*

Numerous studies have investigated haemostatic responses to acute psychosocial stressors applied in a laboratory setting, including different speech tasks, mental arithmetic, and the Stroop colour–word conflict test, in healthy individuals (Table 6.2). These studies show that acute psychosocial stress increases the activity of pro-coagulant factors (i.e. FXII:C, FVII:C, FVIII:C, fibrinogen, VWF) and of pro-fibrinolytic t-PA, indicating concomitant activation of coagulation and fibrinolysis pathways[8,25,27,36,64-66]. In an extensive review, Thrall et al. found that effects of physical exercise on coagulation and fibrinolysis were intensity-dependent.[27] The few studies on effects of mild exercise (≤55% VO$_2$ max) suggest activation of fibrinolysis, whereas coagulation seems unchanged. Studies on moderately intense physical activity (56–75% VO$_2$ max) produced inconsistent results with increased, unchanged, or even decreased fibrinolytic potential. A pro-thrombotic state (i.e. pro-coagulant changes outweighing concomitant fibrinolysis activation) was most consistently observed with high-intensity physical activity (>75% VO$_2$ max). This is mostly due to increased thrombin generation, platelet hyper-reactivity, and increased activity of several coagulation factors, especially factor VIII and von Willebrand factor, particularly in untrained individuals.[58] Since the coagulation activation markers TAT and D-dimer increase, stress-induced activation of virtually all haemostasis components may result in net hypercoagulability, especially in the presence of endothelial dysfunction.[8,27] Importantly, while strenuous exercise induces a pro-thrombotic state, regular exercisers exhibit lower baseline coagulation activity than individuals with sedentary behavior; this is thought to be one mechanism through which regular physical activity reduces atherothrombotic risk in the long run.[58]

6.5.3   Factors That Modulate Pro-coagulant Responses
to Acute Stress

Age was positively associated with the increase in D-dimer from pre-stress to immediately and 20 min after stress, suggesting that acute stress might increase vulnerability in the elderly for haemostasis-associated CVD.[67] Young men may experience slightly greater net stress-hypercoagulability than women because increases in FVII:C were particularly pronounced in men and t-PA activity was more apparent in women.[64,65]

The pro-thrombotic response to acute stress seems to be exaggerated in patients with established CHD partly because of decreased release of t-PA and altered haemodynamic forces related to endothelial dysfunction. Increased platelet responsiveness in CHD patients has been mentioned above. Compared to normotensive controls, individuals with primary hypertension showed reduced fibrinolytic responses to acute stress.[68] Patients with stable angina had elevated tPA:Ag (all patients) and PAI-1 activity (men only) at rest, as well as reduced tPA:Ag responses to exercise which independently predicted the risk of suffering MI or CV death during long-term follow-up.[69] Elderly subjects with a history of CHD showed greater D-dimer responses to a speech stressor than those with no CHD.[70] Patients with CHD also experienced delayed recovery of the stress-induced decline in anti-thrombin III compared to normal controls.[71]

Chronic psychosocial stress and negative affect may both exaggerate the acute pro-coagulant stress response. Elderly Alzheimer caregivers experience chronic stress due to the burden of providing informal care to a spouse with Alzheimer's disease. In dementia caregivers the number of negative life events during the preceding month correlated directly with changes in a pro-coagulability score comprising TAT, D-dimer, VWF:Ag, t-PA:Ag and PAI-1:Ag during speech stress.[72] Dementia severity of the care recipient showed a graded association with stress-induced D-dimer changes in caregivers independently of their age.[73] In elderly subjects, anxiety and depression were associated with greater stress-induced D-dimer formation, though only the anxiety effect withheld co-variate adjustment.[74] In caregivers, but not in controls, depressive and anxiety symptoms were associated with increased reactivity and delayed recovery of platelet P-selectin expression when controlling for age, sex, aspirin use, antidepressant use, and history of CHD.[51] Hostility was positively associated with increased platelet secretion of β-thromboglobulin following a Type A structured interview and speech stress in men with and without CHD independently of anti-platelet medication.[75] Hostility was associated with increased wound-induced platelet activation in both CHD patients and matched controls.[76]

Conversely, positive affect and social support may mitigate the pro-coagulant stress response. Happiness, as assessed by ecological momentary assessment over a working day, was associated with reduced fibrinogen responses to stress in middle-aged individuals after adjustment for a range of potential confounders.[77] We found higher levels of social support to be associated with lower concentrations of fibrinogen and D-dimer, but not FVII:C, both before and after stress when controlling for age, body mass index, and blood pressure.[78] Whether exaggerated coagulation responses to acute stress are prognostic for poor cardiovascular outcome has not been investigated. Similarly, it is as yet unknown whether mitigation of the acute pro-coagulant stress response by for instance positive affect and social support is protective in terms of future cardiovascular events.

6.6 Chronic Stress and Haemostasis

Different domains of chronic psychosocial stress (e.g. job stress, stress of dementia caregiving) and of psychological distress (e.g. depression, anxiety) have been associated with changes in haemostasis (Table 6.2). Psychological distress can be conceptualized as a maladaptive behavioural response in the form of negative affect to chronic stress.[79] Hence, negative affect is associated with haemostatic changes similar to those observed with chronic psychosocial stress, and result in a low-grade hypercoagulable state.

In agreement with responses to acute stress, pro-coagulant factors such as fibrinogen, D-dimer, FVII:C, and VWF:Ag are increased by chronic stress.[8] Importantly, however, the effects on fibrinolytic activity are opposite those seen with acute stress because chronic stress seems to impair fibrinolytic activity; this is evidenced by increased PAI-1 (activity and antigen) and t-PA:Ag, on the one hand, and decreased t-PA activity on the other. Taken together, chronic psychosocial stress appears to shift the balance between coagulation and fibrinolysis towards a hypercoagulable state that exceeds the physiologic net hypercoagulable changes seen with acute stress in healthy individuals.

6.6.1 Low Socio-Economic Status

There is substantial evidence supporting a relationship between low socio-economic status, as measured by different constructs (e.g. education, occupational class, and social class), and elevated levels of fibrinogen, FVII:C, and VWF:Ag.[8] Demographic variables, major CV risk factors, and health-related behaviours were important co-variates. However, a meta-analysis revealed higher fibrinogen levels in unemployed men and women than in employed workers, as well as in individuals with less education, even after controlling for many CV risk factors.[80]

6.6.2 Job Stress

Job stress is most often defined as a mismatch between job demands and decision latitude (i.e. job control) or as an imbalance between effort spent and reward obtained at work; this is moderated by a personality trait of over-commitment to work. There is evidence for an association between high job stress and a pro-thrombotic milieu with elevated fibrinogen and FVII:C and a reduced fibrinolytic capacity (i.e. decreased t-PA activity and increased PAI-1:Ag).[8] Elevated plasma fibrinogen might be an important mediator linking job stress with increased risk of CHD in both sexes, whereby low job control seems to be more consistently related to fibrinogen than job demand.[81,82] While most of this literature is cross-sectional, one prospective study found increased FVII:C, FVIII:C and fibrinogen levels, as well as exaggerated ADP- and thrombin-induced platelet aggregation in accountants during a period of increased work load compared to a calm period.[83]

6.6.3 Stress of Caregiving

Providing in-home care to a demented spouse is a model of chronic human stress. In elderly Alzheimer caregivers, we found higher resting D-dimer levels than in age- and sex-matched non-caregiving controls, even when controlling for CHD, CV risk factors, lifestyle, and medications.[84] Interestingly, the elevations of D-dimer levels among caregivers were associated with perturbed sleep, as measured by poly-somnography.[85,86] Applying a longitudinal design, we found that after the demented spouse was deceased or placed in a long-term care facility, D-dimer levels were not reduced until between 6 and 30 months after the transition in the caregiving situation. In contrast, there was immediate psychological recovery from placement and bereavement. Therefore, pro-thrombotic responses to chronic stress might impact CV health long after the stress has resolved.[87] Over a 5-year study period caregivers also demonstrated greater increases in t-PA:Ag, compatible with impaired fibrinolysis, than non-caregiving controls after controlling for age, sex, body mass index, blood pressure, and medications. Caregivers were predicted to reach t-PA:Ag levels that had been associated with increased CHD risk in a meta-analysis 11 years earlier than non-caregivers.[88]

6.6.4 Depression

There is an interesting association between depression and a worsened prognosis for patients with CHD, but the mechanisms involved and effects of treatments for depression need further clarification (see Chap. 12, Hoen et al.). Serotonin is a modulator of platelet function, and platelets store almost all serotonin present in whole blood.[14] Treatment with non-selective or serotonin-selective re-uptake inhibitors (SSRIs) will deplete the platelet serotonin stores, and such treatment may increase the risk of bleeding.[89] It is thus an attractive hypothesis that platelets could be involved in the relationship between depression and CV morbidity.

Depression appears to be associated with increased platelet activity and elevated fibrinogen levels. However, the findings on platelet hyperactivity are not uniform.[90,91] Flow cytometric studies have consistently found increased expression of platelet activation markers (e.g., activated GPIIb/IIIa, fibrinogen binding, P-selectin expression) in patients with major depressive disorder,[92,93] as well as in patients with depressive symptoms without CHD.[94] Platelet secretion markers in plasma were also higher in depressed than in non-depressed individuals.[93] In contrast, platelet aggregation studies show no change or even decreased aggregability in depression[90,91]; such contrasts between different platelet function indices have also been noted above. Interestingly, platelet activation was greater in CHD patients with depression than in those without.[95,96]

Treatment with SSRIs would be expected to reduce platelet activation in depressed CHD patients due to, both, amelioration of depressive symptoms and the depletion of platelet serotonin. Small placebo-controlled studies evaluating platelet biomarkers in plasma during SSRI treatment of CHD patients have[97] or have not[98] been able to show this. Of interest, improvement of depressive symptoms in patients without CHD was associated with reduced platelet activity whether the treatment was pharmacological (mainly SSRIs) or non-pharmacological (psychotherapy).[94] Thus, amelioration of symptoms may be the key to improvement of platelet function in depression. Outcome studies comparing the effects of different antidepressant treatments in depressed CHD patients are lacking, and the platelet link in the association between depression and CHD remains speculative.

Depressive symptoms and clinical depression have been associated with elevated fibrinogen levels in several studies.[99-102] In addition, there was a correlation between higher depressive symptom scores and fibrinogen levels across annual assessments over a 5-year period in women,[103] and across two assessments in healthy teachers over a 2-year period.[104] The latter study showed that changes in fibrinogen predicted changes in depression scores, whereas changes in depression failed to predict changes in fibrinogen.[104] Studies have also found positive associations between depressive mood and FVII:C in elderly individuals,[101] and PAI-1:Ag and t-PA:Ag in women,[103] and in individuals with and without CHD.[105] Only in the latter study did the association between depression scores and PAI-1 remain significant after co-variate adjustment.

6.6.5 Anxiety

The literature on haemostasis and anxiety is comparably scant and partially inconclusive.[8] Hypercoagulability with a predominant activation of inhibitors of fibrinolysis has been found in psychiatric patients with phobic anxiety.[106] In factory workers panic-like anxiety was associated with higher D-dimer and lower fibrinogen levels, whereas PAI-1:Ag did not differ significantly.[107] Investigations in healthy individuals found direct relationships between anxiety symptoms and fibrinogen levels which remained significant after adjustment for co-variates in one study[108] but not in another one.[101]

A recent study[109] found that serotonin-induced platelet activation (using 4–10 μM serotonin combined with 4 μM adrenaline to facilitate serotonin responses) was related to anxiety rather than depression ratings in CHD patients treated with aspirin and clopidogrel. Both agonists were, however, used at supraphysiological concentrations, as plasma levels of both adrenaline (see above) and serotonin[14] are in the nanomolar range. The hypothesis of a platelet–serotonin link in the increased cardiovascular risk associated with anxiety is only speculative without considerably more evidence.

6.6.6 Vital Exhaustion

'Vital exhaustion' designates a state of undue mental fatigue, increased irritability, and demoralization that may manifest as a consequence of long-term psychosocial stress.[110] Vital exhaustion has been associated with elevations of fibrinogen[101,111] and PAI-1:Ag[101,112,113] in healthy populations, and with activated FVII:C levels in women with stable CHD.[41]

6.7 Conclusions and Perspective

Acute psychosocial stress results in mild platelet activation and net hypercoagulability as part of the 'fight or flight' response. Compatible with an evolutionary paradigm, stress-induced platelet activation and hypercoagulability seem to be physiologic phenomena that are unlikely to harm a healthy individual, but may protect the organism from excessive blood loss when injury occurs. An open wound of the skin will usually stop bleeding within several minutes. Thereafter, a hypercoagulable state would no longer be functional, and studies indeed show that coagulation and platelet activity return to pre-stress levels within 20–45 min.[16,38,53] Several factors may exaggerate hypercoagulable responses to acute stress. Activation of platelets and coagulation may contribute to the triggering of MI, even if modest haemostatic responses are seen in laboratory studies of mental stress. However, acute real-life (perhaps threatening) stress cannot be recreated in the laboratory, and may elicit larger responses. Studies during exercise show more pronounced platelet activation which is not attenuated by anti-platelet treatment, but also that increasing physical fitness has a protective effect regarding haemostatic activation.[58] A causative role for haemostatic activation in the triggering of acute events remains speculative in the absence of large prospective studies relating findings in the laboratory to clinical outcomes.

While not ultimately imposing harm to a healthy individual, in CHD patients with impaired endothelial function and vulnerable plaques, increased platelet activity as well as increased and prolonged hypercoagulability might accelerate coronary thrombus growth ensuing the rupture of an atherosclerotic plaque. Frequent episodes of acute stress with haemostatic activation may even foster the development of atherosclerosis.[3,4]

Chronic psychosocial stress and negative affect kindle chronic low-grade hypercoagulability that is no longer protective but contributes to atherosclerosis progression and co-determines the degree of hypercoagulability during acute coronary events. The sympatho-adrenal system may be involved in haemostatic changes during acute stress, whereas the HPA axis and vagal function seem more important in modulating haemostatic activity during chronic stress. Increased inflammatory activity during chronic stress and in patients with CHD may also enhance pro-thrombotic mechanisms. Given the important role of a hypercoagulable state for CHD, randomized controlled trials seem warranted to investigate whether restoring stress-related hypercoagulability by behavioural interventions such as stress management may restore normal haemostatic function to ultimately decrease CHD risk.

References

1. Libby P, Ridker PM, Hansson GK. Inflammation in atherosclerosis. *JACC*. 2009;54:2129-2138.
2. Huo Y, Schober A, Bradley Forlow S, et al. Circulating activated platelets exacerbate atherosclerosis in mice deficient in apolipoprotein E. *Nat Med*. 2003;9:61-67.
3. Gawaz M, Langer H, May AE. Platelets in inflammation and atherogenesis. *J Clin Invest*. 2005;115:3378-3384.
4. Langer HF, Bigalke B, Seizer P, et al. Interaction of platelets and inflammatory endothelium in the development and progression of coronary artery disease. *Semin Thromb Hemost*. 2010;36: 131-138.
5. Michelson AD, ed. *Platelets*. 2nd ed. San Diego: Academic; 2007.
6. Deanfield JE, Halcox JP, Rabelink JP. Endothelial function and dysfunction: testing and clinical relevance. *Circulation*. 2007;115:1285-1295.
7. Antman EM, Bennett JS, Daugherty A, et al. Use of nonsteroidal antiinflammatory drugs – an update for clinicians; a scientific statement from the American Heart Association. *Circulation*. 2007;115:1634-1642.
8. von Känel R, Mills PJ, Fainman C, Dimsdale JE. Effects of psychological stress and psychiatric disorders on blood coagulation and fibrinolysis: a biobehavioral pathway to coronary artery disease? *Psychosom Med*. 2001;63:531-544.
9. Angiolillo DJ, Capodanno D, Goto S. Platelet thrombin receptor antagonism and atherothrombosis. *Eur Heart J*. 2010;31:17-28.
10. Harrrison P, Frelinger AL, Furman MI, Michelson AD. Measuring antiplatelet drug effects in the laboratory. *Thromb Res*. 2007;120:323-336.
11. Cattaneo M. Resistance to antiplatelet drugs: molecular mechanisms and laboratory detection. *J Thromb Haemost*. 2007;5(suppl 1):230-237.
12. Li N, Goodall AH, Hjemdahl P. A sensitive flow cytometric assay for circulating platelet-leukocyte aggregates. *Br J Haematol*. 1997;99:808-816.
13. Li N, Goodall A, Hjemdahl P. Efficient flow cytometric assay for platelet-leukocyte aggregates in whole blood using fluorescence signal triggering. *Cytometry*. 1999;35:154-161.
14. Beck O, Wallén NH, Bröijersén A, et al. On the accurate determination of serotonin in human plasma. *Biochem Biophys Res Commun*. 1993;196:260-266.

15. Patrono C, Garcia Rodriguez LA, Landolfi R, Baigent C. Low-dose aspirin for the prevention of atherothrombosis. *N Engl J Med*. 2005;353:2373-2383.
16. von Känel R, Preckel D, Zgraggen L, et al. The effect of natural habituation on coagulation responses to acute mental stress and recovery in men. *Thromb Haemost*. 2004;92:1327-1335.
17. Wiman B, Hamsten A. Impaired fibrinolysis and risk of thromboembolism. *Prog Cardiovasc Dis*. 1991;34:179-192.
18. Herren T, Stricker H, Haeberli A, et al. Fibrin formation and degradation in patients with arteriosclerotic disease. *Circulation*. 1994;90:2679-2686.
19. Allen MT, Patterson SM. Hemoconcentration and stress: a review of physiological mechanisms and relevance for cardiovascular disease risk. *Biol Psychol*. 1995;41:1-27.
20. Bacon SL, Ring C, Lip GY, Carroll D. Increases in lipids and immune cells in response to exercise and mental stress in patients with suspected coronary artery disease: effects of adjustment for shifts in plasma volume. *Biol Psychol*. 2004;65:237-250.
21. von Känel R, Kudielka BM, Haeberli A, et al. Prothrombotic changes with acute psychological stress: combined effect of hemoconcentration and genuine coagulation activation. *Thromb Res*. 2009;123:622-630.
22. von Känel R, Preckel D, Kudielka BM, Fischer JE. Responsiveness and habituation of soluble ICAM-1 to acute psychosocial stress in men: determinants and effect of stress-hemoconcentration. *Physiol Res*. 2007;56:627-639.
23. Hjemdahl P, Larsson PT, Wallén H. Effects of stress and ß-blockade on platelet function. *Circulation*. 1991;84(suppl 6):VI-44-VI-61.
24. von Känel R, Dimsdale JE. Effects of sympathetic activation by adrenergic infusions on hemostasis in vivo. *Eur J Haematol*. 2000;65:357-369.
25. Preckel D, von Känel R. Regulation of hemostasis by the sympathetic nervous system: any contribution to coronary artery disease? *Heartdrug*. 2004;4:123-130.
26. Brydon L, Magid K, Steptoe A. Platelets, coronary heart disease, and stress. *Brain Behav Immun*. 2005;20:113-119.
27. Thrall G, Lane D, Carroll D, Lip GYH. A systematic review of the effects of acute psychological stress and physical activity on haemorheology, coagulation, fibrinolysis and platelet reactivity: implications for the pathogenesis of acute coronary syndromes. *Thromb Res*. 2007;120: 819-847.
28. Larsson PT, Hjemdahl P, Olsson G, et al. Platelet aggregability: contrasting *in vivo* and *in vitro* findings during sympatho-adrenal activation and relationship to serum lipids. *Eur J Clin Invest*. 1990;20:398-405.
29. Larsson PT, Wallén NH, Egberg N, Hjemdahl P. α-Adrenoceptor blockade by phentolamine inhibits adrenaline-induced platelet activation *in vivo* without affecting resting measurements. *Clin Sci*. 1992;82:369-376.
30. Larsson PT, Olsson G, Angelin B, et al. Metoprolol does not reduce platelet aggregability during sympatho-adrenal stimulation. *Eur J Clin Pharmacol*. 1992;42:413-421.
31. Larsson PT, Wallén NH, Martinsson A, et al. Significance of platelet ß-adrenoceptors for platelet responses *in vivo* and *in vitro*. *Thromb Haemost*. 1992;68:687-693.
32. Larsson PT, Wallén NH, Hjemdahl P. Norepinephrine-induced human platelet activation in vivo is only partly counteracted by aspirin. *Circulation*. 1994;89:1951-1957.
33. Hjemdahl P, Chronos N, Wilson D, et al. Epinephrine sensitizes human platelets in vivo and in vitro as studied by fibrinogen binding and P-selectin expression. *Arterioscler Thromb*. 1994;14:77-84.
34. Li N, Wallén NH, Hjemdahl P. Evidence for prothrombotic effects of exercise and limited protection by aspirin. *Circulation*. 1999;100:1374-1379.
35. Ikarugi H, Taka T, Nakajima S, et al. Norepinephrine, but not epinephrine, enhances platelet reactivity and coagulation after exercise in humans. *J Appl Physiol*. 1999;86:133-138.
36. Larsson PT, Wiman B, Olsson G, et al. Influence of metoprolol treatment on sympatho-adrenal activation of fibrinolysis. *Thromb Haemost*. 1990;63:482-487.
37. von Känel R, Dimsdale JE, Adler KA, et al. Effects of nonspecific beta-adrenergic stimulation and blockade on blood coagulation in hypertension. *J Appl Physiol*. 2003;94:1455-1459.

38. von Känel R, Mills PJ, Ziegler MG, Dimsdale JE. Effect of beta2-adrenergic receptor function-ing and increased norepinephrine on the hypercoagulable state with mental stress. *Am Heart J.* 2002;144:68-72.
39. Wirtz PH, Ehlert U, Emini L, et al. Anticipatory cognitive stress appraisal and the acute procoagulant stress response in men. *Psychosom Med.* 2006;68:851-858.
40. von Känel R, Kudielka BM, Abd-el-Razik A, et al. Relationship between overnight neuroen-docrine activity and morning haemostasis in working men. *Clin Sci (Lond).* 2004;107:89-95.
41. von Känel R, Mausbach BT, Kudielka BM, Orth-Gomér K. Relation of morning serum cortisol to prothrombotic activity in women with stable coronary artery disease. *J Thromb Thrombolysis.* 2008;25:165-172.
42. Lippi G, Franchini M, Salvagno GL, et al. Higher morning serum cortisol level predicts increased fibrinogen but not shortened APTT. *J Thromb Thrombolysis.* 2008;26:103-105.
43. von Känel R, Nelesen RA, Ziegler MG, et al. Relation of autonomic activity to plasminogen activator inhibitor-1 plasma concentration and the role of body mass index. *Blood Coagul Fibrinolysis.* 2007;18:353-359.
44. von Känel R, Orth-Gomér K. Autonomic function and prothrombotic activity in women after an acute coronary event. *J Womens Health (Larchmt).* 2008;17:1331-1337.
45. von Känel R, Thayer JF, Fischer JF. Night-time vagal cardiac control and plasma fibrinogen levels in a population of working men and women. *Ann Noninvasive Electrocardiol.* 2009;14: 176-184.
46. Jae SY, Carnethon MR, Ahn ES, et al. Association between heart rate recovery after exercise testing and plasminogen activator inhibitor 1, tissue plasminogen activator, and fibrinogen in apparently healthy men. *Atherosclerosis.* 2008;197:415-419.
47. Wallén NH, Goodall AH, Li N, Hjemdahl P. Activation of hemostasis by exercise, mental stress and epinephrine; effects on platelet sensitivity to thrombin and thrombin generation. *Clin Sci.* 1999;97:27-35.
48. Wallén NH, Held C, Rehnqvist N, Hjemdahl P. Effects of mental and physical stress on platelet function in patients with stable angina pectoris and healthy controls. *Eur Heart J.* 1997;18: 807-815.
49. Grignani G, Pacchiarini L, Zucchella M, et al. Effect of mental stress on platelet function in normal subjects and in patients with coronary artery disease. *Haemostasis.* 1992;22:138-146.
50. Reid GJ, Seidelin PH, Kop WJ, et al. Mental stress-induced platelet activation among patients with coronary artery disease. *Psychosom Med.* 2009;71:438-445.
51. Aschbacher K, Mills PJ, von Känel R, et al. Effects of depressive and anxious symptoms on norepinephrine and platelet P-selectin responses to acute psychological stress among elderly caregivers. *Brain Behav Immun.* 2008;22:493-502.
52. Steptoe A, Magid K, Edwards S, et al. The influence of psychological stress and socioeconomic status on platelet activation in men. *Atherosclerosis.* 2003;168:57-63.
53. Strike PC, Magid K, Brydon L, et al. Exaggerated platelet and hemodynamic reactivity to mental stress in men with coronary artery disease. *Psychosom Med.* 2004;66:492-500.
54. Wang J-S. Intense exercise increases shear-induced platelet aggregation in men through enhancement of von Willebrand factor binding, glycoprotein IIb/IIIa activation, and P-selectin expression on platelets. *Eur J Appl Physiol.* 2004;91:741-747.
55. Aurigemma C, Fattorossi A, Sestito A, et al. Relationship between changes in platelet reactiv-ity and changes in platelet receptor expression induced by physical exercise. *Thromb Res.* 2007;120:901-909.
56. Wang J-S, Liao C-H. Moderate-intensity exercise suppresses platelet activation and polymor-phonuclear leukocyte interaction with surface-adherent platelets under shear flow in men. *Thromb Haemost.* 2004;91:587-594.
57. Wang J-S, Li Y-S, Chen J-C, Chen Y-W. Effects of exercise training and deconditioning on platelet aggregation induced by alternating shear stress in men. *Arterioscler Thromb Vasc Biol.* 2005;25:454-460.
58. Lippi G, Mafulli N. Biological influence of physical exercise on hemostasis. *Semin Thromb Hemost.* 2009;35:269-276.

59. Wang J-S, Li Y-S, Yang C-M. Warm-up exercise suppresses platelet-eosinofi/neutrophil aggregation and platelet-promoted release of eosinofi/neutrophil oxidant products enhanced by severe exercise in men. *Thromb Haemost.* 2006;95:490-498.

60. Perneby C, Wallén NH, Hu H, et al. Prothrombotic responses to exercise are little influenced by clopidogrel treatment. *Thromb Res.* 2004;114:135-143.

61. Perneby C, Hofman-Bang C, Wallén NH, et al. Effect of clopidogrel treatment on stress-induced platelet activation and myocardial ischemia in aspirin-treated patients with stable coronary artery disease. *Thromb Haemost.* 2007;98:1316-1322.

62. Li N, He S, Blombäck M, Hjemdahl P. Platelet activity, coagulation, and fibrinolysis during exercise in healthy males: effects of thrombin inhibition by argatroban and enoxaparin. *Arterioscler Thromb Vasc Biol.* 2007;27:407-412.

63. Wallén NH, Held C, Rehnqvist N, Hjemdahl P. Platelet aggregability in vivo is attenuated by verapamil but not by metoprolol in patients with stable angina pectoris. *Am J Cardiol.* 1995; 75:1-6.

64. Jern C, Eriksson E, Tengborn L, et al. Changes of plasma coagulation and fibrinolysis in response to mental stress. *Thromb Haemost.* 1989;62:767-771.

65. Jern C, Manhem K, Eriksson E, et al. Hemostatic response to mental stress during the menstrual cycle. *Thromb Haemost.* 1991;66:614-618.

66. Jern C, Selin L, Jern S. In vivo release of tissue-type plasminogen activator across the human forearm during mental stress. *Thromb Haemost.* 1994;72:285-291.

67. Wirtz PH, Redwine LS, Baertschi C, et al. Coagulation activity before and after acute psychosocial stress increases with age. *Psychosom Med.* 2008;70:476-481.

68. Palermo A, Bertalero P, Pizza N, et al. Decreased fibrinolytic response to adrenergic stimulation in hypertensive patients. *J Hypertens.* 1989;7(suppl):S162-S163.

69. Held C, Hjemdahl P, Rehnqvist N, et al. Prognostic implications of fibrinolytic variables in patients with stable angina pectoris treated with verapamil or metoprolol. Results from the APSIS study. *Circulation.* 1997;95:2380-2386.

70. von Känel R, Dimsdale JE, Ziegler MG, et al. Effect of acute psychological stress on the hypercoagulable state in subjects (spousal caregivers of patients with Alzheimer's disease) with coronary or cerebrovascular disease and/or systemic hypertension. *Am J Cardiol.* 2001; 87:1405-1408.

71. Canevari A, Tacconi F, Zucchella M, et al. Antithrombin III biological activity and emotional stress in patients with coronary artery disease. *Haematologica.* 1992;77:180-182.

72. von Känel R, Dimsdale JE, Patterson TL, Grant I. Acute procoagulant stress response as a dynamic measure of allostatic load in Alzheimer caregivers. *Ann Behav Med.* 2003; 26:42-48.

73. Aschbacher K, von Känel R, Dimsdale JE, et al. Dementia severity of the care receiver predicts procoagulant response in Alzheimer caregivers. *Am J Geriatr Psychiatry.* 2006;14:694-703.

74. von Känel R, Dimsdale JE, Adler KA, et al. Effects of depressive symptoms and anxiety on hemostatic responses to acute mental stress and recovery in the elderly. *Psychiatry Res.* 2004; 126:253-264.

75. Markovitz JH, Matthews KA, Kiss J, Smitherman TC. Effects of hostility on platelet reactivity to psychological stress in coronary heart disease patients and in healthy controls. *Psychosom Med.* 1996;58:143-149.

76. Markovitz JH. Hostility is associated with increased platelet activation in coronary heart disease. *Psychosom Med.* 1998;60:586-591.

77. Steptoe A, Wardle J, Marmot M. Positive affect and health-related neuroendocrine, cardiovascular, and inflammatory processes. *Proc Natl Acad Sci USA.* 2005;102:6508-6512.

78. Wirtz PH, Redwine LS, Ehlert U, von Känel R. Independent association between lower level of social support and higher coagulation activity before and after acute psychosocial stress. *Psychosom Med.* 2009;71:30-37.

79. von Känel R. Psychological distress and cardiovascular risk: what are the links? *J Am Coll Cardiol.* 2008;52:2163-2165.

80. Kaptoge S, White IR, Thompson SG, et al. Fibrinogen Studies Collaboration: associations of plasma fibrinogen levels with established cardiovascular disease risk factors, inflammatory markers, and other characteristics: individual participant meta-analysis of 154,211 adults in 31 prospective studies: the fibrinogen studies collaboration. *Am J Epidemiol.* 2007;166:867-879.
81. Kittel F, Leynen F, Stam M, et al. Job conditions and fibrinogen in 14226 Belgian workers: the Belstress study. *Eur Heart J.* 2002;23:1841-1848.
82. Theorell T. Job stress and fibrinogen. *Eur Heart J.* 2002;23:1799-1801.
83. Frimerman A, Miller HI, Laniado S, Keren G. Changes in hemostatic function at times of cyclic variation in occupational stress. *Am J Cardiol.* 1997;79:72-75.
84. von Känel R, Dimsdale JE, Mills PJ, et al. Effect of Alzheimer caregiving stress and age on frailty markers interleukin-6, C-reactive protein, and D-dimer. *J Gerontol A Biol Sci Med Sci.* 2006;61:963-969.
85. von Känel R, Dimsdale JE, Ancoli-Israel S, et al. Poor sleep is associated with higher plasma proinflammatory cytokine interleukin-6 and procoagulant marker fibrin D-dimer in older caregivers of people with Alzheimer's disease. *J Am Geriatr Soc.* 2006;54:431-437.
86. Mausbach BT, Ancoli-Israel S, von Känel R, et al. Sleep disturbance, norepinephrine, and D-dimer are all related in elderly caregivers of people with Alzheimer disease. *Sleep.* 2006;29:1347-1352.
87. Mausbach BT, Aschbacher K, Patterson TL, et al. Effects of placement and bereavement on psychological well-being and cardiovascular risk in Alzheimer's caregivers: a longitudinal analysis. *J Psychosom Res.* 2007;62:439-445.
88. Mausbach BT, von Känel R, Aschbacher K, et al. Spousal caregivers of patients with Alzheimer's disease show longitudinal increases in plasma level of tissue-type plasminogen activator antigen. *Psychosom Med.* 2007;69:816-822.
89. Halperin D, Reber G. Influence of antidepressants on hemostasis. *Dialogues Clin Neurosci.* 2007;9:47-59.
90. von Känel R. Platelet hyperactivity in clinical depression and the beneficial effect of antidepressant drug treatment: how strong is the evidence? *Acta Psychiatr Scand.* 2004;110: 163-177.
91. Parakh K, Sakhuja A, Bhat U, Ziegelstein RC. Platelet function in patients with depression. *South Med J.* 2008;101:612-617.
92. Musselman DL, Tomer A, Manatunga AK, et al. Exaggerated platelet reactivity in major depression. *Am J Psychiatry.* 1996;153:1313-1317.
93. Walsh MT, Dinan TG, Condren RM, et al. Depression is associated with an increase in the expression of the platelet adhesion receptor glycoprotein Ib. *Life Sci.* 2002;70:3155-3165.
94. Morel-Kopp M-C, McLean L, Tofler GH, et al. The association of depression with platelet activation: evidence for a treatment effect. *J Thromb Haemost.* 2009;7:573-581.
95. Pollock BG, Laghrissi-Thode F, Wagner WR. Evaluation of platelet activation in depressed patients with ischemic heart disease after paroxetine or nortriptyline treatment. *J Clin Psychopharmacol.* 2000;20:137-140.
96. Laghrissi-Thode F, Wagner WR, Pollock BG, et al. Elevated platelet factor 4 and beta-thromboglobulin plasma levels in depressed patients with ischemic heart disease. *Biol Psychiatry.* 1997;42:290-295.
97. Serebruany VL, Glassman AH, Malinin AI, Sertraline AntiDepressant Heart Attack Randomized Trial Study Group, et al. Platelet/endothelial biomarkers in depressed patients treated with the selective serotonin reuptake inhibitor sertraline after acute coronary events: the Sertraline AntiDepressant Heart Attack Randomized Trial (SADHART) Platelet Substudy. *Circulation.* 2003;108:939-944.
98. van Zyl LT, Lespérance F, Frasure-Smith N, et al. Platelet and endothelial activity in comorbid major depression and coronary artery disease patients treated with citalopram: the Canadian Cardiac Randomized Evaluation of Antidepressant and Psychotherapy Efficacy Trial (CREATE) biomarker sub-study. *J Thromb Thrombolysis.* 2009;27:48-56.

99. Folsom AR, Qamhieh HT, Flack JM, et al. Plasma fibrinogen: levels and correlates in young adults. The Coronary Artery Risk Development in Young Adults (CARDIA) Study. *Am J Epidemiol.* 1993;138:1023-1036.

100. Maes M, Delange J, Ranjan R, et al. Acute phase proteins in schizophrenia, mania and major depression: modulation by psychotropic drugs. *Psychiatry Res.* 1997;66:1-11.

101. Kop WJ, Gottdiener JS, Tangen CM, et al. Inflammation and coagulation factors in persons >65 years of age with symptoms of depression but without evidence of myocardial ischemia. *Am J Cardiol.* 2002;89:419-424.

102. Panagiotakos DB, Pitsavos C, Chrysohoou C, ATTICA study, et al. Inflammation, coagulation, and depressive symptomatology in cardiovascular disease-free people; the ATTICA study. *Eur Heart J.* 2004;25:492-499.

103. Matthews KA, Schott LL, Bromberger J, et al. Associations between depressive symptoms and inflammatory/hemostatic markers in women during the menopausal transition. *Psychosom Med.* 2007;69:124-130.

104. von Känel R, Bellingrath S, Kudielka BM. Association between longitudinal changes in depressive symptoms and plasma fibrinogen levels in school teachers. *Psychophysiology.* 2009;46:473-480.

105. Lahlou-Laforet K, Alhenc-Gelas M, Pornin M, et al. Relation of depressive mood to plasminogen activator inhibitor, tissue plasminogen activator, and fibrinogen levels in patients with versus without coronary heart disease. *Am J Cardiol.* 2006;97:1287-1291.

106. Geiser F, Meier C, Wegener I, et al. Association between anxiety and factors of coagulation and fibrinolysis. *Psychother Psychosom.* 2008;77:377-383.

107. von Känel R, Kudielka BM, Schulze R, et al. Hypercoagulability in working men and women with high levels of panic-like anxiety. *Psychother Psychosom.* 2004;73:353-360.

108. Pitsavos C, Panagiotakos DB, Papageorgiou C, et al. Anxiety in relation to inflammation and coagulation markers, among healthy adults: the ATTICA study. *Atherosclerosis.* 2006; 185:320-326.

109. Zafar MU, Paz-Yepes M, Shimbo D, et al. Anxiety is a better predictor of platelet reactivity in coronary artery disease patients than depression. *Eur Heart J.* 2010;31:1573-1582.

110. Appels A. Exhaustion and coronary heart disease: the history of a scientific quest. *Patient Educ Couns.* 2004;55:223-229.

111. Kudielka BM, Bellingrath S, von Känel R. Circulating fibrinogen but not D-dimer level is associated with vital exhaustion in school teachers. *Stress.* 2008;11:250-258.

112. Raikkonen K, Lassila R, Keltikangas-Jarvinen L, Hautanen A. Association of chronic stress with plasminogen activator inhibitor-1 in healthy middle-aged men. *Arterioscler Thromb Vasc Biol.* 1996;16:363-367.

113. von Känel R, Frey K, Fischer J. Independent relation of vital exhaustion and inflammation to fibrinolysis in apparently healthy subjects. *Scand Cardiovasc J.* 2004;38:28-32.

Chapter 7
Stress, Inflammation, and Coronary Heart Disease

Andrew Steptoe

Keywords Stress • Inflammation • Coronary heart disease • Atherosclerosis • Acute coronary disease • Immune function • Hypertension • Acute inflammatory stress responses

7.1 Introduction

This chapter focuses on the contribution of inflammatory and immune processes to the links between stress and coronary heart disease (CHD). The aim is to demonstrate that the impact of stress on CHD development and prognosis is likely to be mediated in part through activation of innate and adaptive immune pathways, with inflammatory responses playing a major role. Understanding of these pathways may have implications for prevention and for the management of patients with established CHD. The first section of the chapter draws on our previous review to outline the contribution of inflammation to atherosclerosis and prognosis following acute cardiac events.[1] The accumulating evidence that stress and psychosocial factors such as low socioeconomic status and depression stimulate inflammation is described in later sections, with findings emerging from both epidemiological and experimental studies. Implications for the prevention of CHD and the management of patients with advanced disease are also drawn.

A. Steptoe
Department of Epidemiology and Public Health,
University College London,
London, UK
e-mail: a.steptoe@ucl.ac.uk

P. Hjemdahl et al. (eds.), *Stress and Cardiovascular Disease*,
DOI 10.1007/978-1-84882-419-5_7, © Springer-Verlag London Limited 2012

7.2 Inflammation in Atherosclerosis

Coronary atherosclerosis, the disease underlying CHD, is a complex process that develops gradually over many years or even decades, only coming to clinical attention at an advanced stage. The response to injury hypothesis proposed that the first step in atherosclerosis was endothelial denudation and that the major events in the development of atherosclerosis were the passive accumulation of lipids within the artery wall and proliferation of smooth muscle cells. Research over the past three decades has increased understanding of the atherosclerosis process, with growing awareness that inflammation plays a pivotal role. Ross's 1999 *New England Journal of Medicine* review ushered in this new perspective,[2] and it has since been elaborated by several authorities.[3,4] It is now known that the vascular endothelium is an active tissue which normally promotes cardiovascular health by producing antiplatelet and vasodilating substances (nitric oxide and prostacyclin), as well as anticlotting and fibrinolytic factors that protect against atherothrombosis. Endothelial dysfunction is caused by a variety of factors including high levels of circulating modified low density lipoprotein (LDL)-cholesterol, physical shear stress, elevated levels of free radicals and vasoactive amines, infectious micro-organisms, and, as we shall see, psychological stress; it leads to a breakdown in these cardioprotective properties and development of a pro-inflammatory and pro-thrombotic environment. A dysfunctional endothelium becomes permeable to LDL-cholesterol which accumulates in the subendothelial matrix. Oxidative modification of LDL-cholesterol by reactive oxygen species produced by vascular cells results in minimally oxidised LDL species (mOx LDL) with proinflammatory activity. mOxLDL stimulates endothelial cells to express cell adhesion molecules which bind leukocytes and platelets, thereby promoting their recruitment to the vessel wall. Interactions between complementary adhesion molecules expressed on leukocytes, platelets and endothelial cells, ensure firm adhesion of leukocytes to the vessel wall, while chemokines, specialised chemo-attractant cytokines, stimulate the migration of monocytes into the intimal layer of the arterial wall.

Upon entering the intimal layer, platelets, monocytes, and T lymphocytes participate in local pro-inflammatory and pro-thrombotic responses that develop the lesion. Activated platelets release a wealth of adhesive and proinflammatory factors, including cytokines, chemokines, vasoactive amines and growth factors, which they deposit on the surface of leukocytes and endothelial cells through P-selectin-mediated interactions.[5] The pro-inflammatory cytokine interleukin (IL)-1β and platelet factor (PF)-4, secreted by activated platelets, further promote leukocyte recruitment by upregulating endothelial cell expression of cell adhesion molecules and stimulating endothelial release of the chemokine monocyte chemotactic protein (MCP)-1, which recruits and activates monocytes. The monocytes rapidly proliferate and differentiate into macrophages. Macrophages express scavenger receptors which allow them to ingest highly oxidised LDL (Ox-LDL), leading to formation of macrophageous foam cells, thus promoting the accumulation of LDL in the arterial lesion.

Activated T lymphocytes also contribute to the progression of atherosclerosis, and are present at all stages of plaque development. Several classes of lymphocyte are involved, notably CD4+ type 1 helper (Th1) cells, regulatory T cells, and CD8+ cytolytic T cells.[4] These cells become activated upon recognition of protein antigens, which are processed and presented to them by macrophages or dendritic cells (a special type of macrophage). The antigens include oxidised lipoproteins, bacterial endotoxins and apoptic cell fragments. Activated Th1 cells secrete the cytokines interferon (IFN)γ, IL-2, tumour necrosis factor (TNF)α and TNFβ, which stimulate macrophage production of oxygen free radicals and proinflammatory cytokines and upregulate cell adhesion molecule expression on endothelial cells, thereby accelerating the inflammatory process.

The early stage of atherosclerosis, characterised by an accumulation of lipid-laden macrophages, together with some platelets and T lymphocytes, is often referred to as a fatty streak. The transition from fatty streak to a more complex lesion is characterised by migration of smooth muscle cells from the medial to intimal layers. Their migration and proliferation is stimulated by cytokines and growth factors released by activated platelets, macrophages, T cells and endothelial cells. These factors also promote smooth muscle cell production of fibrous elements (collagen and fibrin), leading to the formation of a dense extracellular matrix of fibrous tissue known as the fibrous cap.

As these inflammatory processes continue over years, the atherosclerotic plaque grows into an advanced lesion. Some lesions are occluding, meaning that the plaque protrudes into the arterial lumen and obstructs the flow of blood to the working heart muscle, resulting in ischaemia. However, the majority are non-occluding, because the vessel compensates by dilating or remodelling so that the thickening of the arterial wall does not immediately result in narrowing of the vessel lumen. Eventually, however, the artery can no longer compensate by dilation and the lesion may then intrude into the lumen and inhibit blood flow. Non-occluding lesions are typically rich in inflammatory cells and lipids, are covered with a thin fibrous cap, and are vulnerable to rupture. Acute cardiac events occur when the supply of blood through the coronary arteries to the working muscle of the heart is reduced or stopped altogether. Although this can happen with progressive narrowing of the lumen of the artery, more commonly acute cardiac events involve rupture of vulnerable plaque, exposing the underlying layers to circulating platelets, which then aggregate to form a blood clot (thrombus). Inflammatory processes are pivotal with regard to plaque rupture, as it appears that the degree of inflammatory activity and associated morphologic instability of a plaque, rather than the amount of occlusion or stenosis, defines its propensity to cause an acute coronary syndrome (ACS).[6]

7.2.1 Inflammatory Markers and CHD

Much of the evidence about atherogenesis has accumulated from cell biology studies, and work on genetic strains such as the Apo-E deficient mouse. However, human population studies corroborate biological science in documenting prospective associations between inflammatory markers and CHD. The marker that has been most extensively studied in this respect is the acute phase reactant C-reactive protein, which is measured by a high-sensitivity assay that discriminates CRP levels in the 'normal' range (hsCRP). Several large scale prospective studies have shown that baseline level of hsCRP in apparently healthy individuals is a strong independent predictor of future cardiovascular mortality and ACS.[7] However, the functional role of C-reactive protein itself is uncertain. Mendelian randomisation studies that compare cardiovascular risk in people with genetic polymorphisms associated with different levels of C-reactive protein cast doubt on its direct role,[8] and other lines of evidence suggest that it may be a marker rather than contributing directly.[9] C-reactive protein production by the liver is stimulated by IL-6 and TNFα. Prospective studies have shown that elevated plasma IL-6 is independently associated with an increased risk of CHD in apparently healthy middle-aged and elderly people.[10] TNFα responses are short-lasting and thus more difficult to evaluate than alterations in IL-6. Nevertheless, at least one study has found an association between elevated plasma TNFα and future risk of coronary events in apparently healthy elderly people.[11] The acute phase reactant fibrinogen has both haemostatic and inflammatory properties. A meta-analysis of 31 prospective studies found significant independent associations between plasma fibrinogen levels and the risks of suffering CHD, stroke, other vascular mortality and non-vascular mortality in healthy middle-aged adults.[12] Other inflammatory markers associated with cardiovascular risk in prospective population studies include plasma levels of the soluble forms of intercellular adhesion molecule (sICAM)-1, soluble P-selectin, and von Willebrand factor antigen.[13-15] Measures of these inflammatory markers do not consistently add to the prediction of future cardiovascular disease by conventional risk factors.[16] This does not negate their role in the aetiology of cardiovascular disease, but rather indicates that standard risk factors activate the same pathophysiological processes to which inflammation contributes.

7.2.2   Inflammation in Acute Coronary Disease

In addition to studies relating inflammation to the long-term development of CHD, there is a growing literature indicating that acute inflammatory conditions (such as those induced by infectious illness) may trigger cardiac events. Smeeth et al.[17] showed in a large primary care database that the risk of acute myocardial infarction (MI) and stroke was markedly increased during the first 3 days after the diagnosis of upper respiratory tract infection. It is possible that vaccination against influenza reduces the risk of acute MI, although evidence is inconclusive at present.[18] Chronic infection is accompanied by systemic inflammation and impaired vascular endothelial function, a response that can be reversed by treatment of the chronic infection.[19]

Acute coronary syndromes (acute MI and unstable angina) cause extensive tissue damage and themselves elicit very large inflammatory responses.[20] The magnitude of the acute inflammatory response during ACS is predictive of poor cardiac outcome. For example, Biasucci et al.[21] showed in unstable angina patients that increases in IL-1Ra and IL-6 measured 48 h after hospital admission were associated with greater risk of in-hospital cardiac events, while elevated C-reactive protein predicts 14 day mortality in unstable angina and non-Q wave MI independently of troponin responses.[22] Further studies have confirmed this positive association in non ST-segment elevation ACS patients and acute MI patients.[23,24] A meta-analysis of 20 cohort and randomised controlled trials showed that C-reactive protein levels >10 mg/L measured within 72 h of ACS onset were associated with a relative risk of 2.18 (95% C.I. 1.77–2.68) for recurrent cardiovascular events or death compared with values ≤3 mg/L.[25] Another acute-phase reactant, serum amyloid A, is also elevated in CHD patients compared with healthy controls, and is predictive of mortality in patients with unstable angina. Conversely, raised levels of the anti-inflammatory cytokine IL-10 are associated with a more favourable prognosis in ACS patients.[26] Most of these studies controlled for age, sex, cardiac enzyme levels, ejection fraction, heart failure and other markers of risk, suggesting that the impact of acute inflammation is independent of multiple risk indicators.

7.2.3 Inflammation, Immune Function, and Hypertension

Immune processes and inflammation also appear to be involved in the development of hypertension. Population-based studies have shown that prehypertension is associated with elevated plasma inflammatory markers,[27] that raised hsCRP levels predict future hypertension,[28] and that periodontal infections are related to hypertension.[29] Mechanistic studies are beginning to uncover the processes responsible. Harrison et al.[30] have proposed that small elevations in blood pressure lead to T cell activation through the formation of neoantigens. The activated T cells enter the vasculature and kidneys and express signals such as IL-17 that promote the entry of macrophages. These in turn release cytokines that cause vasoconstriction and sodium and water absorption. Sympathetic nervous system activation may contribute to the early stages of this process, along with stimuli such as angiotensin II acting in the central nervous system, particularly in the circumventricular organs that are critically involved in blood pressure regulation.[31]

7.3 Stress and Inflammation

The previous section outlined the role played by inflammation and immune processes at many stages of the cardiovascular disease process. The question that arises is what causes the inflammation and immune dysregulation, and whether stress makes a contribution. There are other important influences on inflammation in CHD, including genetic factors, oxidative stress, and infectious processes.[18,32]

As will be apparent from other chapters in this book, there are many ways of investigating stress, ranging from cell biological and animal research through experimental and clinical studies of humans, to population-based epidemiological work. The emphasis here is on human research at the experimental, clinical and epidemiological levels. Each approach has strengths and limitations.[33] Experimental studies are valuable in documenting the impact of stress in inflammation under controlled conditions; clinical studies help to address the issue of whether stress-related inflammatory processes are disturbed in people with documented CHD; while epidemiological studies can show whether stress affects CHD risk and the development of clinical disease through disturbances in inflammatory and immune processes in a longitudinal fashion. The psychosocial processes discussed here include not only exposure to life stress, but also protective factors in the social environment (social connectedness and social support), and psychological factors such as hostility, depression, and positive affect.

7.4 Experimental Studies of Stress and Inflammation

Psychophysiological or mental stress testing is a valuable method of investigating stress and inflammation in relation to CHD, as noted in Chap. 1. It is particularly suited to investigating inflammatory and immune variables, since blood samples can be repeatedly drawn and rapidly processed. However, the studies are acute, so that only short-term responses are observed, and typically involve reactions to artificial stimuli that rarely occur in the real world.

The early work on stress focused on lymphocyte counts and other enumerative measures, and simple functional tests such as natural killer cell activity.[34] However, effects of acute stress on inflammatory responses were seldom observed, since in the typical psychophysiological study blood is drawn at baseline and immediately after tasks. It turns out that inflammatory cytokine responses are slower to evolve, often not becoming apparent until 60–90 min after stress.[35] For example, our first study showed that plasma IL-6, TNFα and IL-1 receptor antagonist (IL-1Ra) concentrations increased around 2 h following stress, and similar effects have been observed in other laboratories.[36] Although leukocytosis may contribute, another factor underlying the temporal pattern of increase in plasma levels may be gene expression. Brydon et al.[37] showed that acute stress is associated with IL-1β gene expression in mononuclear cells 30 min after stress. IL-1β stimulates IL-6 production, and increased levels of IL-1β gene expression were positively correlated with plasma IL-6 responses to stress. This suggests that stress-induced increases in mononuclear IL-1β may contribute to the plasma IL-6 response. In animals, a variety of stressors including physical restraint, social disruption, restraint stress and open-field exposure stimulate increased levels of IL-6, IL-1 and TNFα.[38] Von Känel et al.[39] have added to our understanding of mechanisms by demonstrating that individuals treated with low-dose aspirin had attenuated increases in circulating IL-6 following mental stress compared to those who were not; propranolol treatment was not associated with any difference. Aspirin can inhibit the transcription nuclear factor κB (NF- κB) and prostaglandin E2, both of which are involved in IL-6 synthesis. Acute mental stress also leads to upregulation of other inflammatory factors such as sICAM-1,[40] enhancement of mononuclear cell chemotaxis,[41] and transient endothelial dysfunction.[42]

Experimental studies have not only demonstrated that stress can stimulate inflammatory responses, but also that the magnitude of responses varies with psychosocial risk factors for CHD. For example, low socioeconomic status (SES) is a risk factor for CHD,[43] and both lifestyle behavioural factors and psychobiological processes contribute.[44,45] Low SES individuals show greater plasma IL-6 responses to standardised challenging tasks than do more affluent individuals.[46] Work stress is associated with greater C-reactive protein responses,[47] while another study found that men reporting low job control had larger stress-induced increases in fibrinogen than those with high control at work.[48] Other forms of chronic stress have not been investigated extensively. However, Redwine et al.[49] observed greater inhibition of lymphocyte chemotaxis in response to a public speaking task in people under chronic stress (Alzheimer caregivers) compared with controls. Hostility is consistently associated with increased CHD risk,[50] and Gottdiener et al.[51] found that stress-induced inhibition of endothelial function was greater in more hostile individuals. Interestingly, depression is linked with endothelial dysfunction, an effect that can be reversed by blockade of cortisol synthesis with metyrapone.[52]

Very few studies of stress-induced inflammation in patients with CHD have been reported. One recent study from our group measured plasma IL-6 responses to behavioural tasks in survivors of ACS.[53] We found that the magnitude of IL-6 responses was positively correlated with hostility, with larger changes in more hostile individuals independently of age, body mass, smoking, medication at the time of testing, and baseline levels. The pattern of results is shown in Fig. 7.1, where positive associations between hostility and IL-6 measured both 75 and 120 min after stress can be seen. Effects are moderate, with hostility accounting for around 9–10% of the variance in IL-6 levels. Interestingly, hostility was also positively correlated with systolic and diastolic blood pressure stress responses.

7.4.1 Clinical Significance of Acute Inflammatory Stress Responses

Little is yet known about the clinical significance of variations in the magnitude of acute inflammatory responses to mental stress. It is possible that these responses are scientifically interesting but irrelevant to the real world, since they are measured under artificial laboratory conditions. Prospective studies are needed to test whether individuals who show large inflammatory stress responses are at greater risk of CHD. No such studies have yet been done. However, we were able to retest 153 individuals who had undergone psychophysiological stress testing 3 years earlier.[54] On both occasions, participants carried out ambulatory blood pressure monitoring,

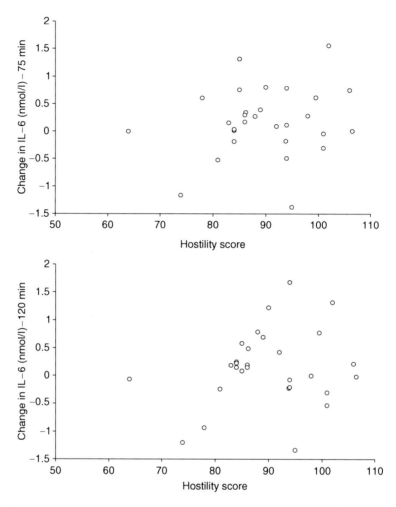

Fig. 7.1 Scatter plots of stress-related changes in plasma IL-6 between baseline and 75 min after stress (upper panel, $p = 0.009$) and 120 min after stress (lower panel, $p = 0.006$) in relation to hostility scores in cardiac patients. The associations were significant after adjustment for age, body mass, smoking status, medication at the time of testing, and baseline IL-6 (Adapted from Brydon et al.[53])

with measures taken every 20 min over the day and evening. We found that larger increases in ambulatory systolic pressure were predicted by greater acute fibrinogen and IL-6 stress responses. These effects were independent of previous ambulatory blood pressure level, acute blood pressure responses to stress, age, sex, body mass and smoking. IL-6 and fibrinogen appear to be involved in the arterial remodelling that underlies hypertension.[30] Thus stress could conceivably promote hypertension through stimulating these proteins.

In another analysis, we evaluated the relationship between inflammatory cytokine responses to stress and arterial stiffness measured 3 years later with

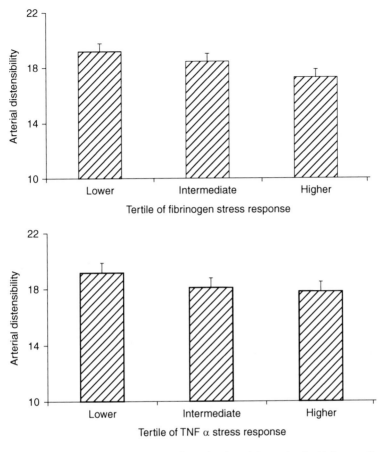

Fig. 7.2 Mean distensibility coefficient (10^{-3} kPa^{-1}) of participants in the higher, medium and lower fibrinogen stress response tertiles (upper panel, $p=0.037$ for trend across categories) and TNFα stress response tertiles (lower panel, $p=0.036$ for trend across categories), adjusted statistically for age, gender, socioeconomic status, smoking, body mass, waist/hip ratio, blood pressure, lipids and C-reactive protein. Error bars are standard errors of the mean (Adapted from Ellins et al.[55])

carotid ultrasound.[55] Results are summarized in Fig. 7.2. The measure of arterial stiffness was the distensibility coefficient. It can be seen that individuals who displayed greater TNFα and fibrinogen stress responses had stiffer arteries 3 years later, independently of potential confounders including age, gender, SES, smoking, body mass, abdominal adiposity, blood pressure, lipids and C-reactive protein. No significant relationship was found for IL-6. Of course, these findings do not demonstrate a causal relationship, since arterial stiffness was not measured at the time of stress testing as well, but they do suggest that acute inflammatory responses to stress are meaningful, and may be relevant to the understanding of CHD development.

7.5 Population Studies

Psychophysiological studies assess the dynamic responses of inflammatory and immune measures to externally applied stressors. By contrast, population studies typically involve correlating values obtained from single blood samples with psychosocial factors on the one hand, and clinical outcomes on the other hand. The strength of these methods lies not in evaluating dynamic processes, but in investigating psychoneuroimmunological mechanisms in relation to real-life challenges and experiences. Since measures of fibrinogen, C-reactive protein, and inflammatory cytokines are relatively inexpensive, it is possible to obtain data from large samples, allowing quite small associations to be detected. Effects can therefore be modest in absolute terms, but important as far as population health is concerned. For example, the relationship between inflammation and low SES or depressive symptoms may be small, but have considerable impact in the light of the high prevalence of these factors in the population at large. Additionally, population sampling can be employed, avoiding the selection factors that operate when small convenience samples are recruited.

Cross-sectional observational studies cannot determine the direction of causality, so it is impossible to conclude that psychosocial factors stimulate inflammation, or that inflammation contributes to psychosocial disturbance. Measures of inflammation are influenced by a host of factors that need to be taken into account, ranging from demographic characteristics (age, ethnicity, gender), lifestyle factors (smoking, alcohol consumption, physical activity), and anthropometric characteristics (body mass, abdominal adiposity). Therefore, an association between psychosocial factors and an inflammatory response may be secondary to other influences. More valuable data comes from large scale population-based studies that have a longitudinal element, so that relationships with the development of CHD risk profiles, or manifest clinical disease can be analysed.

The most consistent evidence from population studies relates to low SES, as defined by wealth, education or occupational status. Lower SES is associated with higher plasma fibrinogen, plasma hsCRP, IL-6, MCP-1 and von Willebrand factor antigen levels, after adjusting for age, adiposity, smoking, blood pressure and other covariates.[56–61] These associations have been observed both in younger and older adults in many countries. Life course studies indicate that SES earlier in life may contribute to adult inflammatory profiles. For example, Tabassum et al.[62] computed a cumulative score of SES at birth, age 23, and age 42 in a British birth cohort. Both hsCRP and fibrinogen at age 42 were positively related to the cumulative SES score after adjustment for body mass, smoking, and physical activity.

There is growing evidence that adversity in early life has an impact on inflammation in adults. An analysis of participants in the Coronary Artery Risk Development in Young Adults (CARDIA) study showed that retrospective ratings of early life stress were associated with hsCRP levels in middle age.[63] Stronger evidence has emerged from the Dunedin birth cohort study, in which harsh experience in early life was assessed contemporaneously.[64] It was found that maltreated children had elevated hsCRP and fibrinogen levels when aged 32, and that these effects were independent of childhood and adult SES, adult health behaviours and depression. These findings are interesting in the light of evidence that childhood adversity may be a predictor of CHD in adult life.[65]

Evidence linking work stress with CHD has been discussed in Chap. 11 (Kivimäki et al.). Several studies have investigated relationships between work stress and inflammatory markers.[57] A study of healthy Belgian men found that job control was inversely associated with fibrinogen after adjusting for age, education, body mass, smoking, alcohol consumption, and treatment of high blood pressure and hyperlipidaemia,[66] while associations between high work stress and von Willebrand factor have been shown in healthy Swedish women.[58] However, population studies have not found consistent relationships between IL-6 or hsCRP and work stress.[66] Nevertheless, other forms of chronic stress relate to inflammation. For example, Kiecolt-Glaser et al.[67] monitored informal carers for dementing relatives and matched controls over a 6 year period. Caregivers showed a progressive increase in plasma IL-6 over the years that was around four times greater than that recorded from controls. This effect was not due to differences in body mass, smoking, sleep quality, physical activity or alcohol consumption. An analysis from the Multi-Ethnic Study of Atherosclerosis (MESA) found that chronic life stress was positively related to IL-6 and hsCRP levels.[68] It is not clear why work stress does not show consistent associations, but one possibility is that more severe forms of life stress are needed before changes in C-reactive protein or IL-6 can be detected.

Social support and social networks are thought to protect against CHD. A limited amount of population work has shown relationships with inflammatory markers. Thus both in Swedish women and in the British Whitehall II cohort, fibrinogen levels were elevated in socially isolated compared with well integrated individuals.[48,58] Social integration was associated with lower fibrinogen in a study of high functioning older men aged 70–79 years, but there was no effect in women.[69]

The psychosocial risk factor that has been researched most thoroughly in relation to inflammation is depression and psychological distress, which are discussed in Chap. 12 (Hoen) and Chap. 19 (Linden). Several studies have documented cross-sectional associations between depression and circulating inflammatory markers such as hsCRP and IL-6.[70] We recently identified a relationship between fibrinogen and psychological distress in a nationally representative sample of young adults that was independent of age, gender, ethnicity, body mass index, lipids, smoking, alcohol and medication use.[71] There is likely to be a two-way link between depressive symptoms and inflammation, since peripheral inflammation may induce fatigue and somatic features of depression through its influence on sickness behaviour.[72] In the Whitehall II study, hsCRP and IL-6 predicted distress 12 years later, while baseline distress did not predict inflammation on follow-up, suggesting that inflammation precedes emotional distress.[73]

It can be seen from this brief summary that the evidence from population studies relating inflammatory markers with psychosocial risk factors for CHD is limited. Some of the factors that one might expect to be associated with inflammation (such as work stress) show only weak associations. A related question is whether inflammation contributes to the associations between psychosocial factors and CHD. Few studies have tested this possibility, since it requires prospective analysis of large samples of individuals initially free of CHD. A longitudinal analysis from the Whitehall II study found that both inflammation and psychological distress predicted future CHD over a 12 year follow-up after taking standard risk factors into account, but that these effects were independent of one another.[74] An analysis of the Women's Ischemia Syndrome Evaluation (WISE) study showed that hsCRP and IL-6 could account for a small but significant proportion of the association between depression and the incidence of cardiovascular events.[75]

7.6 Stress and Inflammation in Patients with Cardiovascular Disease

Evidence concerning the relationship between psychosocial factors and inflammation in patients with cardiovascular diseases is limited at present. Lesperance et al.[76] assessed 481 outpatients 2 months after hospitalisation for ACS with diagnostic psychiatric interviews. Depressed participants had higher levels of sICAM-1 and those who were not taking statins (which reduce inflammation) had raised hsCRP, but there was no association with IL-6. Frasure-Smith et al.[77] followed up 741 patients for 2 years after ACS for recurrent cardiac events, and showed that elevated hsCRP and depression ratings 2 months after the initial hospitalisation were both associated with increased risk to a similar extent. By contrast, a comparison of matched depressed and nondepressed MI patients found no differences in hsCRP, IL-6, TNFα or soluble TNF receptors,[78] while an analysis from the Heart and Soul study observed an inverse relationship between depression and inflammation in chronic CHD patients.[79]

Effects may be stronger in heart failure, where depressive symptoms have been positively associated with TNFα levels in two studies,[80,81] and negatively with the anti-inflammatory cytokine IL-10. Mommersteeg et al. recently reported that poor quality of life in heart failure patients predicted raised soluble TNF receptor 1 levels 12 months later.[82] Cytokines have also been implicated in associations between cardiovascular morbidity and Type D personality in patients with heart failure. Type D is a psychological trait identified by Denollet that consists of a tendency to experience negative emotions coupled with the inhibition of self-expression (see also Chap. 19, Linden). Denollet et al.[83] showed that Type D personality was associated with elevated levels of TNFα and soluble TNFα receptors (both types 1 and 2) in patients with congestive heart failure. These associations were confirmed in a later larger study that also reported that Type D patients had higher IL-6/IL-10 ratios.[84] In a similar vein, circulating levels of sICAM-1 predicted the severity of depressive symptoms 12 months later in heart failure patients, independently of cardiovascular risk factors, medication and baseline severity of heart failure.[85]

The links observed in these studies between inflammatory factors and affective state in patients with cardiovascular disease suggest that a two way process is in operation. Although stress and depression can stimulate inflammation, inflammation also has an effect on the central nervous system.[72] A parallel can be drawn with the animal research literature on sickness behaviour.[86,87] Sickness behaviour refers to a cluster of symptoms affecting both behavioural and affective states, triggered by the release of pro-inflammatory cytokines commonly observed in response to a systemic infection. Sickness behaviour in animals is reflected in social withdrawal, decreased locomotion and exploratory activity, and reduced food and water intake. In humans, these actions are accompanied by malaise, increased negative mood, listlessness and fatigue. This is reminiscent of the somatic symptoms of depression, including lassitude, fatigue and dysphoric mood. Sickness behaviour is regarded as adaptive in organising bodily responses that fight infection, promote cellular (T-helper 1) immunity, and target intracellular organisms through activation of macrophages, cytotoxic T lymphocytes and natural killer cells. However, in advanced cardiovascular diseases such as CHD and heart failure, the damaged cardiac tissue may cause large inflammatory responses capable of triggering sickness behaviours in vulnerable individuals. The result may be fatigue and even depression in some cases.[88]

One useful model in which these mechanisms can be explored is during acute inflammation induced by vaccination with *Salmonella typhi* or *Salmonella abortus equi* endotoxin. Hingorani et al.[89] demonstrated that typhoid vaccination leads to an acute impairment of endothelial-dependent vasodilation, and that responses correlated with increases in serum IL-6 and IL-1Ra. Interestingly, we found that the same stimulus led to mild impairment of mood,[90] and that the negative mood response was mediated by increases in IL-6.[91] In a functional magnetic resonance imaging (fMRI) study, it was also shown that the deterioration in mood induced by inflammation correlated with enhanced activity in the anterior cingulate cortex, a brain region involved in the development of depression, and with the connections between this region and the amygdala.[92] The combination of acute mental stress and inflammation resulting from typhoid vaccination was associated with activation of the anterior cingulate cortex and the right dorsal prefrontal cortex, areas implicated in cognitive control and in the regulation of internal bodily states.[93] It is possible that the links between cardiovascular function, inflammation, mood and central nervous system activation identified in these acute experiments mirror the processes linking depression with inflammation in CHD.[72]

7.7 Conclusions

Research on stress, inflammation and CHD is rapidly evolving, with new findings that challenge our understanding of the pathways linking psychosocial factors with cardiovascular disease. Much of the research in humans is observational, so causal conclusions are difficult to draw. This is frustrating in a field in which two way links exist, though light can be cast on causal mechanisms through experimental and clinical interventions.[94] It is likely that this field will yield behavioural and pharmacological interventions over the next decade that will help improve the emotional adaptation and quality of life of cardiac patients.

References

1. Steptoe A, Brydon L. Psychosocial factors and coronary heart disease: the contribution of psychoneuroimmunological processes. In: Ader R, ed. *Psychoneuroimmunology.* 4th ed. San Diego: Academic Press; 2007:945-974.
2. Ross R. Atherosclerosis – an inflammatory disease. *N Engl J Med.* 1999;340:115-126.
3. Hansson GK. Inflammation, atherosclerosis, and coronary artery disease. *N Engl J Med.* 2005;352:1685-1695.
4. Libby P, Ridker PM, Hansson GK. Inflammation in atherosclerosis: from pathophysiology to practice. *J Am Coll Cardiol.* 2009;54:2129-2138.
5. Huo Y, Ley KF. Role of platelets in the development of atherosclerosis. *Trends Cardiovasc Med.* 2004;14:18-22.
6. Naghavi M, Libby P, Falk E, et al. From vulnerable plaque to vulnerable patient: a call for new definitions and risk assessment strategies: part II. *Circulation.* 2003;108:1772-1778.
7. Kaptoge S, Di Angelantonio E, Lowe G, et al. C-reactive protein concentration and risk of coronary heart disease, stroke, and mortality: an individual participant meta-analysis. *Lancet.* 2010;375:132-140.
8. Elliott P, Chambers JC, Zhang W, et al. Genetic loci associated with C-reactive protein levels and risk of coronary heart disease. *JAMA.* 2009;302:37-48.
9. Danesh J, Pepys MB. C-reactive protein and coronary disease: is there a causal link? *Circulation.* 2009;120:2036-2039.
10. Danesh J, Kaptoge S, Mann AG, et al. Long-term interleukin-6 levels and subsequent risk of coronary heart disease: two new prospective studies and a systematic review. *PLoS Med.* 2008;5:e78.
11. Cesari M, Penninx BW, Newman AB, et al. Inflammatory markers and onset of cardiovascular events: results from the Health ABC study. *Circulation.* 2003;108:2317-2322.
12. Danesh J, Lewington S, Thompson SG, et al. Plasma fibrinogen level and the risk of major cardiovascular diseases and nonvascular mortality: an individual participant meta-analysis. *JAMA.* 2005;294:1799-1809.
13. Blankenberg S, Barbaux S, Tiret L. Adhesion molecules and atherosclerosis. *Atherosclerosis.* 2003;170:191-203.
14. Merten M, Thiagarajan P. P-selectin in arterial thrombosis. *Z Kardiol.* 2004;93:855-863.
15. Spiel AO, Gilbert JC, Jilma B. von Willebrand factor in cardiovascular disease: focus on acute coronary syndromes. *Circulation.* 2008;117:1449-1459.
16. Tousoulis D, Antoniades C, Stefanadis C. Assessing inflammatory status in cardiovascular disease. *Heart.* 2007;93:1001-1007.
17. Smeeth L, Thomas SL, Hall AJ, Hubbard R, Farrington P, Vallance P. Risk of myocardial infarction and stroke after acute infection or vaccination. *N Engl J Med.* 2004;351:2611-2618.
18. Warren-Gash C, Smeeth L, Hayward AC. Influenza as a trigger for acute myocardial infarction or death from cardiovascular disease: a systematic review. *Lancet Infect Dis.* 2009;9:601-610.
19. Tonetti MS, D'Aiuto F, Nibali L, et al. Treatment of periodontitis and endothelial function. *N Engl J Med.* 2007;356:911-920.
20. Kushner I, Broder ML, Karp D. Control of the acute phase response. Serum C-reactive protein kinetics after acute myocardial infarction. *J Clin Invest.* 1978;61:235-242.
21. Biasucci LM, Liuzzo G, Fantuzzi G, et al. Increasing levels of interleukin (IL)-1Ra and IL-6 during the first 2 days of hospitalization in unstable angina are associated with increased risk of in-hospital coronary events. *Circulation.* 1999;99:2079-2084.
22. Morrow DA, Rifai N, Antman EM, et al. C-reactive protein is a potent predictor of mortality independently of and in combination with troponin T in acute coronary syndromes: a TIMI 11A substudy. *J Am Coll Cardiol.* 1998;31:1460-1465.
23. Kosuge M, Ebina T, Hibi K, et al. Value of serial C-reactive protein measurements in non ST-segment elevation acute coronary syndromes. *Clin Cardiol.* 2008;31:437-442.

24. Suleiman M, Khatib R, Agmon Y, et al. Early inflammation and risk of long-term development of heart failure and mortality in survivors of acute myocardial infarction predictive role of C-reactive protein. *J Am Coll Cardiol*. 2006;47:962-968.
25. He LP, Tang XY, Ling WH, Chen WQ, Chen YM. Early C-reactive protein in the prediction of long-term outcomes after acute coronary syndromes: a meta-analysis of longitudinal studies. *Heart*. 2010;96:339-346.
26. Fichtlscherer S, Heeschen C, Zeiher AM. Inflammatory markers and coronary artery disease. *Curr Opin Pharmacol*. 2004;4:124-131.
27. Chrysohoou C, Pitsavos C, Panagiotakos DB, Skoumas J, Stefanadis C. Association between prehypertension status and inflammatory markers related to atherosclerotic disease: the ATTICA study. *Am J Hypertens*. 2004;17:568-573.
28. Sesso HD, Buring JE, Rifai N, Blake GJ, Gaziano JM, Ridker PM. C-reactive protein and the risk of developing hypertension. *JAMA*. 2003;290:2945-2951.
29. Tsakos G, Sabbah W, Hingorani AD, et al. Is periodontal inflammation associated with raised blood pressure? Evidence from a National US survey. *J Hypertens*. 2010;28(12):2386-2393.
30. Harrison DG, Guzik TJ, Lob HE, et al. Inflammation, immunity, and hypertension. *Hypertension*. 2011;57:132-140.
31. Marvar PJ, Lob H, Vinh A, Zarreen F, Harrison DG. The central nervous system and inflammation in hypertension. *Curr Opin Pharmacol*. 2011;11(2):156-161.
32. Espinola-Klein C, Rupprecht HJ, Blankenberg S, et al. Impact of infectious burden on extent and long-term prognosis of atherosclerosis. *Circulation*. 2002;105:15-21.
33. Steptoe A. Tools of psychosocial biology in health care research. In: Bowling A, Ebrahim S, eds. *Handbook of Health Research Methods*. Maidenhead: Open University Press; 2005:471-493.
34. Segerstrom SC, Miller GE. Psychological stress and the human immune system: a meta-analytic study of 30 years of inquiry. *Psychol Bull*. 2004;130:601-630.
35. Steptoe A, Hamer M, Chida Y. The effects of acute psychological stress on circulating inflammatory factors in humans: a review and meta-analysis. *Brain Behav Immun*. 2007;21:901-912.
36. von Kanel R, Kudielka BM, Preckel D, Hanebuth D, Fischer JE. Delayed response and lack of habituation in plasma interleukin-6 to acute mental stress in men. *Brain Behav Immun*. 2006;20:40-48.
37. Brydon L, Edwards S, Jia H, et al. Psychological stress activates interleukin-1 beta gene expression in human mononuclear cells. *Brain Behav Immun*. 2005;19:540-546.
38. Dhabhar FS, McEwen BS. Bi-directional effects of stress on immune function: possible explanations for salubrious as well as harmful effects. In: Ader R, ed. *Psychoneuroimmunology*. 4th ed. San Diego: Academic Press; 2007:723-760.
39. von Kanel R, Kudielka BM, Metzenthin P, et al. Aspirin, but not propranolol, attenuates the acute stress-induced increase in circulating levels of interleukin-6: a randomized, double-blind, placebo-controlled study. *Brain Behav Immun*. 2008;22:150-157.
40. Goebel MU, Mills PJ. Acute psychological stress and exercise and changes in peripheral leukocyte adhesion molecule expression and density. *Psychosom Med*. 2000;62:664-670.
41. Redwine L, Snow S, Mills P, Irwin M. Acute psychological stress: effects on chemotaxis and cellular adhesion molecule expression. *Psychosom Med*. 2003;65:598-603.
42. Ghiadoni L, Donald A, Cropley M, et al. Mental stress induces transient endothelial dysfunction in humans. *Circulation*. 2000;102:2473-2478.
43. Adler NE, Rehkopf DH. U.S. disparities in health: descriptions, causes, and mechanisms. *Annu Rev Public Health*. 2008;29:235-252.
44. Stringhini S, Sabia S, Shipley M, et al. Association of socioeconomic position with health behaviors and mortality. *JAMA*. 2010;303:1159-1166.
45. Steptoe A, Marmot M. The role of psychobiological pathways in socio-economic inequalities in cardiovascular disease risk. *Eur Heart J*. 2002;23:13-25.
46. Brydon L, Edwards S, Mohamed-Ali V, Steptoe A. Socioeconomic status and stress-induced increases in interleukin-6. *Brain Behav Immun*. 2004;18:281-290.

47. Hamer M, Williams E, Vuonovirta R, Giacobazzi P, Gibson EL, Steptoe A. The effects of effort-reward imbalance on inflammatory and cardiovascular responses to mental stress. *Psychosom Med.* 2006;68:408-413.
48. Steptoe A, Kunz-Ebrecht S, Owen N, et al. Influence of socioeconomic status and job control on plasma fibrinogen responses to acute mental stress. *Psychosom Med.* 2003;65:137-144.
49. Redwine L, Mills PJ, Sada M, Dimsdale J, Patterson T, Grant I. Differential immune cell chemotaxis responses to acute psychological stress in Alzheimer caregivers compared to non-caregiver controls. *Psychosom Med.* 2004;66:770-775.
50. Chida Y, Steptoe A. The association of anger and hostility with future coronary heart disease: a meta-analytic review of prospective evidence. *J Am Coll Cardiol.* 2009;53:936-946.
51. Gottdiener JS, Kop WJ, Hausner E, McCeney MK, Herrington D, Krantz DS. Effects of mental stress on flow-mediated brachial arterial dilation and influence of behavioral factors and hypercholesterolemia in subjects without cardiovascular disease. *Am J Cardiol.* 2003;92:687-691.
52. Broadley AJ, Korszun A, Abdelaal E, et al. Inhibition of cortisol production with metyrapone prevents mental stress-induced endothelial dysfunction and baroreflex impairment. *J Am Coll Cardiol.* 2005;46:344-350.
53. Brydon L, Strike PC, Bhattacharyya MR, et al. Hostility and physiological responses to laboratory stress in acute coronary syndrome patients. *J Psychosom Res.* 2010;68:109-116.
54. Brydon L, Steptoe A. Stress-induced increases in interleukin-6 and fibrinogen predict ambulatory blood pressure at 3-year follow-up. *J Hypertens.* 2005;23:1001-1007.
55. Ellins E, Halcox J, Donald A, et al. Arterial stiffness and inflammatory response to psychophysiological stress. *Brain Behav Immun.* 2008;22:941-948.
56. Ramsay S, Lowe GD, Whincup PH, Rumley A, Morris RW, Wannamethee SG. Relationships of inflammatory and haemostatic markers with social class: results from a population-based study of older men. *Atherosclerosis.* 2008;197:654-661.
57. Brunner E, Davey Smith G, Marmot M, Canner R, Beksinska M, O'Brien J. Childhood social circumstances and psychosocial and behavioural factors as determinants of plasma fibrinogen. *Lancet.* 1996;347:1008-1013.
58. Wamala SP, Murray MA, Horsten M, et al. Socioeconomic status and determinants of hemostatic function in healthy women. *Arterioscler Thromb Vasc Biol.* 1999;19:485-492.
59. Nazmi A, Victora CG. Socioeconomic and racial/ethnic differentials of C-reactive protein levels: a systematic review of population-based studies. *BMC Public Health.* 2007;7:212.
60. Loucks EB, Sullivan LM, Hayes LJ, et al. Association of educational level with inflammatory markers in the Framingham Offspring study. *Am J Epidemiol.* 2006;163:622-628.
61. Friedman EM, Herd P. Income, education, and inflammation: differential associations in a national probability sample (the MIDUS study). *Psychosom Med.* 2010;72:290-300.
62. Tabassum F, Kumari M, Rumley A, Lowe G, Power C, Strachan DP. Effects of socioeconomic position on inflammatory and hemostatic markers: a life-course analysis in the 1958 British birth cohort. *Am J Epidemiol.* 2008;167:1332-1341.
63. Taylor SE, Lehman BJ, Kiefe CI, Seeman TE. Relationship of early life stress and psychological functioning to adult C-reactive protein in the coronary artery risk development in young adults study. *Biol Psychiatry.* 2006;60:819-824.
64. Danese A, Pariante CM, Caspi A, Taylor A, Poulton R. Childhood maltreatment predicts adult inflammation in a life-course study. *Proc Natl Acad Sci USA.* 2007;104:1319-1324.
65. Dong M, Giles WH, Felitti VJ, et al. Insights into causal pathways for ischemic heart disease: adverse childhood experiences study. *Circulation.* 2004;110:1761-1766.
66. Clays E, De Bacquer D, Delanghe J, Kittel F, Van Renterghem L, De Backer G. Associations between dimensions of job stress and biomarkers of inflammation and infection. *J Occup Environ Med.* 2005;47:878-883.
67. Kiecolt-Glaser JK, Preacher KJ, MacCallum RC, Atkinson C, Malarkey WB, Glaser R. Chronic stress and age-related increases in the proinflammatory cytokine IL-6. *Proc Natl Acad Sci USA.* 2003;100:9090-9095.
68. Ranjit N, Diez-Roux AV, Shea S, et al. Psychosocial factors and inflammation in the multi-ethnic study of atherosclerosis. *Arch Intern Med.* 2007;167:174-181.

69. Loucks EB, Berkman LF, Gruenewald TL, Seeman TE. Social integration is associated with fibrinogen concentration in elderly men. *Psychosom Med.* 2005;67:353-358.
70. Howren MB, Lamkin DM, Suls J. Associations of depression with C-reactive protein, IL-1, and IL-6: a meta-analysis. *Psychosom Med.* 2009;71:171-186.
71. Goldman-Mellor S, Brydon L, Steptoe A. Psychological distress and circulating inflammatory markers in healthy young adults. *Psychol Med.* 2010;40:2079-2087.
72. Poole L, Dickens C, Steptoe A. The puzzle of depression and acute coronary syndrome: reviewing the role of acute inflammation. *J Psychosom Res.* 2011;71:61-68.
73. Gimeno D, Kivimaki M, Brunner EJ, et al. Associations of C-reactive protein and interleukin-6 with cognitive symptoms of depression: 12-year follow-up of the Whitehall II study. *Psychol Med.* 2009;39:413-423.
74. Nabi H, Singh-Manoux A, Shipley M, Gimeno D, Marmot MG, Kivimaki M. Do psychological factors affect inflammation and incident coronary heart disease: the Whitehall II study. *Arterioscler Thromb Vasc Biol.* 2008;28:1398-1406.
75. Vaccarino V, Johnson BD, Sheps DS, et al. Depression, inflammation, and incident cardiovascular disease in women with suspected coronary ischemia: the National Heart, Lung, and Blood Institute-sponsored WISE study. *J Am Coll Cardiol.* 2007;50:2044-2050.
76. Lesperance F, Frasure-Smith N, Theroux P, Irwin M. The association between major depression and levels of soluble intercellular adhesion molecule 1, interleukin-6, and C-reactive protein in patients with recent acute coronary syndromes. *Am J Psychiatry.* 2004;161:271-277.
77. Frasure-Smith N, Lesperance F, Irwin MR, Sauve C, Lesperance J, Theroux P. Depression, C-reactive protein and two-year major adverse cardiac events in men after acute coronary syndromes. *Biol Psychiatry.* 2007;62:302-308.
78. Schins A, Tulner D, Lousberg R, et al. Inflammatory markers in depressed post-myocardial infarction patients. *J Psychiatr Res.* 2005;39:137-144.
79. Whooley MA, Caska CM, Hendrickson BE, Rourke MA, Ho J, Ali S. Depression and inflammation in patients with coronary heart disease: findings from the Heart and Soul study. *Biol Psychiatry.* 2007;62:314-320.
80. Ferketich AK, Ferguson JP, Binkley PF. Depressive symptoms and inflammation among heart failure patients. *Am Heart J.* 2005;150:132-136.
81. Parissis JT, Adamopoulos S, Rigas A, et al. Comparison of circulating proinflammatory cytokines and soluble apoptosis mediators in patients with chronic heart failure with versus without symptoms of depression. *Am J Cardiol.* 2004;94:1326-1328.
82. Mommersteeg PM, Kupper N, Schoormans D, Emons W, Pedersen SS. Health-related quality of life is related to cytokine levels at 12 months in patients with chronic heart failure. *Brain Behav Immun.* 2010;24:615-622.
83. Denollet J, Conraads VM, Brutsaert DL, De Clerck LS, Stevens WJ, Vrints CJ. Cytokines and immune activation in systolic heart failure: the role of type D personality. *Brain Behav Immun.* 2003;17:304-309.
84. Denollet J, Schiffer AA, Kwaijtaal M, et al. Usefulness of type D personality and kidney dysfunction as predictors of interpatient variability in inflammatory activation in chronic heart failure. *Am J Cardiol.* 2009;103:399-404.
85. Wirtz PH, Redwine LS, Linke S, et al. Circulating levels of soluble intercellular adhesion molecule-1 (sICAM-1) independently predict depressive symptom severity after 12 months in heart failure patients. *Brain Behav Immun.* 2010;24:366-369.
86. Raison CL, Capuron L, Miller AH. Cytokines sing the blues: inflammation and the pathogenesis of depression. *Trends Immunol.* 2006;27:24-31.
87. Dantzer R, O'Connor JC, Freund GG, Johnson RW, Kelley KW. From inflammation to sickness and depression: when the immune system subjugates the brain. *Nat Rev Neurosci.* 2008;9: 46-56.
88. Dantzer R, Kelley KW. Twenty years of research on cytokine-induced sickness behavior. *Brain Behav Immun.* 2007;21:153-160.
89. Hingorani AD, Cross J, Kharbanda RK, et al. Acute systemic inflammation impairs endothelium-dependent dilatation in humans. *Circulation.* 2000;102:994-999.

90. Strike PC, Wardle J, Steptoe A. Mild acute inflammatory stimulation induces transient negative mood. *J Psychosom Res*. 2004;57:189-194.

91. Wright CE, Strike PC, Brydon L, Steptoe A. Acute inflammation and negative mood: mediation by cytokine activation. *Brain Behav Immun*. 2005;19:345-350.

92. Harrison NA, Brydon L, Walker C, Gray MA, Steptoe A, Critchley HD. Inflammation causes mood changes through alterations in subgenual cingulate activity and mesolimbic connectivity. *Biol Psychiatry*. 2009;66:407-414.

93. Harrison NA, Brydon L, Walker C, et al. Neural origins of human sickness in interoceptive responses to inflammation. *Biol Psychiatry*. 2009;66:415-422.

94. Crossman DC, Morton AC, Gunn JP, et al. Investigation of the effect of interleukin-1 receptor antagonist (IL-1ra) on markers of inflammation in non-ST elevation acute coronary syndromes (the MRC-ILA-HEART study). *Trials*. 2008;9:8.

Chapter 8
Brain Imaging of Stress and Cardiovascular Responses

Marcus Gray, Yoko Nagai, and Hugo D. Critchley

Keywords Brain imaging • Stress • Cardiovascular responses • Neuroimaging techniques • Acute stress challenges • Arrhythmogenic mechanisms • Humoral axes of stress

8.1 Overview

Neuroimaging studies in humans can provide valuable insight into the central mechanisms through which stress can impact on cardiovascular health. Functional brain imaging has become a major investigative tool within neuroscience that is extensively applied to the characterisation of regional activity patterns associated with cognitive and emotional processing. Neuroimaging approaches have also been applied to examine the control of bodily state, including the generation of adaptive and maladaptive cardiovascular responses.[1] Emerging from the combination of these are sophisticated insights into how mental and physiological stress can give rise to potentially pathological short-term changes affecting cardiovascular function.

M. Gray
Department of Experimental Neuropsychology Research Unit, School of Psychology and
Psychiatry, Faculty of Medicine Nursing and Health Sciences, Monash University,
Clayton, VIC, Australia
e-mail: marcus.gray@monash.edu

Y. Nagai • H.D. Critchley (✉)
Department of Psychiatry, Brighton and Sussex Medical School,
University of Sussex, Brighton, East Sussex, UK
e-mail: y.nagai@bsms.ac.uk, h.critchley@bsms.ac.uk,

P. Hjemdahl et al. (eds.), *Stress and Cardiovascular Disease*,
DOI 10.1007/978-1-84882-419-5_8, © Springer-Verlag London Limited 2012

In combination with perspectives from structural neuroimaging studies of clinical and 'analogue' populations, functional neuroimaging is enhancing the mechanistic understanding of how stress impacts long-term cardiovascular well-being. Ultimately, information regarding the translation of psychological stress into physiological change offers the prospect of establishing markers for vulnerability and treatment within 'individualised medicine', and may inform the development of novel preventive strategies and interventions for cardiovascular health.[2]

This chapter draws together some of the evidence from functional imaging studies that has contributed to the understanding of brain systems that mediate interactions between stress and cardiovascular health.

8.2 Neuroimaging Techniques

Human brain imaging research techniques permit (largely noninvasive) quantification in vivo of brain activity, metabolism, neurochemistry and structure. Magnetic Resonance Imaging (MRI), in particular, offers the potential for the same scanner to generate a range of biological measurements within the same individual to give convergent information about brain processes. For imaging brain function, the dominant technique is functional MRI (fMRI) which indexes local activity from blood flow changes coupled to changes in neural firing. There are specific constraints on the spatial and temporal resolution of fMRI (millimetres and seconds) as a consequence of this indirect approach which reflect the extent and lag of regional haemodynamic responses. However, in these respects, fMRI is an improvement on Single Photon Emission Tomography (SPET) and Positron Emission Tomography (PET) techniques for measuring regional cerebral blood flow and metabolism, since in SPECT and PET, radioisotopes are used to label specific molecules, including water, glucose or neurotransmitter analogues. PET uses the source localization of radioactive decay to provide three-dimensional, absolute rather than relative, measures of metabolic activity (e.g., glucose uptake and utilization) or blood flow (e.g., using ^{15}O-labelled water). PET remains the unrivalled technique for quantifying in vivo in humans the distribution of neurotransmitter/neuromodulator and receptor activity and to detect pathological proteins such as amyloid. These scanner-based approaches are complemented by electrical, magnetic and optical imaging methodologies that provide information on synchronization of neural (primarily cortical) function with much higher temporal resolution, but often at the cost of much poorer spatial resolution. Finally, structural brain imaging, which is used clinically for diagnosis of brain conditions (e.g., detecting space-occupying lesions or pathological neurodegeneration), can also be used in group studies of apparently neurologically intact people. Computerised techniques such as voxel-based morphometry can be used to identify brain structures whose size correlates with distinct traits that effect the relative growth or loss of (healthy) neural tissue. Individual differences in genetics, life experiences and personality traits can thus be related to distinct brain systems among healthy people.[3,4] Both functional and structural neuroimaging techniques are used to probe brain mechanisms of stress and possible consequences for cardiovascular health.[1]

8.3   Brain Responses to Acute Stress Challenges

Certain types of task, typically evoking pain, anxiety or involving intense behavioural demand, elicit reactive changes in autonomic and humoral state that may be adaptive in the short term, but maladaptive if excessive or sustained. Such tasks can be used as experimental challenges for studying stress, bridging the gap between experimental acute stress exposures that can be conducted in animals, and the psychological and physiological reactions associated with real-world stress in humans. Functional imaging studies of experimental challenges provide insight into brain mechanisms mediating maladaptive stress responses that ultimately impact on cardiovascular function.

Provocation studies often evoke characteristic patterns of brain activation[5]: Commonly seen is an enhancement of activity within the dorsal anterior cingulate cortex, bilateral (right predominant) insula cortex, and, perhaps less consistently, subcortical activation within centres including amygdala and head of caudate, and brainstem (typically dorsal pons). Brain regions including ventromedial orbital and subgenual cingulate cortices are deactivated. Both early and more recent examples of such neuroimaging experiments include symptom provocation in people with obsessive compulsive disorder[6,7] or posttraumatic stress,[8] psychological challenges including mental stress,[9,10] social rejection,[11] experienced pain,[12] empathy for pain,[13] anxiety or fear induction (e.g., threat of pain[14,15]) and the anticipation of public speaking.[16-18] Physical stress provocations used, occasionally in combination with demanding mental tasks, include exercise, cold pressor tests, and respiratory and inflammatory challenges.[9,19-22] There are modality-specific differences in the patterns of brain activity produced by these different stressors, but the commonalities described above seem to represent a signature of arousal associated with demand. An important interpretive issue is that the findings of these stress studies typically differ only in magnitude from 'normal' patterns of regional brain activity that are recruited when a participant engages in any attention or emotion-demanding behaviour.[5] Unpicking the physiological axis of these responses and identifying a unique mechanistic signature of stress with confidence remains a goal (Fig. 8.1).

8.4   Neural Systems Governing Cardiovascular Control

Functional neuroimaging studies have found their most favoured application in the study of brain mechanisms supporting mind stuff, i.e., thoughts and emotions, that are especially associated with the human condition and which have previously been elusive to organic understanding. In vivo visualization of the brain in action, although usually not immediate, has narrowed this physical–mental divide. Parallel to these cognitive studies are investigations of how the brain regulates bodily states including cardiovascular control. In these studies, the focus is on changes in autonomic activity elicited by one or more tasks (often those used clinically as autonomic function tests and acute stress challenges). Progress in this field has been

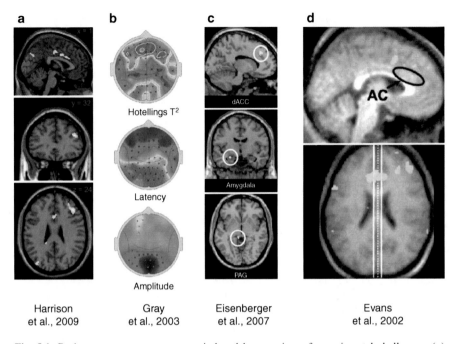

a **b** **c** **d**

Hotellings T²

Latency

Amplitude

dACC

Amygdala

PAG

AC

| Harrison | Gray | Eisenberger | Evans |
| et al., 2009 | et al., 2003 | et al., 2007 | et al., 2002 |

Fig. 8.1 Brain responses to acute stress induced by a variety of experimental challenges. (a) Neural activity associated with the interaction of a cognitive stressor task and acute inflammatory stress induced by typhoid vaccination.[22] (b) Steady State Probe Topography during anticipation of electrical stimulation.[15] (c) Neural correlates of social exclusion which correlated with momentary social distress during daily social interactions.[11] (d) Neural correlates of stress associated with acute air hunger[21] (Figures modified from originals and reproduced with permission)

relatively slow, in part due to methodological difficulties of implementing subject monitoring, but also practical concerns about confounding the brain signal with physiological noise and interpretation of correlated dependent variables.[23] Relatively early examples of studies probing cardiac control without simultaneous physiological monitoring include brain responses to the Valsalva manoeuvre (breathing against a closed glottis), isometric handgrip exercise, deep inspiration, mental stress (arithmetic) and cold pressor tests. Increased activity in anterior and posterior insula, medial prefrontal cortex and ventroposterior thalamus was observed during respiratory, Valsalva and exercise challenges using fMRI[24] (see Fig. 8.2a(ii)). Another group observed increased activity in ventral and medial prefrontal cortex, anterior cingulate, insula, medial temporal lobe, medial thalamus, cerebellum midbrain and pons during Valsalva manoeuvres and cold pressor challenge.[25] In such experiments, activity within brainstem sites encompassing periaqueductal grey matter (PAG) and dorsal raphé nucleus may distinguish respiratory autonomic challenge (maximum inspiration, Valsalva) from isometric exercise.[26] (See Fig. 8.2a(i)). Unfortunately standard human neuroimaging experiments have yet to attain the level of detail regarding the contributions of discrete brainstem nuclei to the proximate neural control of the cardiovascular system. Encouragingly, there is increasing progress with functional brainstem imaging from autonomic perspectives.[27-30]

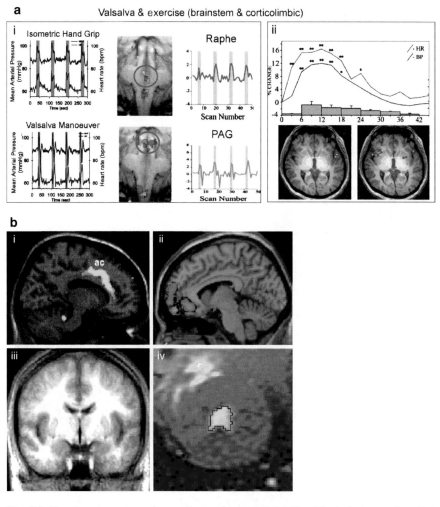

Fig. 8.2 Neural systems governing cardiovascular control. (**a**) Physiological stress tasks which induce changes in heart rate and blood pressure including Valsalva manoeuvre and isometric exercise activate both (i) brainstem regions including the PAG and raphe,[26] and (ii) corticolimbic regions such as the insula.[24] (**b**) Additionally, during acute stress, neural activity directly correlates with changes in cardiovascular function; (i) ACC correlations with mean arterial pressure (MAP).[9](ii) Subgenual cingulate correlations with heart rate (HR).[38] (iii) Amygdala activity correlating with increasing ventricular contractility, measured via (iv) direct cardiac imaging.[43] (**c**) Stress responses are tied to the balance of activity within the autonomic nervous system. (i) High-frequency heart rate variability (parasympathetic branch) is associated with (ii) neural activity during emotional induction task[37] and (iii) neural activity predicting pain induced alterations in blood pressure.[29] (**d**) The degree to which the activity within discrete neural structures during social evaluative threat stressor mediate the accompanying increase in heart rate was investigated statistically. Increased rostrodorsal (rdACC) and decreased subgenual cingulate/ventromedial prefrontal cortex (vmPFC) activity during stress of preparing a speech were associated with thalamic and PAG activity correlating with the cardiovascular responses induced by the acute stress.[18] The numbers reflect the strength of significant partial correlations between the brain structures predicting the heart rate changes, indicating the two pathways through which heart rate is influenced. Significance is shown by *asterisks* (Figures modified from originals and reproduced with permission)

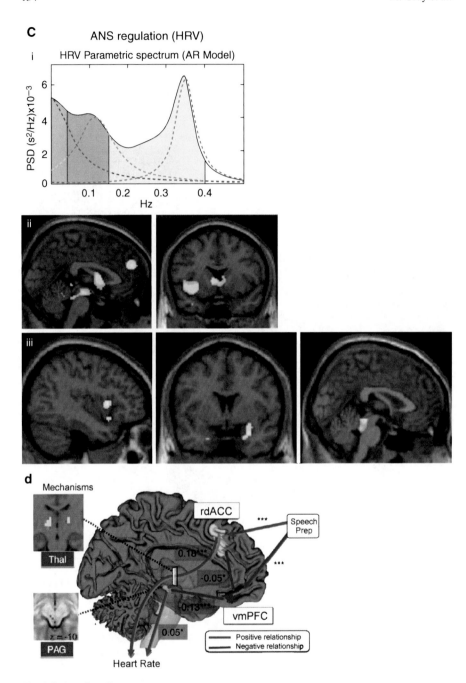

Fig. 8.2 (continued)

In one PET study examining neural centres supporting cardiovascular control, increases in heart rate and blood pressure were induced by effortful mental arithmetic and physical exercise tasks. Corresponding brains states were contrasted with activity patterns during non-effortful control tasks[9] (Fig. 8.2b(i)). The experiment was designed to specifically examine arousal-related commonalities engendered by the cognitive and exercise conditions while excluding task-specific inner-speech (prefrontal and speech-related frontotemporal cortices) and musculature-related (somatomotor cortices) activity. Performance of both effortful tasks increased heart rate and blood pressure and was associated with increased activity within the mid cingulate and dorsal pons. More specifically, across both cognitive and exercise conditions, increases in blood pressure correlated with increased activity within right anterior cingulate, right insula and pons while decreases were observed in medial temporal and prefrontal regions. This study pointed toward a role of dorsal anterior cingulate in generating cardiovascular responses to effortful, potentially stressful behaviours. The study also suggested a laterality of sympathetic responses to the right hemisphere which accords with an earlier proposal based upon stimulation of human insular cortices.[31] This relationship between right anterior cingulate activity and increases in blood pressure was later confirmed in an older group of healthy subjects, and supported by evidence from patients with anterior cingulate cortex lesions and patients with pure autonomic failure.[32,33]

This basic approach was extended into fMRI, combined with heart rate variability (HRV) measures of cardiovascular autonomic control during paced exercise and cognitive (working memory) tasks.[33] *HRV reflects the sympatho-vagal balance in the neurogenic heart rate control.* Increases in the low-frequency, presumably sympathetic, component of HRV was associated with increased dorsal anterior cingulate, somatomotor and insular activity. This contrasts with increases in activity relating to predominantly parasympathetic components of HRV putatively mediated by the subgenual cingulate cortex, anterior temporal lobe and basal ganglia[34,35] (see Fig. 8.2c(i)). These findings reinforce earlier observations implicating dorsal and mid anterior cingulate cortex in cardiovascular autonomic arousal, notably sympathetic autonomic drive to the heart during high-demand behaviour.[36]

Other studies combining functional brain imaging with HRV measures highlight parasympathetic cardiac control centres. Two PET studies[34,37] report that the activity of medial prefrontal and insular cortices correlated with parasympathetic HRV measures as participants watched emotional films. Areas including caudate nucleus and insula and periaqueductal grey matter (PAG) were recruited when HRV changes accompanied emotional processing. In a PET study of a much larger group, activity within insula, anterior cingulate and parietal cortices was enhanced during mental challenge (working memory) and correlated with increased heart rate, and activity within regions including ventromedial prefrontal cortex and amygdala correlated with HRV measures of parasympathetic cardiac influences.[38] This same group later demonstrated linear bilateral correlation of activity within perigenual and mid anterior cingulate cortex with stress-induced increases in blood pressure evoked by a Stroop colour–word interference task.[39]

These studies, coupled with observations in patient groups (see below), argue for a contribution of dorsal anterior cingulate cortex to the control of cardiovascular sympathetic responses during behaviour. The engagement of other brain regions including insula, ventromedial prefrontal and subgenual cingulate cortices and amygdala appears more contextual in influencing states of cardiovascular arousal.[5,36] Mediation analyses of neuroimaging data have recently helped unpick some of the causality. During psychological stress, induced through preparation for public speaking, cardiovascular changes were attributable to two discrete loci of cortical activity changes: a pregenual anterior cingulate region where increased activity predicted increased heart rate, and a medial orbitofrontal/ventromedial prefrontal region where decreased activity predicted increases in heart rate; the latter effect was further mediated via PAG[17,18] (see Fig. 8.2(d)).

Although much animal work, and later human studies, suggest a prominent role for amygdala in mediating acute stress reactions and responses to real or perceived threat, amygdala activity is generally a poor predictor of heart rate fluctuation, for example during social stress.[17,18] Amygdala activity correlated negatively with heart rate in a PET study[9] yet, during processing of emotional faces, amygdala activation covaried positively with emotion-induced changes in heart rate[40] and, in other studies, other autonomic responses.[41,42] Most strikingly the magnitude of amygdala activity during anxiety provocation has been linked to direct autonomic modulation of the myocardium[43] (see Fig. 8.2b(iii)). Simultaneous functional imaging of the heart and brain is difficult, so the relationship was inferred in separate sessions. The magnitude of cardiac contractility (based on MRI measurements of end-diastolic volumes of the heart) was modulated by inducing states of heightened anxiety with the threat of electric shock. Repeating the anxiety-inducing conditions while performing fMRI of the brain showed that activity changes in the amygdala and in prefrontal and insula cortices correlated closely with these cardiac changes. This study paves the way for future use of combined brain and cardiac MR techniques within the same experiment. In sum, there is strong evidence in particular contexts for a contribution of activity in the amygdala to adaptive and maladaptive cardiovascular neural responses to stress. However, its role is by no means consistent, suggesting a task dependence not observed as much in regions such as dorsal anterior cingulate or insula cortices.

Changes in the control of blood pressure occur in response to both acute and chronic stress. Mechanistically, baroreceptor reflexes emanating from the high and low pressure sides of the cardiovascular system provide continuous control of arterial pressure in response to changes in arterial pressure and orthostatic volume shifts, respectively. The brainstem sites responsible for this mechanism are well characterized in animals and involve baroreceptor afferents to the nucleus of the solitary tract (NTS) that modulate efferent autonomic pressor tone generated and maintained within rostral ventrolateral medulla. Neuroimaging correlates of central responses to blood pressure manipulations have been examined in both animal and humans. In anaesthetized cats, decreases in arterial pressure (induced by sodium nitroprusside) evoke decreases in fMRI signal within the medullary/NTS pathway and also cerebellum, pons and right insula.[44] The same regions respond to increases in arterial pressure induced by phenylephrine. Interestingly, amygdala activity is enhanced by decreases, not increases, in blood pressure. In humans, low pressure (volume) baroreceptor reflex activity can be induced experimentally using lower body negative pressure, which causes increases in heart rate and muscle sympathetic nerve activity to maintain blood pressure. Kimmerly and co-workers[45] used this technique with fMRI. They showed that low pressure baroreflex responses were associated with enhanced activity in the posterior insula and lateral prefrontal cortex. Decreased activity occurred in the genual (not dorsal) anterior cingulate cortex, amygdala and anterior insula, suggesting these latter areas suppress, or are suppressed by, sympathoexcitatory tone at rest.

Natural baroreceptor activation within the cardiac cycle gates the efferent sympathetic nerve traffic to vessels supplying skeletal muscle (Muscle Sympathetic Nerve Activity, MSNA). This (effect) phasic arterial baroreflex activity modulates bodily reactions to painful somatosensory stimulation. The delivery of electrical shocks to skin during cardiac systole inhibits MSNA.[46] In an fMRI study, combining triggered shock delivery at systole and diastole with beat-to-beat blood pressure monitoring, natural baroreceptor activation at systole inhibited blood pressure reactions to pain delivery; the effect was associated with differences in evoked activity within the right insula, amygdala and dorsal pons/PAG.[29] Individual differences in resting and evoked parasympathetic activity further predict the magnitude of these baroreceptor effects in the brain (see Fig. 8.2c(iii)). This study has direct relevance to the understanding of cardiovascular control, particularly in response to aversive physical stimulation. The findings also have broader relevance; the brain regions implicated are sensitive to cognitive and emotional stress and, baroreceptor gating of pain is proposed as a mechanism through which hypertension may develop through conditioning (associative learning). Attenuation of experiential and physical reactions to pain by baroreceptor activation[47] favours the development of an 'analgesic' hypertensive state, particularly in the context of hypersensitive negative emotional states such as stress.[48]

8.5 Neuroimaging Studies Relating to Cardiovascular Risk

Cardiovascular reactivity (i.e., heart and blood pressure responsiveness to stress) is a constitutional psychophysiological predictor of cardiovascular morbidity and mortality.[49-51] Individual differences in blood pressure reactivity during performance of a demanding cognitive task (a tailored version of the Stroop colour–word challenge) are predicted by differences in magnitude of activation within the posterior cingulate cortex[38,39] (see Fig. 8.3a). Further, the functional connectivity between subgenual cingulate and autonomic nuclei within the pons during stress predicts blood pressure reactivity, as does grey matter volume and amygdala–pons connectivity[10] (see Fig. 8.3b). Cardiovascular risk is also enhanced by psychosocial stressors, including grief, depression and socioeconomic status.[52,53] Low vagal (parasympathetic) tone and exaggerated stress-induced sympathetic (blood pressure

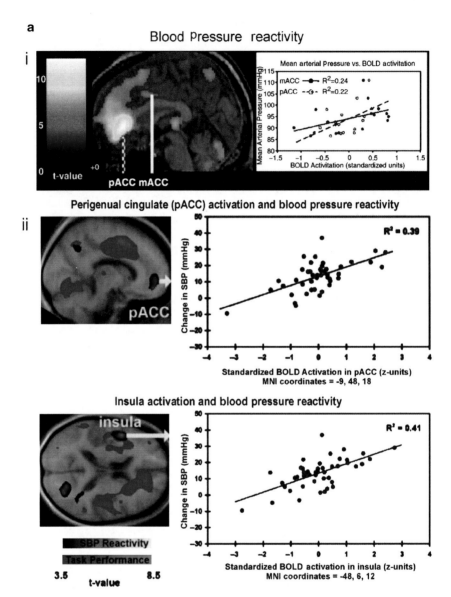

Fig. 8.3 Neuroimaging of cardiovascular risk. (**a**) Increased blood pressure reactivity during acute stress may highlight increased risk of adverse cardiovascular events. (i) Anterior cingulate activity correlated with increased mean arterial pressure.[39] (ii) Cingulate and insula activity correlated with degree of change in systolic blood pressure.[58] (**b**) Increased stress associated blood pressure reactivity is also associated with increased connectivity between pons and (i) genual cingulate and (ii) amygdala.[10] (**c**) Additionally, grey matter volume within the genual cingulate is associated with social predictors of cardiovascular risk such as perceived social standing.[57] The panels *A*, *B* and *C* show left parasagittal, coronal and right parasagittal views (*x* and *y* coordinates in mm relative to anterior commissure) of the regions showing lower volumes across individuals reporting lower social standing, the strength of the regression indicated by the *T* value colour bar (Figures modified from originals and reproduced with permission)

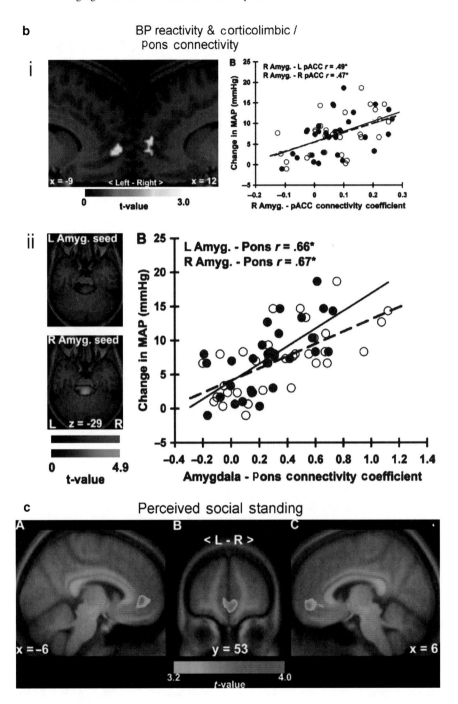

Fig. 8.3 (continued)

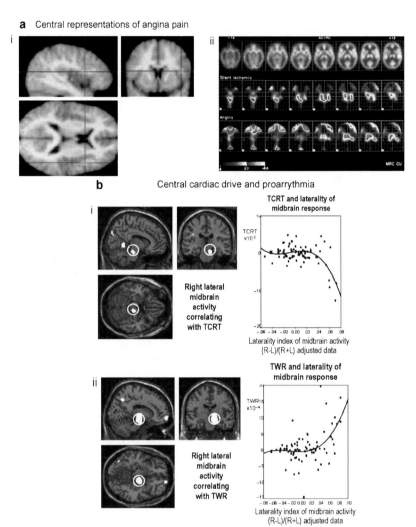

Fig. 8.4 Neural activity associated with acute cardiovascular dysfunction. (**a**) Dobutamine-induced angina associated with increased neural activity within (i) right anterior insula within cardiac syndrome X patients,[62] (ii) changes in regional cerebral blood flow in a group of coronary artery disease patients with no ischaemia (*top*), ischaemic ECG changes (*middle*) and angina accompanying ischaemic ECG changes (*lower line* of brain images).[61] Impaired heart perfusion is accompanied by subcortical activation. Cortical activation accompanies reported angina pain. (**b**) Unsymmetrical activation of brainstem autonomic nuclei during acute stress predicted electrocardiographic measures illustrating proarrythmic risk within cardiac outpatients, indicating (i) decreased global evenness and (ii) increased local variability in ventricular repolarization, indexed by two measures of T-wave morphology: T-wave residual (TWR) and total-cosine R to T (TCRT) increasing TWR and decreasing TCRT suggests a more proarrhythmic state.[69] (**c**) In a similar cardiac outpatient population, heart beat evoked potentials (HBEP on figure) reflected cardiac function during acute stress, specifically reflecting both (i) increased cardiac output (CO) and (ii) inhomogeneity in ventricular repolarization, measured here using the Hill parameter applied to T-wave morphology[70] (Figures modified from originals and reproduced with permission)

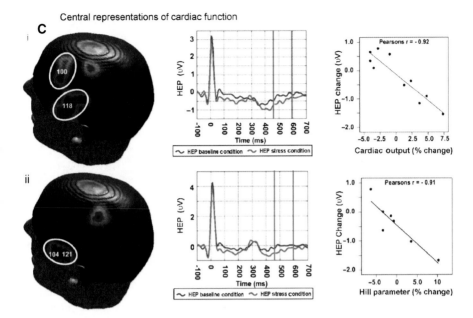

Fig. 8.4 (continued)

and heart rate) responses are potential physiological mediators to link psychosocial factors to cardiac risk[50,52,54] Functional abnormalities within the subgenual cingulate cortex are observed in at-risk people who have recently been bereaved. These abnormalities correspond to withdrawal of the protective parasympathetic vagal influence on the heart.[55] Subgenual cingulate and ventromedial prefrontal dysfunction are commonly reported in depressed patients who also manifest similar predisposing attenuation of parasympathetic tone.[55] Interestingly, the structural morphology of these brain regions in healthy individuals relates to social predictors of cardiac risk, including perceived life stress and social standing[56,57](see Fig. 8.3c).

8.6 Arrythmogenic Mechanisms

Mental and physical stress associated with everyday living can undermine cardiac health[58,59] precipitate sudden cardiac death.[60] Acute stress challenges applied to cardiac patients during neuroimaging have provided insight into mechanisms underlying the acute morbidity and mortality associated with stress in patients with pre-existing cardiac dysfunction. Changes in brain activity patterns during cardiac ischaemia were noted in relatively early neuroimaging studies where subcortical changes accompanied electrocardiographic evidence of cardiac ischaemia and activation extended to cortical areas with perception of angina[61] (see Fig. 8.4a(ii)). Cingulate deactivation and shifts in the symmetry of brain activity have also been observed in patients developing myocardial ischaemia during mental stress challenge.[62] Further studies have highlighted the enhancement of right anterior insula activity during patients' experience of cardiac chest pain in cardiac Syndrome X[63] (see Fig. 8.4a(i)). These findings suggest that cardiac afferent information during ischemia is represented within subcortical and cortical regions, and that disturbances in the central representation of cardiac afferents may underlie silent myocardial ischemia.

Equally, top down regulation of cardiovascular function may also be disturbed during stress. Sudden death is usually due to an abnormal heart rhythm and potential brain mechanisms are suggested from observations in neurological conditions, where epilepsy, subarachnoid haemorrhage and cerebrovascular disease are associated with an enhanced risk of suffering potentially fatal arrhythmia.[31,64-66] ECG changes may also be elicited by stimulation of specific brain regions.[64,65] Patients with pre-existing cardiovascular disease are at a particularly high risk of suffering stress-induced neurogenic arrhythmia, reflecting the reactivity of a compromised myocardium.[52,67]

One suggested mechanism by which mental stress triggers arrhythmia is via the ipsilateral peripheral channelling of lateralized cortical and subcortical activation during the central processing of stress, resulting in lateralized imbalance of autonomic neural drive to the heart.[68] The coordinated propagation of the excitation of cardiac muscle from the ventricular pacemaker is influenced by sympathetic and parasympathetic nerves, predominantly through their effect on the refractory (recovery) period of the cardiac cycle. Electrical recovery is speeded by enhanced sympathetic activity and decreased parasympathetic activity. Different regions of ventricular myocardium are supplied by left and right autonomic nerves, so if the left/right balance of autonomic input is disrupted, this may lead to a proarrhythmic state when some parts of the heart muscle are ready to contract before other parts. The smoothness and coherence in cardiac electrical recovery can be measured from the morphology and distribution of T-waves using 12-lead electrocardiography. Inhomogeneity of T-waves suggests a proarrhythmic state.

Mental stress shifts the electrical activity of the heart toward this proarrhythmic state, even in healthy people[69] perhaps representing a descending overspill from asymmetrical cortical activity during emotional processing.[68] An afferent–efferent loop in cardiac autonomic control exists such that, in health, feedback from the heart regulates the efferent autonomic drive. In patients with ischaemic heart disease, the situation may be further exacerbated by abnormal feedback from the heart. In a PET study, changes in regional brain activity induced by mental and physical stress (mental and exercise pressor tasks) were correlated to proarrhythmic changes in cardiac repolarization in patients with heart disease.[70] Specifically, stress tasks enhanced sympathetic drive to the heart and evoked proarrhythmic ECG changes which were correlated with a right-lateralized shift in dorsal pons and midbrain activity (in the region of the parabrachial nucleus). Moreover, the degree of right lateralization predicted the extent to which proarrhythmic changes occurred, and which patients were at greatest risk (Fig. 8.4a). These findings were consistent with lateralization of efferent autonomic drive at the level of a brainstem relay to the heart, endorsing the model of acute cardiac pathology from lateralised overspill of stress-related cortical activity.

In addition, pre-existing cardiac disease may be an amplifying factor whereby afferent feedback of abnormal cardiac responses during stress contributes to disordered central regulation of cardiovascular function. An electroencephalographic study tested this notion by first identifying a signature of afferent cardiac activity (a heart beat evoked potential) that reflected the integrity of effective cardiac function during mental arithmetic in cardiac patients who varied in the degree to which they could mount an effective cardiac output response to the stress challenge. Significant overlap was observed in the spatial distribution and related features of this potential and the ECG-derived proarrhythmic changes induced by stress.[71] The observation that a central representation of the stress-induced cardiac response predicts a proarrhythmic state highlights the dynamic relationship between peripheral and central factors in mechanisms underpinning the risk for stress-induced cardiac sudden death (Fig. 8.4b).

8.7   Humoral Axes of Stress

The focus of this chapter is the effect of experimental stress on neurally mediated cardiovascular reactions. Nevertheless there is a wealth of clinical and basic scientific data regarding the hypothalamic-pituitary-adrenal (HPA) axis and the role of humoral factors, notably cortisol, in responses to stress.[11,16,72-75] Cortisol is strongly implicated in metabolic risk factors for cardiovascular disease and is an important mediator of negative cardiovascular effects of chronic stress (see Chap. 15). A number of neuroimaging studies have examined neural correlates of cortisol responses to stress. For example, during an emotion induction task, intentionally increasing negative affect was associated with increased prefrontal (ventrolateral, dorsolateral and dorsomedial cortex) and amygdala activity.[76] Importantly, when intentionally decreasing negative affect, participants with greater prefrontal (dorsolateral and dorsomedial cortex) and lower amygdala activity also exhibited a steeper natural decline in cortisol levels over the day. Studies using a mental stress challenge in the context of negative social evaluation (Montreal Imaging Stress Task) show decreased activity within the medial temporal lobe, especially the hippocampus, in response to stress.[77] The degree of deactivation correlated with the cortisol response to stress. Similarly, cortisol elevations elicited by the Trier Social Stress Task correlated with increased dorsal anterior cingulate and dorsal medial prefrontal activation during a social rejection task performed during fMRI scanning.[11] Further, during acute psychosocial stress, prefrontal cortical activities in Brodmann areas 9 and 10 were negatively associated with stress-induced increases in salivary cortisol, and with activity within the amygdala–hippocampal complex, regions known to be involved in HPA axis regulation.[78] Injections of cortisol impact on emotional memory, again through effects mediated at the level of the hippocampus.[79,80] In healthy individuals, inverse correlations are observed between hippocampal volume and cortisol responses to a neuroimaging stress task,[81] an effect replicated in a prospective study of chronic life stress.[58] Neuroimaging techniques are increasingly contributing to elucidating neural systems associated with stress and their association with markers of HPA axis function such as cortisol. It is increasingly recognised that neural activity associated with humoral stress responses is also tied to cardiovascular responses during stress.

8.8   Conclusions

The neuroimaging studies highlighted here focus on brain correlates of acute stress challenge and central aspects of cardiovascular control. They lie within a wider body of relevant work on stress and its addressing broader pathoaetiological role in the development and maintenance of chronic cardiovascular health problems. The basic premise is that specific autonomic changes (sympathetic hyper-responsivity, reduced vagal tone and exaggerated parasympathetic withdrawal) bridge central neural to peripheral cardiovascular reactions to stress. One experimental problem is that dissection of discrete psychological processes using functional neuroimaging typically relies on subtleties in experimental design and analysis, while psychological stress and its physiological consequences are arguably most effectively engendered by challenges that combine multiple high-demand psychological and emotional processes beyond the threshold of optimal performance sustainability. The precision attained by imaging experiments neatly dissecting aspects of decision, control and monitoring is arguably compromised in studies of stress by multiple interacting psychological, affective, physiological arousal processes. Nevertheless, simultaneous measurements of physiological and neuroimaging parameters enable a direct perspective on the psychophysiological effects of stress. Even greater progress is anticipated from longitudinal studies of individual differences in stress responses or cardiovascular pathology related to genetic,[82] experimental,[10,71] metabolic[83] and temperamental[84] vulnerabilities/resilience to stress. Within neuroimaging, there is ongoing exploration and development of new applications, beyond studies of disease and treatment effects. For example, fMRI may be used in neurofeedback experiments to facilitate the establishment of new response patterns to challenges such as pain.[85] Together, functional and structural neuroimaging is contributing to the understanding of stress mechanisms and how they impact on cardiovascular health. Clinically, neuroimaging may find future applications within health screening and individualised medicine.

References

1. Lane RD, Wager TD. The new field of Brain-Body Medicine: what have we learned and where are we headed? *Neuroimage*. 2009;47:1135-1140.
2. Lane RD, Waldstein SR, Critchley HD, et al. The rebirth of neuroscience in psychosomatic medicine, part II: clinical applications and implications for research. *Psychosom Med*. 2009;71: 135-151.
3. Maguire EA, Spiers HJ, Good CD, Hartley T, Frackowiak RS, Burgess N. Navigation expertise and the human hippocampus: a structural brain imaging analysis. *Hippocampus*. 2003; 13:250-259.
4. Modinos G, Mechelli A, Ormel J, Groenewold NA, Aleman A, McGuire PK. Schizotypy and brain structure: a voxel-based morphometry study. *Psychol Med*. 2009;17:1-9.
5. Critchley HD. Psychophysiology of neural, cognitive and affective integration: fMRI and autonomic indicants. *Int J Psychophysiol*. 2009;73:88-94.

6. Rauch SL, Jenike MA, Alpert NM, et al. Regional cerebral blood flow measured during symptom provocation in obsessive-compulsive disorder using oxygen 15-labeled carbon dioxide and positron emission tomography. *Arch Gen Psychiatry*. 1994;51:62-70.

7. Rotge JY, Guehl D, Dilharreguy B, et al. Provocation of obsessive-compulsive symptoms: a quantitative voxel-based meta-analysis of functional neuroimaging studies. *J Psychiatry Neurosci*. 2008;33:405-412.

8. Pannu Hayes J, Labar KS, Petty CM, McCarthy G, Morey RA. Alterations in the neural circuitry for emotion and attention associated with posttraumatic stress symptomatology. *Psychiatry Res*. 2009;172:7-15.

9. Critchley HD, Corfield DR, Chandler MP, Mathias CJ, Dolan RJ. Cerebral correlates of autonomic cardiovascular arousal: a functional neuroimaging investigation. *J Physiol*. 2000; 523:259-270.

10. Gianaros PJ, Sheu LK, Matthews KA, Jennings JR, Manuck SB, Hariri AR. Individual differences in stressor-evoked blood pressure reactivity vary with activation, volume, and functional connectivity of the amygdala. *J Neurosci*. 2008;28:990-999.

11. Eisenberger NI, Gable SL, Lieberman MD. Functional magnetic resonance imaging responses relate to differences in real-world social experience. *Emotion*. 2007;7:745-754.

12. Tracey I, Becerra L, Chang I, et al. Noxious hot and cold stimulation produce common patterns of brain activation in humans: a functional magnetic resonance imaging study. *Neurosci Lett*. 2000;288:159-162.

13. Singer T, Seymour B, O'Doherty J, Kaube H, Dolan RJ, Frith CD. Empathy for pain involves the affective but not sensory components of pain. *Science*. 2004;303:1157-1162.

14. Kalisch R, Wiech K, Critchley HD, et al. Anxiety reduction through detachment: subjective, physiological, and neural effects. *J Cogn Neurosci*. 2005;17:874-883.

15. Gray M, Kemp AH, Silberstein RB, Nathan PJ. Cortical neurophysiology of anticipatory anxiety: an investigation utilizing steady state probe topography (SSPT). *Neuroimage*. 2003;20: 975-986.

16. Dedovic K, Rexroth M, Wolff E, et al. Neural correlates of processing stressful information: an event-related fMRI study. *Brain Res*. 2009;1293:49-60.

17. Wager TD, Waugh CE, Lindquist M, Noll DC, Fredrickson BL, Taylor SF. Brain mediators of cardiovascular responses to social threat: part I: reciprocal dorsal and ventral sub-regions of the medial prefrontal cortex and heart-rate reactivity. *Neuroimage*. 2009;47:821-835.

18. Wager TD, van Ast VA, Hughes BL, Davidson ML, Lindquist MA, Ochsner KN. Brain mediators of cardiovascular responses to social threat, part II: prefrontal-subcortical pathways and relationship with anxiety. *Neuroimage*. 2009;47:836-851.

19. Frankenstein UN, Richter W, McIntyre MC, Rémy F. Distraction modulates anterior cingulate gyrus activations during the cold pressor test. *Neuroimage*. 2001;14:827-836.

20. Harper RM, Gozal D, Bandler R, Spriggs D, Lee J, Alger J. Regional brain activation in humans during respiratory and blood pressure challenges. *Clin Exp Pharmacol Physiol*. 1998;25:483-486.

21. Evans KC, Banzett RB, Adams L, McKay L, Frackowiak RS, Corfield DR. BOLD fMRI identifies limbic, paralimbic, and cerebellar activation during air hunger. *J Neurophysiol*. 2002; 88:1500-1511.

22. Harrison NA, Brydon L, Walker C, et al. Neural origins of human sickness in interoceptive responses to inflammation. *Biol Psychiatry*. 2009;66:415-422.

23. Gray MA, Minati L, Harrison NA, Gianaros PJ, Napadow V, Critchley HD. Physiological recordings: basic concepts and implementation during functional magnetic resonance imaging. *Neuroimage*. 2009;47:1105-1115.

24. King AB, Menon RS, Hachinski V, Cechetto DF. Human forebrain activation by visceral stimuli. *J Comp Neurol*. 1999;413:572-582.

25. Harper RM, Bandler R, Spriggs D, Alger JR. Lateralized and widespread brain activation during transient blood pressure elevation revealed by magnetic resonance imaging. *J Comp Neurol*. 2000;417:195-204.

26. Topolovec JC, Gati JS, Menon RS, Shoemaker JK, Cechetto DF. Human cardiovascular and gustatory brainstem sites observed by functional magnetic resonance imaging. *J Comp Neurol.* 2004;471:446-461.

27. Corfield DR, Murphy K, Josephs O, et al. Cortical and subcortical control of tongue movement in humans: a functional neuroimaging study using fMRI. *J Appl Physiol.* 1999;86: 1468-1477.

28. McAllen RM, Farrell M, Johnson JM, et al. Human medullary responses to cooling and rewarming the skin: a functional MRI study. *Proc Natl Acad Sci USA.* 2006;103:809-813.

29. Gray MA, Rylander K, Harrison NA, Wallin BG, Critchley HD. Following one's heart: cardiac rhythms gate central initiation of sympathetic reflexes. *J Neurosci.* 2009;29:1817-1825.

30. Macefield VG, Henderson LA. Real-time imaging of the medullary circuitry involved in the generation of spontaneous muscle sympathetic nerve activity in awake subjects. *Hum Brain Mapp.* 2010;31:539-549.

31. Oppenheimer SM, Gelb A, Girvin JP, Hachinski VC. Cardiovascular effects of human insular cortex stimulation. *Neurology.* 1992;42:1727-1732.

32. Critchley HD, Mathias CJ, Dolan RJ. Neural correlates of first and second-order representation of bodily states. *Nat Neurosci.* 2001;4:207-212.

33. Critchley HD, Josephs O, O'Doherty J, et al. Human cingulate cortex and autonomic cardiovascular control: converging neuroimaging and clinical evidence. *Brain.* 2003;216:2139-2156.

34. Lane RD, Reiman EM, Ahern GL, Thayer JF. Activity in the medial prefrontal cortex correlates with vagal component of heart rate variability. *Brain Cogn.* 2001;47:97-100.

35. Matthews SC, Paulus MP, Simmons AN, Nelesen RA, Dimsdale JE. Functional subdivisions within anterior cingulate cortex and their relationship to autonomic nervous system function. *Neuroimage.* 2004;22:1151-1156.

36. Critchley HD. Neural mechanisms of autonomic, affective, and cognitive integration. *J Comp Neurol.* 2005;493:154-166.

37. Lane RD, McRae K, Reiman EM, Chen K, Ahern GL, Thayer JF. Neural correlates of heart rate variability during emotion. *Neuroimage.* 2009;44:213-222.

38. Gianaros PJ, Van Der Veen FM, Jennings JR. Regional cerebral blood flow correlates with heart period and high-frequency heart period variability during working-memory tasks: implications for the cortical and subcortical regulation of cardiac autonomic activity. *Psychophysiology.* 2004;41:521-530.

39. Gianaros PJ, Derbyshire SW, May JC, Siegle GJ, Gamalo MA, Jennings JR. Anterior cingulate activity correlates with blood pressure during stress. *Psychophysiology.* 2005;42:627-635.

40. Critchley HD, Rotshtein P, Nagai Y, O'Doherty J, Mathias CJ, Dolan RJ. Activity in the human brain predicting differential heart rate responses to emotional facial expressions. *Neuroimage.* 2005;24:751-762.

41. Williams LM, Phillips ML, Brammer MJ, et al. Arousal dissociates amygdala and hippocampal fear responses: evidence from simultaneous fMRI and skin conductance recording. *Neuroimage.* 2001;14:1070-1079.

42. Phelps EA, O'Connor KJ, Gatenby JC, Gore JC, Grillon C, Davis M. Activation of the left amygdala to a cognitive representation of fear. *Nat Neurosci.* 2001;4:437-441.

43. Dalton KM, Kalin NH, Grist TM, Davidson RJ. Neural-cardiac coupling in threat-evoked anxiety. *J Cogn Neurosci.* 2005;17:969-980.

44. Henderson LA, Richard CA, Macey PM, et al. Functional magnetic resonance signal changes in neural structures to baroreceptor reflex activation. *J Appl Physiol.* 2004;96:693-703.

45. Kimmerly DS, O'Leary DD, Menon RS, Gati JS, Shoemaker JK. Cortical regions associated with autonomic cardiovascular regulation during lower body negative pressure in humans. *J Physiol.* 2005;569:331-345.

46. Donadio V, Kallio M, Karlsson T, Nordin M, Wallin BG. Inhibition of human muscle sympathetic activity by sensory stimulation. *J Physiol.* 2002;544:285-292.

47. Dworkin BR, Elbert T, Rau H, et al. Central effects of baroreceptor activation in humans: attenuation of skeletal reflexes and pain perception. *Proc Natl Acad Sci USA.* 1994;91:6329-6333.

48. Rau H, Elbert T. Psychophysiology of arterial baroreceptors and the etiology of hypertension. *Biol Psychol.* 2001;57:179-201.
49. Treiber FA, Kamarck T, Schneiderman N, Sheffield D, Kapuku G, Taylor T. Cardiovascular reactivity and development of preclinical and clinical disease states. *Psychosom Med.* 2003;65: 46-62.
50. Jennings JR, Kamarck TW, Everson-Rose SA, Kaplan GA, Manuck S, Salonen JT. Exaggerated blood pressure responses during mental stress are prospectively related to enhanced carotid atherosclerosis in middle-aged Finnish men. *Circulation.* 2004;110:2198-2203.
51. Matthews KA, Zhu S, Tucker DC, Whooley MA. Blood pressure reactivity to psychological stress and coronary calcification in the coronary artery risk development in young adults study. *Hypertension.* 2006;47:391-395.
52. Lown B. Sudden cardiac death: biobehavioral perspective. *Circulation.* 1987;76:186-196.
53. Strike PC, Steptoe A. Psychosocial factors in the development of coronary artery disease. *Prog Cardiovasc Dis.* 2004;4:337-347.
54. Carroll D, Smith GD, Shipley MJ, Steptoe A, Brunner EJ, Marmot MG. Blood pressure reactions to acute psychological stress and future blood pressure status: a 10-year follow-up of men in the Whitehall II study. *Psychosom Med.* 2001;63:737-743.
55. O'Connor MF, Gündel H, McRae K, Lane RD. Baseline vagal tone predicts BOLD response during elicitation of grief. *Neuropsychopharmacology.* 2007;32:2184-2189.
56. Gianaros PJ, Jennings JR, Sheu LK, Greer PJ, Kuller LH, Matthews KA. Prospective reports of chronic life stress predict decreased grey matter volume in the hippocampus. *Neuroimage.* 2007;35:795-803.
57. Gianaros PJ, Horenstein JA, Cohen S, et al. Perigenual anterior cingulate morphology covaries with perceived social standing. *Soc Cogn Affect Neursci.* 2007;2:161-173.
58. Gianaros PJ, Jennings JR, Sheu LK, Derbyshire SW, Matthews KA. Heightened functional neural activation to psychological stress covaries with exaggerated blood pressure reactivity. *Hypertension.* 2007;49:134-140.
59. Steptoe A, Feldman PJ, Kunz S, Owen N, Willemsen G, Marmot M. Stress responsivity and socioeconomic status: a mechanism for increased cardiovascular disease risk? *Eur Heart J.* 2002;23:1757-1763.
60. Fries R, Konig J, Schafers HJ, Bohm M. Triggering effect of physical and mental stress on spontaneous ventricular tachyarrhythmias in patients with implantable cardioverter-defibrillators. *Clin Cardiol.* 2002;25:474-478.
61. Rosen SD, Paulesu E, Nihoyannopoulos P, et al. Silent ischemia as a central problem: regional brain activation compared in silent and painful myocardial ischemia. *Ann Intern Med.* 1996; 124:939-949.
62. Soufer R, Bremner JD, Arrighi JA, et al. Cerebral cortical hyperactivation in response to mental stress in patients with coronary artery disease. *Proc Natl Acad Sci USA.* 1998;95:6454-6459.
63. Rosen SD, Paulesu E, Wise RJ, Camici PG. Central neural contribution to the perception of chest pain in cardiac syndrome X. *Heart.* 2002;87:513-519.
64. Oppenheimer SM, Cechetto DF, Hachinski VC. Cerebrogenic cardiac arrhythmias. Cerebral electrocardiographic influences and their role in sudden death. *Arch Neurol.* 1990;47: 513-519.
65. Oppenheimer SM. Neurogenic cardiac effects of cerebrovascular disease. *Curr Opin Neurol.* 1994;7:20-24.
66. Nei M, Ho RT, Abou-Khalil BW, et al. EEG and ECG in sudden unexplained death in epilepsy. *Epilepsia.* 2004;45:338-345.
67. Lampert R, Jain D, Burg MM, Batsford WP, McPherson CA. Destabilising effect of mental stress on ventricular arrhythmias in patients with implantable cardioverter-defibrillators. *Circulation.* 2000;101:158-164.
68. Lane RD, Jennings JR. Hemispheric asymmetry autonomic asymmetry and the problem of sudden cardiac death. In: Davidson RJ, Hugdahl K, eds. *Brain Asymmetry.* Cambridge: The MIT Press; 1995:271-304.

69. Taggart P, Sutton P, Redfern C, et al. The effect of mental stress on the non-dipolar components of the T wave: modulation by hypnosis. *Psychosom Med*. 2005;67:376-383.
70. Critchley HD, Taggart P, Sutton PM, et al. Mental stress and sudden cardiac death: asymmetric midbrain activity as a linking mechanism. *Brain*. 2005;128:75-85.
71. Gray MA, Taggart P, Sutton PM, et al. A cortical potential reflecting cardiac function. *Proc Natl Acad Sci USA*. 2007;104:6818-6823.
72. Dedovic K, Renwick R, Mahani NK, Engert V, Lupien SJ, Pruessner JC. The Montreal Imaging Stress Task: using functional imaging to investigate the effects of perceiving and processing psychosocial stress in the human brain. *J Psychiatry Neurosci*. 2005;30:319-325.
73. Pruessner M, Pruessner JC, Hellhammer DH, Bruce Pike G, Lupien SJ. The associations among hippocampal volume, cortisol reactivity, and memory performance in healthy young men. *Psychiatry Res*. 2007;155:1-10.
74. Taylor SE, Burklund LJ, Eisenberger NI, Lehman BJ, Hilmert CJ, Lieberman MD. Neural bases of moderation of cortisol stress responses by psychosocial resources. *J Pers Soc Psychol*. 2008;95:197-211.
75. Wang J, Rao H, Wetmore GS, et al. Perfusion functional MRI reveals cerebral blood flow pattern under psychological stress. *Proc Natl Acad Sci USA*. 2005;102:17804-17809.
76. Urry HL, van Reekum CM, Johnstone T, et al. Amygdala and ventromedial prefrontal cortex are inversely coupled during regulation of negative affect and predict the diurnal pattern of cortisol secretion among older adults. *J Neurosci*. 2006;26:4415-4425.
77. Pruessner JC, Dedovic K, Khalili-Mahani N, et al. Deactivation of the limbic system during acute psychosocial stress: evidence from positron emission tomography and functional magnetic resonance imaging studies. *Biol Psychiatry*. 2008;63:234-240.
78. Kern S, Oakes TR, Stone CK, McAuliff EM, Kirschbaum C, Davidson RJ. Glucose metabolic changes in the prefrontal cortex are associated with HPA axis response to a psychosocial stressor. *Psychoneuroendocrinology*. 2008;33:517-529.
79. King AP, Liberzon I. Assessing the neuroendocrine stress response in the functional neuroimaging context. *Neuroimage*. 2009;47:1116-1124.
80. Lovallo WR, Robinson JL, Glahn DC, Fox PT. Acute effects of hydrocortisone on the human brain: an fMRI study. *Psychoneuroendocrinology*. 2010;351:15-20.
81. Pruessner JC, Baldwin MW, Dedovic K, et al. Self-esteem, locus of control, hippocampal volume, and cortisol regulation in young and old adulthood. *Neuroimage*. 2005;28:815-826.
82. Zhou Z, Zhu G, Hariri AR, et al. Genetic variation in human NPY expression affects stress response and emotion. *Nature*. 2008;452:997-1001.
83. Soreca I, Rosano C, Jennings JR, et al. Gain in adiposity across 15 years is associated with reduced gray matter volume in healthy women. *Psychosom Med*. 2009;71:485-490.
84. Ganzel BL, Kim P, Glover GH, Temple E. Temperamental after 9/11: multimodal neuroimaging evidence for stress-related change in the healthy adult brain. *Neuroimage*. 2008;40:788-795.
85. deCharms RC. Reading and controlling human brain activation using real-time functional magnetic resonance imaging. *Trends Cogn Sci*. 2007;11:473-481.

Part II
Acute Stress and Triggering

Chapter 9
Psychological Triggers for Plaque Rupture

Geoffrey H. Tofler, Alexandra O'Farrell, and Thomas Buckley

Keywords Psychological triggers • Plaque rupture • Acute cardiovascular disease • Triggers and mechanisms of myocardial infarction (TRIMM) • Anger • Anxiety • Acute depression • Bereavement • Population stress

9.1 Introduction

Emotional stress has long been suspected as a trigger for myocardial infarction (MI) and sudden cardiac death. An early description of MI published by Obraztsov and Strazhesko in 1910 noted that 'Direct events often precipitated the disease; the infarct began in one case on climbing a high staircase, in another during an unpleasant conversation, and in a third during emotional stress associated with a heated card game'.[1] However, this link has been regarded with some suspicion, and only with recent advances in understanding of the mechanisms of onset and treatment of acute cardiovascular disease has it become accepted that psychological factors, both acute and chronic, play a significant role in onset of MI, sudden cardiac death and stroke. This chapter will focus on the role of acute psychological stress in the onset of cardiovascular disease.

G.H. Tofler (✉)
Department of Preventative Cardiology, University of Sydney, Sydney, NSW, Australia

Department of Cardiology, Royal North Shore Hospital, Sydney, NSW, Australia
e-mail: gtofler@nsccahs.health.nsw.gov.au

A. O'Farrell
Department of Cardiology, Royal North Shore Hospital, Sydney, NSW, Australia

T. Buckley
Department of Cardiology, Royal North Shore Hospital, Sydney, NSW, Australia

Sydney Nursing School, University of Sydney, Sydney, NSW, Australia

P. Hjemdahl et al. (eds.), *Stress and Cardiovascular Disease*,
DOI 10.1007/978-1-84882-419-5_9, © Springer-Verlag London Limited 2012

9.2 Evidence for Psychological Triggers of Acute Cardiovascular Disease

Evidence for psychological triggers is based on the following points. First, MI usually results from plaque rupture or erosion and thrombosis.[2] Second, thrombotic occlusion frequently occurs at coronary artery sites that did not have severe stenosis prior to the acute plaque rupture.[3] Third, a morning peak in frequency of MI, sudden cardiac death and stroke[4-8] coincides with heightened blood pressure, heart rate, vasoconstriction and prothrombotic changes.[9] Fourth, emotional stressors cause similar acute physiological changes to those seen in the morning period, and can transiently increase the risk of plaque rupture and thrombosis, and decrease the threshold for ventricular fibrillation.[10] Fifth, epidemiological studies, stimulated by the development of the case-crossover study design, have confirmed and characterised several acute triggers of MI and sudden cardiac death, including individual and population exposure to psychological stress.[11-20] Finally, cardio-protective agents, such as aspirin and beta-blockers, modify the physiological responses to acute stressors and have been shown to reduce the likelihood of morning and trigger-induced MI.[21-24]

9.3 Terminology

For discussion, it is useful to consider the following terms: *Trigger*: An activity that produces acute physiologic changes that may lead directly to onset of acute cardiovascular disease.[25] *Acute risk factor*: A transient physiologic change, such as a surge in arterial pressure or heart rate, an increase in coagulability, or vasoconstriction, follows a trigger and may result in disease onset. *Hazard period*: The time interval after trigger initiation associated with an increased risk of disease onset due to the trigger. The onset and offset times of the hazard period, which could also be designated a 'vulnerable period' may be sharply defined, as in heavy exertion, or less well defined as with respiratory infection. The duration of the hazard period may also vary, from less than 1 h during heavy physical exertion, to weeks to months with bereavement. *Triggered acute risk prevention*: Cardiovascular risk reduction that focuses on the transient increase in risk associated with a trigger.[25]

9.4 Triggers That Have Been Identified

In the Multicenter Investigation of Limitation of Infarct Size (MILIS) study, almost half (48%) of the patients reported a possible trigger, of whom 13% reported a combination of two or more possible triggers[26] (Fig. 9.1). The activities most commonly reported were emotional upset (18%), moderate physical activity (14%), heavy physical activity (9%), and lack of sleep (8%). This analysis and others like it[27,28] are

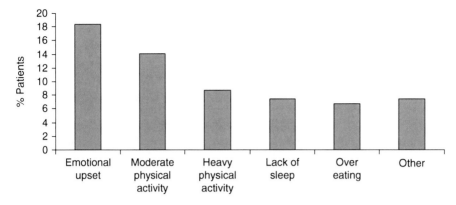

Fig. 9.1 Possible triggers of acute myocardial infarction. A possible trigger was reported by 412 of 849 patients (48.5%) from the Multicenter Investigation of Limitation of Infarct Size (*MILIS*). 109 patients (13%) reported two or more possible triggers (Adapted from Tofler et al.[26])

limited by a lack of control data, since exposure to potential triggers is common, yet MI occurs rarely. Development of the case-crossover study design helped to address this and other limitations in the study of triggering.[11,29]

9.5 Triggers of Acute Cardiovascular Disease

Although the focus of this chapter is psychological triggers, the identification of non-psychological triggers has provided support for the presence of acute psychological triggers, and is worth brief mention. In addition, while much of the recent studies have focused on MI, triggers appear similar for sudden cardiac death and stroke.

Heavy physical exertion (≥6 metabolic equivalents [METS]) was reported by 4.4% of patients in the Determinants of Onset of Myocardial Infarction Study (ONSET),[11] and was associated with a relative risk of 5.9 using a hazard period of 1 h. Triggering of MI by heavy exertion has been observed in other studies, including the Stockholm Heart Epidemiology Program (SHEEP),[19] in which the relative risk for heavy exertion using a 1-h hazard period was 6.1, and the Triggers and Mechanisms of Myocardial Infarction (TRIMM) study,[14] in which the relative risk was 2.1. In ONSET, sedentary individuals had a 107-fold relative risk for heavy exertion triggering MI, whereas the risk was only doubled among individuals active at least five times per week. The modifying effect of regular exertion on triggered risk reinforces the benefit of regular physical activity in reducing risk. An added perspective to note is that even though the relative risk associated with heavy exertion may be high, for instance, 16.9 (95% confidence interval, CI, of 10.5–25.0) for causing sudden death in a study of US male physicians, the absolute risk during any one individual episode of heavy exertion was very low (1 sudden death per 1.51 million episodes of exertion). The low absolute risk to an individual from any single event points to the need to avoid unnecessarily alarming patients into avoiding activities of daily living. This is equally of practical importance for psychological triggers. Indeed, data on triggering can be used in a reassuring manner with regard to sexual activity as a trigger. In ONSET, 3% reported sexual activity within the 2 h before onset of symptoms, with a relative risk of 2.5 (95% CI 1.7–3.7) for MI. Similar results were found in the SHEEP study. In ONSET, the relative risk for sexual activity triggering MI was similar for individuals with prior MI (2.9) or without known prior coronary disease (2.5). The relative risk was significantly reduced by regular usual physical activity, suggesting that physically active individuals are at minimal incremental absolute risk from sexual activity.

Other triggers: Respiratory infection has been associated with an increased relative risk of suffering MI or stroke, which was highest during the first 3 days (relative risk for MI 4.9 [95% CI 4.4–5.5] and for stroke 3.2 [95% CI 2.8–3.6]). Heavy meals have also been associated with a four-fold increase in relative risk for MI. Cocaine intake was associated with a 23-fold increase in the relative risk of suffering MI over baseline in the 1 h following use,[30] while marijuana intake was associated with a 4-fold increased risk over baseline in the 1 h after use.[31] Air pollution has also been identified as an acute trigger of MI and stroke.[32]

9.6 Individual Psychological Triggers

Anger: In ONSET, 2.4% of patients reported episodes of anger (≥5 on an anger scale) during a 2-h period before MI. This level of anger, which corresponds with 'very angry, body tense, clenching fists or teeth' up to 'furious or enraged' was associated with a transient relative risk increase of 2.3 (95% CI 1.2–32) above baseline when the control was usual annual frequency. When the control period was the same 2-h period the day before MI, the relative risk was 4.0 (95% CI 1.9–9.4). The most frequent reported contributors to anger were arguments with family members (25%), conflicts at work (22%) and legal problems (8%).[12] In the SHEEP study, the relative risk was nine-fold for anger as a trigger.[33] Strike and colleagues found that anger was reported by 17.4% of 295 patients using a 2-h hazard period. Compared to the same time period 1 day before, the odds ratio was 2.06 (95% CI 1.12–3.92) while compared with the previous 6 months, the odds ratio was 7.30 (95% CI 5.22–10.19).[34] Koton et al. showed an odds ratio of 14 (95% CI 3–253) for anger triggering stroke in the subsequent 2 h.[35] In patients with Implantable Cardioverter Defibrillators, episodes of anger increases the likelihood of a ventricular arrhythmia requiring shock (odds ratio 1.8, 95% CI 1.04–3.16).[36] In addition, a higher score on the Spielberger Trait Anger questionnaire was a significant predictor of anger-triggered shock.[37] A higher likelihood of anger triggering MI has been associated with socioeconomic deprivation[34] and lower educational attainment.[38] In ONSET, aspirin was associated with a reduced impact of anger as a trigger.[12] The relative risk tended to be lower among men than women, and among regular users of beta-blockers than non-users; however, these differences were not statistically significant.

Anxiety: Acute anxiety episodes are also associated with increased cardiac risk. In ONSET, in the 2 h prior to MI symptom onset, 5% of patients reported anxiety symptoms above the 75th percentile on an anxiety scale. When the hazard period was compared to a control period, 24–26 h earlier, the relative risk was 1.6 (95% confidence interval 1.1–2.2, $p = 0.01$).[12] In addition to the association between anxiety state and cardiac risk, considerable evidence exists that higher symptoms of anxiety are associated with poorer outcome in patients with prior cardiac disease.[39]

Acute depression: Steptoe and colleagues reported that discrete time-limited episodes of depressed mood were present in 18.2% of patients admitted with Acute Coronary Syndrome (ACS).[40] The odds of ACS following depressed mood were 2.5 (95% CI 1.05–6.56) relative to the same 2-h period 24 h earlier. When analysis was restricted to patients who reported moderately to severely depressed mood, the odds ratio was greater 5.08 (95% CI 1.07–47.0). Chronic depression has also been associated with increased MI risk[41,42] (see also Chap. 12 by Hoen et al.). A more complex relationship was noted in the Systolic Hypertension in the Elderly Program (SHEP).[43] In this trial, 4,736 subjects aged 60 years or more with isolated systolic hypertension were followed for an average of 4.5 years, with depressive symptoms being assessed by 6 month questionnaires. Baseline levels of depressive symptoms did not predict future cardiovascular events; however an increasing depression score was associated with higher risk. Another study found that in men, but not women, the recent onset of depression, but not chronic depression, was associated with increased MI risk.[44]

Bereavement: Increased cardiac mortality in bereaved individuals is well described, and has been described as 'the broken heart'.[45-50] In a cohort of middle-aged widowers, a 40% increase in the mortality rate was observed in the first 6 months following bereavement.[47] The risk appears to be maximal in the first weeks.[51] A schema of the pathophysiologic mechanisms by which bereavement and other psychological triggers may lead to MI and sudden cardiac death is described in Fig. 9.2.[51]

Work-related stress: A high pressure work deadline in the prior 24 h was associated with a six-fold increase in the relative risk of suffering MI in the SHEEP study[52] while in ONSET, the relative risk for a high pressure deadline over a 7-day hazard period was 2.3 (1.4–4.0), and 2.2 (1.0–5.0) for firing somebody.[12] The emotional significance of a job stress influenced its contribution to relative risk of MI. Thus, when increased work responsibilities affected men in a very or fairly negative way in the SHEEP study, the relative risk, adjusted for other risk factors, was 6.3 (2.7–14.7) whereas the relative risk was only 1.5 (0.9–2.3) when the increased work responsibilities did not mean very much, and 0.7 (0.5–0.9) when it had a positive effect. Corresponding relative risks among women were 3.8 (1.3–11.0), 0.8 (0.3–2.5), and 1.0 (0.6–1.8).[52] The acute stress link is also complemented by the Whitehall II and INTERHEART studies showing increased MI risk with chronic stress.[42,53]

Fig. 9.2 Potential
mechanism by which
bereavement increases risk of
MI or SCD. Bereavement
may produce responses such
as anxiety, anger, depression
and hopelessness. These
responses may be modified
by factors such as social
support. Contributing
lifestyle changes include
dietary change, smoking and
sleep disturbance. Potentially
adverse physiological
changes include
hemodynamic with a blood
pressure and heart rate surge,
prothrombotic,
vasoconstrictive, autonomic
imbalance, inflammatory,
immune and electrolyte
changes

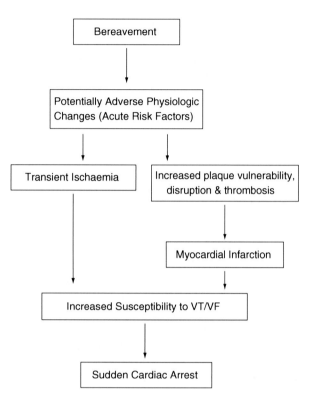

9.7 Population Stressors

Earthquakes[54] and wartime missile attack[55] are associated with acute increases in cardiovascular risk. In the week after the Los Angeles earthquake of 1994, which occurred at 4.31 a.m., there was a 35% increase in nonfatal MI compared to the week before, and a four-fold increase in sudden cardiac death on the day of the earth-quake[54,56] (Fig. 9.3). However, for the 6 days after this spike, the number of sudden deaths was below the baseline suggesting that the sudden deaths may have been moved forward by several days in individuals who were predisposed.[56] The 1989 Loma Prieta, San Francisco Bay earthquake, which occurred at 5.04 p.m., was not associated with increased MI, leading Brown to suggest that the triggering in the 4.31 a.m. Los Angeles earthquake was contributed to by the added stress of abrupt awakening.[57] More recently, Nakagawa and colleagues noted a more long-term effect of the Niigata-Chuetsu earthquake on mortality from MI.[58] During the first week of Iraqi missile attacks on Israel in 1991, Meisel and colleagues found a doubling of nonfatal MI compared to a control period 1 year previously.[55] This was mirrored by a near doubling of sudden out-of-hospital deaths for a 1-month period.[55] Comparing the 60 days before and after September 11, 2001, Allegra et al. found a 49% increase in patients with MI (118 after versus 79 before, $p=0.01$) admitted through 16 Emergency Departments within a 50 mile radius of the World Trade Center.[59]

During the 1999 earthquake in Taiwan, 12 individuals who were undergoing Holter heart rate monitoring showed pronounced increases in heart rate (up to

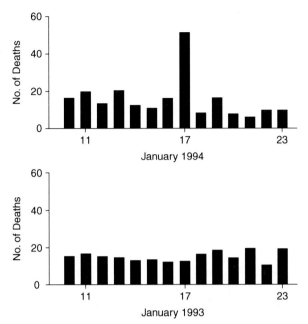

Fig. 9.3 Daily numbers of cardiovascular deaths in Los Angeles County January, 1993 and 1994. On the day of the Northridge earthquake (January 17, 1994), there was a sharp rise in the number of deaths related to atherosclerotic cardiovascular disease (relative risk, 2.6; 95% CI, 1.8–3.7). The daily number of CVD deaths declined in the 6 days after the earthquake ($p = 0.002$) (From Leor et al.[56])

160 beats/min), and an increase in the low-frequency/high-frequency ratio in the minutes after the earthquake compared to the minutes prior.[60] These changes were attenuated in patients who were receiving beta-blockers.

During the first phase of the Gulf war in 1991, in Tel Aviv, during and immediately following the first missile attacks, there was a 58% increase in total mortality from AMI and sudden cardiac death compared to a control period 1 year previously.

Sporting events provide another example of population stress. On the day of the 1996 European football final that Holland narrowly lost to France after penalties, Dutch men had an increased relative risk of MI or stroke of 1.5 (1.1–2.1) whereas there was no increased risk for Dutch women or French men and women.[61,62] A recent study of the World Cup in Germany provided further support to the triggering of events during emotional stress associated with watching sporting events.[63]

Exposure to traffic, related to both pollution and emotional stress, has been associated with an increased relative risk of MI of 2.7 (2.1–3.6).[64] A daily variation in CVD has also been described with a peak incidence on Mondays.[65-68] Holidays such as Christmas and New Years Day have also been associated with increased cardiac mortality, although the findings have not been uniform, and the contribution of psychological versus other behavioural factors is uncertain.[69]

9.8 Pathophysiology

There are several mechanisms by which acute emotional stress might trigger an acute MI (Fig. 9.2). Mental stress produces significant increases in heart rate and blood pressure that may lead to increased myocardial oxygen demand and plaque disruption. In addition to a rise in the rate pressure product, there is also evidence that mental stress may lead to a primary reduction in myocardial oxygen supply in vulnerable individuals. Whereas coronary arteries of normal patients dilate during mental stress, impaired vasodilatation and even constriction has been demonstrated in atherosclerotic arteries.[70] The vasoconstriction induced by stress may not be immediate. In a dog model, profound coronary vasoconstriction could be demonstrated 2–3 min following elicitation of anger.[71] The vasoconstriction persisted well after heart rate and arterial blood pressure had recovered. Myocardial ischemia, as evidenced by ST-segment depression and more sensitive means such as radionuclide ventriculography and positron emission tomography, has been shown to be precipitated by psychologically stressful circumstances (e.g. public speaking).[72] One study, for example, found that among 29 patients with coronary artery disease with exercise induced wall motion abnormalities, 21 (72%) also exhibited wall motion abnormalities following mental stress.[73] The ischemia was usually silent, often without ECG abnormalities.

Although studies have not all shown consistent findings, mental stress has been shown to enhance platelet aggregation, with probable contribution by activation of the sympathetic nervous system, hypothalamic pituitary-adrenal axis and serotonergic pathways.[74-76] There is a compensatory increase in fibrinolytic activity following acute stress, but a diminished fibrinolytic response due to endothelial dysfunction may lead to a prothrombotic imbalance (see also the Chap. 6 on haemostasis by Hjemdahl and von Känel in this book).

The new information on triggering can be incorporated into a hypothesis of the progression of coronary artery disease whereby onset of MI may occur when a vulnerable atherosclerotic plaque disrupts in response to mental stress or anger that produces transient pressure surges and increased shear stress due to increased coronary flow or vasoconstriction.[10] If the plaque disruption is major with extensive exposure of collagen and atheromatous core contents to the lumen, this may lead immediately to occlusive thrombosis, with MI or sudden cardiac death. If the disruption is minor, it may lead to nonocclusive thrombosis which may promote the slow progression of atherosclerosis (see Chap. 6). In this setting, the patient may be asymptomatic or develop unstable angina or non-ST elevation MI. The lesion may gradually heal with smooth muscle cell proliferation and a greater degree of stenosis. Alternatively, a further increase in coagulability or vasoconstriction may precipitate occlusive thrombosis, MI and sudden cardiac death.

9.9   Increased Plaque Vulnerability

An inverse relation probably exists between the degree of plaque vulnerability and the intensity of the trigger required to produce rupture and thrombosis. For instance, an extremely vulnerable plaque or severe stenosis may occlude without a demonstrable trigger whereas someone with less vulnerable lesions or stenosis may

Table 9.1 Potential strategies for triggered acute risk protection

1. Long-term general preventive therapy
2. Long-term trigger-specific preventive therapy
3. Ignore added risk of the trigger since the risk is so low
4. Avoid or modify the trigger
5. Take therapy at the time of trigger

require a major trigger for plaque rupture and thrombosis. While acute treatment would be primarily directed against the effects of the triggering activity, reducing plaque vulnerability would be advantageous when the hazard period of triggers extends over several weeks or months, as seen with bereavement or longer-term work or home stress.[42] Plaque disruption often occurs in more than one coronary artery location in the same individual,[77] which may be due to a general increase in inflammatory activity and correlated with higher CRP levels.[78] These considerations raise the possibility that transient increases in vulnerability of plaques may occur over weeks and months associated with external activities and exposures of the individual.

9.10 Strategy for Triggered Acute Risk Protection

Five broad approaches can be followed to protect against MI triggered by acute emotional stress[25] (Table 9.1). First, one can adopt a long-term behavioural and pharmaceutical approach that emphasises absolute risk reduction. This corresponds to traditional risk factor modification, emphasising optimal blood pressure and lipids, not smoking, being physically active and maintaining optimal weight. By reducing the atherosclerotic burden and the number of vulnerable plaques, such a long-term strategy would reduce the risk that a trigger such as acute emotional stress would produce an acute CVD event. Second, a long-term preventive approach can be directed at a specific trigger. For instance, stress reduction training can be used to limit the responses of anger and anxiety. Third, one could determine that the risk of the trigger is very low and does not require any protection. This approach would be applicable to an individual considered to be at very low risk of having atherosclerotic disease or vulnerable plaques, in whom even a major emotional stress should pose little absolute risk. Nonetheless, even in young individuals without significant atherosclerosis, stressors such as cocaine usage can trigger MI and sudden death[31,79-81] In addition, trigger-related surges in catecholamines may be a mechanism for subclinical plaque disruption and progression of atherosclerosis.[82-84] Fourth, individuals could avoid or modify the specific triggering activity, for instance, avoiding an angry confrontation. Finally, one could potentially take increased protective therapy at the time of or just prior to a recognised trigger, such as severe emotional stress. The evidence for benefit is variable, and highlights areas for future research.

9.11   Potential Triggered Acute Risk Protection Therapy

9.11.1   Beta-Adrenergic Blocking Drugs

Beta-blockers provide the most compelling evidence for protection against the emotional triggers of acute coronary syndromes. Their protective effect against transient ischaemia, MI, and sudden cardiac death is pronounced during the morning peak in frequency of these events, a time associated with daily life challenges.[4,22,24,85-87] Although statistical power is limited for subgroup analyses of triggering studies, trends suggest that beta-blockers reduce the likelihood of MI being triggered by emotional stress.[12,26,88] Beta-blockers reduce peri-operative MI[89] and attenuate morning and stress-related haemodynamic surges.[24] Most transient ischemic episodes are preceded by increases in heart rate and blood pressure[90,91] and propranolol reduced these episodes more than diltiazem or nifedipine.[92] In an analysis of patients who underwent two coronary angiograms within 6 months, higher heart rate was associated with coronary plaque disruption, and beta-blocker use was protective.[84] By reducing flow velocity, turbulence and vortex formation at regions of high circumferential tensile stress,[92] beta-blockers could reduce endothelial damage and plaque rupture. Some studies suggest beneficial effects of beta-blockers on coagulability, although findings have not been consistent.[93-96]

9.11.2   Other Potential Medications

In the Physicians Health study, aspirin preferentially reduced the morning peak of MI that corresponds with a morning peak of platelet reactivity and catecholamine levels.[23] Aspirin inhibits epinephrine-induced platelet aggregation in-vitro, and reduces platelet aggregates in the Folts model of stenosis, although the inhibitory effect was diminished in a high catecholamine state.[97] The links require further investigation.

Heart rate lowering calcium channel agents, such as verapamil and diltiazem, may attenuate stress-related surges in heart rate and reduce platelet reactivity.[98,99]

Statins protect against CVD not only through lipid lowering, but also through reduced inflammation, plaque stabilisation and inhibition of thrombus deposition.[100] While statins are used long-term, evidence suggests an early benefit, both in terms of lipid lowering,[101] and other processes such as ischaemia-reperfusion injury.[102] These rapid effects suggest that statins could play a protective role in triggering situations whose hazard period extends over days and weeks. Emotional stress is associated with higher lipid levels, in part due to hemoconcentration.[103-105]

9.12 Potential Approaches to Protect Against Specific Triggers

9.12.1 Anger or Acute Anxiety

Long-term trigger-specific approach: Recognising potentially inflammatory situations and defusing them before they reach a high level can be helped by stress reduction training and relaxation exercises. At a society level, defibrillators should be made available in sporting arenas, aircraft terminals and other locations where large populations congregate and stress levels may be high.[106]

Avoid or modify: Examples would be avoiding an angry confrontation with a neighbour, writing a letter rather than having a verbal argument, and practising relaxation and breathing exercises when exposed to an acute stressor.

TARP therapy: Beta-blocker and possibly aspirin could be taken at the time of an acute emotional stress, such as prior to watching a grand final sporting game or a stressful meeting. If the individual has the medication in a wallet or handbag, it would be taken immediately following an unexpected stressful event.

9.12.2 Bereavement

Long-term trigger-specific approach: Ensure strong social and community support and possible religious affiliation.

Modify: Provide social support and sensitivity at the time of bereavement.

TARP therapy: Possible use of low-dose beta-blocker and aspirin during early bereavement. Medical review with close attention to risk factors for cardiovascular disease may also be of particular benefit. The role of TARP therapy would be not to interfere with the normal grieving process, but rather to reduce the risk of acute cardiovascular events in the bereaved individuals.

9.12.3 Population Stress (Missile Attack, Earthquake)

Long-term trigger-specific approach: Government and international efforts to prevent reduce risk of war and exposure to civilians or to develop early warning for natural disasters. Ambulances and rescue workers should be trained in cardiac resuscitation and equipped with defibrillators.

Avoid or modify: Leave area of war conflict or provide physical and psychological preparation for individuals.

TARP therapy: Since natural and man-made disasters will continue to occur despite preventive efforts, public health measures and research into how to mitigate the immediate and longer-term consequences of disasters are of increasing importance.[107] Beta-blockade and possibly aspirin may be protective acutely against

CVD while statins and more intensive treatment of other risk factors may be helpful in the subsequent weeks and months.

9.13 Multiple Triggers

One quarter of the individuals reporting a possible trigger in the MILIS study reported two or more possible triggers[26] although in the study by Strike and colleagues, both physical stress and anger were rarely seen as combined triggers.[34] An added cardiovascular risk may be present when multiple potential triggers are concurrent, such as heavy exertion at the time of emotional stress, such as hurrying to catch a plane while stressed and carrying a suitcase.

9.14 Areas for Future Research

The frequency of specific triggers, their relative risks of triggering MI and their attributable risk need to be better evaluated in different populations. There is a need to better characterise the physiological mechanisms by which stressors trigger acute coronary syndromes. It would be useful to investigate the determinants of individual variability to the same stress, including genetic factors. Strike and colleagues compared, at 15 months post-MI, the responses to psychological testing of 14 men who had experienced acute negative emotion in the 2 h before MI with 20 with prior MI not associated with emotional stress. The emotion triggered group had heightened platelet activation and haemodynamic poststress recovery.[108] Psychosocial interventions improve depressive symptoms and reduce social isolation in patients post-MI, but it is not clear whether these benefits translate into improved cardiovascular outcome.[109]

9.15 Absolute Risk

Although the relative risks from triggers may be substantial, the absolute risk from a single triggering event, and likewise the risk reduction from any single episode of therapy, is low. For instance, if the absolute risk of MI in any given hour for an asymptomatic individual aged 50 years was one per million, then an increased relative risk of ten-fold would still lead to a small increase in absolute risk (1 per 100,000).

9.16 Conclusion

An extensive literature supports a role for mental stress as a trigger of MI and for cardiac events after an MI. Since stressors provoking anger are frequently unavoidable, benefit may be gained through efforts to interrupt the link between the stressor and the cardiovascular event by nonpharmacologic and pharmacologic means. Psychosocial treatment or behaviour therapy may prove useful in reducing the adverse consequences of mental stress in triggering cardiovascular events. From a public health perspective, recognition of the increased cardiovascular risk among populations exposed to natural disasters, such as earthquakes and other conditions of extreme stress, may be relevant for preparedness of emergency services as they respond to such disasters. Although the proportion of individuals with plaques that are vulnerable to rupture at any given moment is likely to be very low, the recognition that stressors trigger cardiovascular events also supports the need for availability of cardiac care including defibrillators at large gatherings of individuals who may experience mental stress.

References

1. Obraztsov VP, Strazhesko ND. The symptomatology and diagnosis of coronary thrombosis. In: Vorobeva VA, Konchalovski MP, eds. *Works of the First Congress of Russian Therapists.* Moscow: Comradeship Typography of A.E. Mamontov; 1910:26-43.
2. Davies MJ, Thomas AC. Plaque fissuring – the cause of acute myocardial infarction, sudden ischemic death, and crescendo angina. *Br Heart J.* 1985;53:363-373.
3. Ambrose JA, Tannenbaum MA, Alexopoulos D, et al. Angiographic progression of coronary artery disease and the development of myocardial infarction. *J Am Coll Cardiol.* 1988;12:56-62.
4. Muller JE, Stone PH, Turi ZG, et al. Circadian variation in the frequency of onset of acute myocardial infarction. *N Engl J Med.* 1985;313:1315-1322.
5. Willich SN, Levy D, Rocco MB, Tofler GH, Stone PH, Muller JE. Circadian variation in the incidence of sudden cardiac death in the Framingham Heart Study population. *Am J Cardiol.* 1987;60:801-806.
6. Marler JR, Price TR, Clark GL, et al. Morning increase in onset of ischemic stroke. *Stroke.* 1989;20:473-476.
7. Behar S, Halabi M, Reicher-Reiss H, et al. Circadian variation and possible external triggers of onset of myocardial infarction. SPRINT Study Group. *Am J Med.* 1993;94:395-400.
8. Tofler GH, Muller JE, Stone PH, et al. Modifiers of timing and possible triggers of acute myocardial infarction in the Thrombolysis in Myocardial Infarction Phase II (TIMI II) Study Group. *J Am Coll Cardiol.* 1992;20:1049-1055.
9. Muller JE, Tofler GH, Stone PH. Circadian variation and triggers of onset of acute cardiovascular disease. *Circulation.* 1989;79:733-743.
10. Muller JE, Abela GS, Nesto RW, Tofler GH. Triggers, acute risk factors and vulnerable plaques: the lexicon of a new frontier. *J Am Coll Cardiol.* 1994;23:809-813.
11. Mittleman MA, Maclure M, Tofler GH, et al. Triggering of acute myocardial infarction by heavy physical exertion. Protection against triggering by regular exertion. *N Engl J Med.* 1993; 329:1677-1683.
12. Mittleman MA, Maclure M, Sherwood JB, et al. Triggering of acute myocardial infarction onset by episodes of anger. *Circulation.* 1995;92:1720-1725.
13. Giri S, Thompson PD, Kiernan FJ, et al. Clinical and angiographic characteristics of exertion-related acute myocardial infarction. *JAMA.* 1999;282:1731-1736.
14. Willich SN, Lewis M, Lowel H, et al. Physical exertion as a trigger of acute myocardial infarction. *N Engl J Med.* 1993;329:1684-1690.
15. Davidson KW. Emotional predictors and behavioral triggers of acute coronary syndrome. *Cleveland Clin J Med.* 2008;75:S15-S19.
16. Kloner RA. Natural and unnatural triggers of myocardial infarction. *Prog Cardiovasc Dis.* 2006;48:285-300.

17. Strike PC, Steptoe A. Behavioural and emotional triggers of acute coronary syndromes: a systematic review and critique. *Psychosom Med.* 2005;67:179-186.

18. Culic V, Etorovic D, Miric D. Meta-analysis of possible external triggers of acute myocardial infarction. *Int J Cardiol.* 2005;9:1-8.

19. Hallqvist J, Moller J, Ahlbom A, Diderichsen F, Reuterwall C, de Faire U. Does heavy physical exertion trigger myocardial infarction? A case-crossover analysis nested in a population-based case-referent study. *Am J Epidemiol.* 2000;151:459-467.

20. Desvarieux M, Demmer RT, Rundek T, et al. Periodontal microbiota and carotid intima-media thickness. The oral infections and vascular disease epidemiology study (INVEST). *Circulation.* 2005;111:576-582.

21. Hennekens CH, Buring JE, Sandercock P. Aspirin and other antiplatelet agents in the secondary and primary prevention of cardiovascular disease. *Circulation.* 1989;80:749-756.

22. Peters RW, Muller JE, Goldstein S, Byington R, Friedman LM. Propranolol and the morning increase in the frequency of sudden cardiac death (BHAT Study). *Am J Cardiol.* 1989;63: 1518-1520.

23. Ridker PM, Manson JE, Buring JE, Muller JE, Hennekens CH. Circadian variation of acute myocardial infarction and the effect of low-dose aspirin in a randomized trial of physicians. *Circulation.* 1990;82:897-902.

24. Parker JD, Testa MA, Jimenez AH, et al. Morning increase in ambulatory ischemia in patients with stable coronary artery disease. Importance of physical activity and increased cardiac demand. *Circulation.* 1994;89:604-614.

25. Tofler GH, Muller JE. Triggering of acute cardiovascular disease and potential preventive strategies. *Circulation.* 2006;114:1863-1872.

26. Tofler GH, Stone PH, Maclure M, et al. Analysis of possible triggers of acute myocardial infarction (The MILIS Study). *Am J Cardiol.* 1990;66:22-27.

27. Sumiyoshi T. Evaluation of clinical factors involved in onset of myocardial infarction. *Jpn Circ J.* 1986;50:164-173.

28. Culic V, Eterovic D, Miric D, Rumboldt HI. Gender differences in triggering of acute myocardial infarction. *Am J Cardiol.* 2000;85:753-756.

29. Maclure M. The case-crossover design: a method for studying transient effects on the risk of acute events. *Am J Epidemiol.* 1991;133:144-153.

30. Mittleman MA, Lewis RA, Maclure M, Sherwood JB, Muller JE. Triggering myocardial infarction by marijuana. *Circulation.* 2001;103:2805-2809.

31. Mittleman MA, Mintzer D, Maclure M, Tofler GH, Sherwood JB, Muller JE. Triggering of myocardial infarction by cocaine. *Circulation.* 1999;99:2737-2741.

32. Tsai S-S, Goggins WB, Chiu H-F, Yang C-Y. Evidence for an association between air pollution and daily stroke admissions in Kaohsiung, Taiwan. *Stroke.* 2003;34:2612-2616.

33. Moller J, Hallqvist J, Diderichsen F, Theorell T, Reuterwall C, Ahlbom A. Do episodes of anger trigger myocardial infarction? A case-crossover analysis in the Stockholm Heart Epidemiology Program (SHEEP). *Psychosom Med.* 1999;61:842-849.

34. Strike PC, Perkins-Porras L, Whitehead DL, McEwan J, Steptoe A. Triggering of acute coronary syndromes by physical exertion and anger: clinical and sociodemographic characteristics. *Heart.* 2006;92:1035-1040.

35. Koton S, Tanne D, Bornstein NM, Green MS. Triggring risk factors for kchaemic stroke. A case-crossover study. *Neurology* 2004;63:2006-2010

36. Lampert R, Joska T, Burg MM, Batsford WP, McPherson CA, Jain D. Emotional and physical precipitants of ventricular arrhythmia. *Circulation.* 2002;106:1800-1805.

37. Burg MM, Lampert R, Joska T, Batsford W, Jain D. Psychological traits and emotion-triggering of ICD shock-terminated arrhythmias. *Psychosom Med.* 2004;66:898-902.

38. Mittleman MA, Maclure M, Nachnani M, Sherwood JB, Muller JE, The Determinants of Myocardial Infarction Onset Study Investigators. Educational attainment, anger, and the risk of triggering myocardial infarction onset. *Arch Intern Med.* 1997;157:769-775.

39. Moser DK, Riegel B, McKinley S, Doering LV, An K, Sheahan S. Impact of anxiety and perceived control on in-hospital complications after acute myocardial infarction. *Psychosom Med.* 2007;69:10-16.
40. Steptoe A, Strike PC, Perkins-Porras L, McEwan JR, Whitehead DL. Acute depressed mood as a trigger of acute coronary syndromes. *Biol Psychiatry.* 2006;60:837-842.
41. Wassertheil-Smoller S, Shumaker S, Ockene JTGA, et al. Depression and cardiovascular sequelae in postmenopausal women. The Women's Health Initiative (WHI). *Arch Intern Med.* 2004;164:289-298.
42. Rosengren A, Hawken S, Ounpuu S, et al. Association of psychosocial risk factors with risk of acute myocardial infarction in 11119 cases and 13648 controls from 52 countries (the INTERHEART study): case-control study. *Lancet.* 2004;364:953-962.
43. Wassertheil-Smoller S, Applegate WB, Berge K, et al. Change in depression as a precursor of cardiovascular events. SHEP Cooperative Research Group (Systolic Hypertension in the Elderly). *Arch Intern Med.* 1996;156:553-561.
44. Penninx BW, Guralnik JM, de Leon CF Mendes, et al. Cardiovascular events and mortality in newly and chronically depressed persons >70 years of age. *Am J Cardiol.* 1998;81:988-994.
45. Jacobs S. An epidemiological review of the mortality of bereavement. *Psychosom Med.* 1977; 39:344-357.
46. Stroebe MS. The broken heart phenomenon: an examination of the mortality of bereavement. *J Commun Appl Soc Psychol.* 1994;4:47-61.
47. Young M, Benjamin B, Wallis C. The mortality of widowers. *Lancet.* 1963;2:454-456.
48. O'Connor M, Allen J, Kasniak A. Autonomic and emotion regulation in bereavement and depression. *J Psychosom Res.* 2002;52:183-185.
49. Tennant C. Life stress, social support and coronary heart disease. *Aust NZ J Psychiatry.* 1999; 33:636-641.
50. Rees WD, Lutkins SG. Mortality of bereavement. *Br Med J.* 1967;4:13-16.
51. Buckley T, McKinley S, Tofler GH, Bartrop RP. Cardiovascular risk in early bereavement: a literature review and proposed mechanisms. *Int J Nurs Stud.* 2009;47(2):229-238. Epub 2009 Aug 8. PMID 19665709.
52. Moller I, Theorell T, de Faire U, Ahlbom A, Hallqvist J. Work related stressful life events and the risk of myocardial infarction. Case-control and case-crossover analyses within the Stockholm heart epidemiology programme (SHEEP). *J Epidemiol Community Health.* 2005; 59:23-30.
53. Chandola T, Britton A, Brunner E, et al. Work stress and coronary heart disease: what are the mechanisms? *Eur Heart J.* 2008;29:640-648.
54. Leor J, Kloner RA. The Northridge earthquake as a trigger for acute myocardial infarction. *Am J Cardiol.* 1996;77:1230-1232.
55. Meisel SR, Kutz I, Dayan KI, et al. Effect of Iraqi missile war on incidence of acute myocardial infarction and sudden death in Israeli civilians. *Lancet.* 1991;338:660-661.
56. Leor J, Poole WK, Kloner RA. Sudden cardiac death triggered by an earthquake. *N Engl J Med.* 1996;334:413-419.
57. Brown DL. Disparate effects of the 1989 Loma Prieta and 1994 Northbridge earthquakes on hospital admissions for acute myocardial infarction: importance of superimposition of triggers. *Am Heart J.* 1999;137:830-836.
58. Nakagawa I, Nakamura K, Oyama M, et al. Long-term effects of the Niigata-Chuetsu earthquake in Japan on acute myocardial infarction mortality: an analysis of death certificate data. *Heart.* 2009;95:2009-2013.
59. Allegra JR, Mostashari F, Rothman J, Milano P, Cochrane DG. Cardiac events in New Jersey after the September 11, 2001, terrorist attack. *J Urban Health.* 2005;82:358-363.
60. Huang J, Chiou C, Ting C, Chen Y, Chen S. Sudden changes in heart rate variability during the 1999 Taiwan earthquake. *Am J Cardiol.* 2001;87:245-248.

61. Witte DR, Bois MI, Hoes AW, Grobbee DE. Cardiovascular mortality in Dutch men during 1996 European football championship: longitudinal population study. *Br Med J.* 2000;321: 1552-1554.
62. Toubiana L, Tanslik T, Letrilliart L. French cardiovascular mortality did not increase during football championship. *Br Med J.* 2001;322:1306.
63. Wilbert-Lampen U, Leistner D, Greven S, et al. Cardiovascular events during world cup soccer. *N Engl J Med.* 2008;358:475-483.
64. Peters A, von Klot S, Heier M, et al. Exposure to traffic and the onset of myocardial infarction. *N Engl J Med.* 2004;351:1721-1730.
65. Gnecchi-Ruscone T, Piccaluga E, Guzzetti S, Contini M, Montano N, Nocolis E. Morning and Monday: critical periods for the onset of acute myocardial infarction – the GISSI 2 study experience. *Eur Heart J.* 1994;15:882-887.
66. Peters RW, McQuillan S, Kaye SA, Gold MR. Increased Monday incidence of life-threatening ventricular arrhythmias: experience with a third generation implantable defibrillator. *Circulation.* 1995;94:1346-1349.
67. Kelly-Hayes M, Wolf PA, Kase CS, Brand FN, McGuirk JM, D'Agostino RB. Temporal patterns of stroke onset: the Framingham Study. *Stroke.* 1995;26:1343-1347.
68. Barnett AG, Dobson AJ. Excess in cardiovascular events on Mondays: a meta-analysis and prospective study. *J Epidemiol Community Health.* 2005;59:109-114.
69. Phillips DP, Jarvinen JR, Abramson IS, Phillips RR. Cardiac mortality is higher around Christmas and New Year's that at any other time. *Circulation.* 2004;110:3781-3788.
70. Yeung AC, Vekshtein VI, Krantz DS, et al. The effect of atherosclerosis on the vasomotor response of coronary arteries to mental stress. *N Engl J Med.* 1991;325:1551-1556.
71. Verrier RL, Hagestad EL, Lown B. Delayed myocardial ischemia induced by anger. *Circulation.* 1987;75:249-254.
72. Strike PC, Steptoe A. Systematic review of mental stress-induced myocardial ischaemia. *Eur Heart J.* 2003;24:690-703.
73. Rozanski A, Bairey CN, Krantz DS, et al. Mental stress and the induction of silent myocardial ischemia in patients with coronary artery disease. *N Engl J Med.* 1988;318:1005-1012.
74. Levine SP, Towell BL, Suarez AM, Knieriem LK, Harris MM, George JN. Platelet activation and secretion associated with emotional stress. *Circulation.* 1985;71:1129-1134.
75. Wallen NH, Held C, Rehnqvist N, Hjemdahl P. Effects of mental and physical stress on platelet function in patients with stable angina pectoris and healthy controls. *Eur Heart J.* 1997; 18:807-815.
76. Brydon L, Magid K, Steptoe A. Platelets, coronary artery disease and stress. *Brain Behav Immun.* 2006;20:113-119.
77. Takano M, Inami S, Ishibashi F, et al. Angioscopic follow-up study of coronary ruptured plaques in non culprit lesions. *JACC.* 2005;45:652-658.
78. Kolodgie FD, Virmani R, Burke AP, et al. Pathologic assessment of the vulnerable human coronary plaque. *Heart.* 2004;90:1385-1391.
79. Hollander JE, Hoffman RS, Burstein JL, Shih RD, Thode HCJ, For the Cocaine-Associated Myocardial Infarction Study Group. Cocaine-associated myocardial infarction. *Arch Intern Med.* 1995;155:1081-1086.
80. Rezkalla SH, Hale S, Kloner RA. Cocaine-induced heart diseases. *Am Heart J.* 1990;120: 1403-1408.
81. Siegel AJ, Sholar MB, Mendelson JH, et al. Cocaine-induced erythrocytosis and increase in von Willebrand factor. *Arch Intern Med.* 1999;159:1925-1930.
82. Cardona-Sanclemente LE, Born GV. Adrenaline increases the uptake of low-density lipoproteins in carotid arteries of rabbits. *Atherosclerosis.* 1992;96:215-218.
83. Burke AP, Kolodgie FD, Farb A, et al. Healed plaque ruptures and sudden coronary death: evidence that subclinical rupture has a role in plaque progression. *Circulation.* 2001;103: 934-940.

84. Heidland UE, Strauer BE. Left ventricular muscle mass and elevated heart rate are associated with coronary plaque disruption. *Circulation*. 2001;104:1477-1482.
85. Deedwania PC, Carbajal EV. Role of beta blockade in the treatment of myocardial ischaemia. *Am J Cardiol*. 1997;80:23J-28J.
86. Frishman WH, Furberg DC, Friedewald WT. Beta-adrenergic blockade for survivors of acute myocardial infarction. *N Engl J Med*. 1984;310:830-836.
87. Frishman WH. Multifactorial actions of beta-adrenergic blocking drugs in ischemic heart disease: current concepts. *Circulation*. 1983;67:11-18.
88. Tofler GH, Muller JE, Stone PH, et al. Modifiers of timing and possible triggers of acute myocardial infarction in the Thrombolysis in Myocardial Infarction Phase II (TIMI II) Study Group. *JACC*. 1992;20:1049-1055.
89. Mangano DT, Layug EL, Wallace A, Tateo I, For the Multicenter Study of Perioperative Ischaemia Research Group. Effect of atenolol on mortality and cardiovascular morbidity after noncardiac surgery. *N Engl J Med*. 1996;335:1713-1720.
90. Deedwania PC, Nelson JR. Pathophysiology of silent myocardial ischemia during daily life: hemodynamic evaluation by simultaneous electorcardiographic and blood pressure monitoring. *Circulation*. 1990;82:1296-1304.
91. Andrews TC, Fenton T, Toyosaki N, et al. Subsets of ambulatory myoscardial ischemia based on heart rate activity. *Circulation*. 1993;88:92-100.
92. Richardson PD, Davies MJ, Born GV. Influence of plaque configuration and stress distribution on fissuring of coronary atherosclerotic plaques. *Lancet*. 1989;2(8669):941-944.
93. Frishman WH, Weksler B, Christodoulou JP, Smithen C, Killip T. Reversal of abnormal platelet aggregability and change in exercise tolerance in patients with angina pectoris following oral propranolol. *Circulation*. 1974;50:887-896.
94. Horn EH, Jalihal S, Bruce M, Dean A, Rubin PC. The effect on platelet behaviour of treatment with atenolol and the combination of atenolol and nifedipine in healthy volunteers. *Platelets*. 1992;3:15-21.
95. Willich SN, Pohjola-Sintonen S, Bhatia SJ, et al. Suppression of silent ischemia by metoprolol without alteration of morning increase of platelet aggregability in patients with stable coronary artery disease. *Circulation*. 1989;79:557-565.
96. Kestin AS, Ellis PA, Barnard MR, Errichetti A, Rosner BA, Michelson AD. Effect of strenuous exercise on platelet activation state and reactivity. *Circulation*. 1983;88:1502-1511.
97. Folts JD, Rowe GG. Epinephrine potentiation of in vivo stimuli reverses aspirin inhibition of platelet thrombus formation in stenosed canine coronary arteries. *Thromb Res*. 1988;50:507-516.
98. Gibson RS, Hansen JF, Messerli F, Schechtman KB, Boden WE. Long term effects of diltiazem and verapamil on mortality and cardiac events in non-Q-wave acute myocardial infarction without pulmonary congestion: post hoc subset analysis of the multicenter postinfarction trial and the second Danish verapamil infarction trial studies. *Am J Cardiol*. 2000;86:275-279.
99. Gebara OCE, Jimenez AH, McKenna C, et al. Stress-induced hemodynamic and hemostatic changes in subjects with systemic hypertension: effect of verapamil. *Clin Cardiol*. 1996;19:205-211.
100. Sukhova GK, Williams JK, Libby P. Statins reduce inflammation in atheroma of nonhuman primates independent of effects on serum cholesterol. *Arterioscler Thromb Vasc Biol*. 2002;22:1452-1458.
101. Correia LCL, Sposito AC, Lima JC, et al. Anti-inflammatory effect of atorvastatin (80 mg) in unstable angina pectoris and Non-Q-wave acute myocardial infarction. *Am J Cardiol*. 2003;92:298-301.
102. Mensah K, Mocanu MM, Yellon DM. Failure to protect the myocardium against ischemia/reperfusion injury after chronic atorvastatin treatment is recaptured by acute atorvastatin treatment. *JAMA*. 2005;45:1287-1291.

103. Friedman M, Rosenman RH, Carroll V, Tat RJ. Changes in the serum cholesterol and blood clotting time in men subjected to cyclic variation of occupational stress. *Circulation*. 1958;17: 852-861.

104. Bachen EA, Muldoon MF, Matthews KA, Manuck SB. Effect of hemoconcentration and sympathetic activation on serum lipid responses to brief mental stress. *Psychosom Med*. 2002;64:587-594.

105. Siegrist J, Peter R, Cremer P, Siedel D. Chronic work stress is associated with atherogenic lipids and elevated fibrinogen in middle-aged men. *J Intern Med*. 1997;242:149-156.

106. O'Rourke MF, Donaldson E, Geddes JS. An airline cardiac arrest program. *Circulation*. 1997;96:2849-2853.

107. Galea S. Disasters and the health of urban populations. *J Urban Health*. 2006;82:347-349.

108. Strike PC, Magid K, Whitehead DL, Brydon L, Bhattacharyya MR, Steptoe A. Pathophysiological processes underlying emotional triggering of acute cardiac events. *Proc Natl Acad Sci USA*. 2006;103:4322-4327.

109. Rollman BL, Belnap BH, LeManager MS, et al. Telephone-delivered collaborative care for treating post-CABG depression. *JAMA*. 2009;302:2095-2103.

Chapter 10
Stress Cardiomyopathy

Ilan S. Wittstein

Keywords Stress cardiomyopathy • Takotsubo cardiomyopathy • Left ventricular apical ballooning syndrome • Catecholamines • Sympathetic nervous system • Microvascular dysfunction • Myocardial stunning

10.1   Introduction

Throughout history, human beings have always had an intuitive understanding of the connection between their emotions and their hearts. Descriptions of "heartache" and "dying from a broken heart" have appeared in the literary works of diverse cultures for centuries. Similarly, the medical literature is replete with descriptions of sudden death and myocardial infarction in the setting of fear, anxiety, and bereavement.[1,2] In the modern era, there is considerable epidemiologic evidence supporting the association of acute emotional stress with cardiovascular morbidity and mortality, as discussed by Tofler et al. (Chap. 9) in this book. Large population-based studies have clearly demonstrated increases in sudden death and myocardial infarction following emotionally traumatic events such as natural disasters,[3] acts of war,[4] and even sporting events.[5] Further, well-designed case-crossover studies have shown that acute emotional triggers such as anger and sadness more than double the risk of myocardial infarction.[6,7] These emotional triggers appear to precipitate deleterious cardiac events through a variety of mechanisms that include coronary vasoconstriction,[8] acute plaque rupture,[9] and electrical instability,[10] but until recently, there has been little data to support an association between emotional stress and cardiac contractile function.

I.S. Wittstein
Department of Medicine/Division of Cardiology, Johns Hopkins University School of Medicine,
Baltimore, MD, USA
e-mail: iwittste@jhmi.edu

P. Hjemdahl et al. (eds.), *Stress and Cardiovascular Disease*,
DOI 10.1007/978-1-84882-419-5_10, © Springer-Verlag London Limited 2012

During the past few years, a novel syndrome of heart failure and transient left ventricular systolic dysfunction precipitated by acute emotional or physical stress has been described. Originally reported from Japan and referred to as *takotsubo cardiomyopathy*,[11] this syndrome has now been observed in countries worldwide and has acquired several other names that include *stress cardiomyopathy*,[12] *transient left ventricular apical ballooning syndrome*,[13] and *broken heart syndrome*.[12] Because patients with stress cardiomyopathy (SCM) typically present with chest pain, electrocardiographic abnormalities, and elevated cardiac enzymes, this condition went unrecognized for many years while being frequently mistaken for acute myocardial infarction. But as familiarity with this syndrome has increased, it has become clear that SCM not only has unique clinical characteristics that can readily be distinguished from those of an acute infarction, it also appears to have a distinct pathophysiology. In contrast to the irreversible myocardial injury seen with acute infarction, the myocardial dysfunction of SCM is transient and completely reversible and occurs in a manner that appears to be independent of plaque rupture and coronary thrombosis. While there is evidence that the myocardial stunning of SCM may be sympathetically mediated, the precise mechanism underlying the pathogenesis of this disorder remains poorly understood.

This chapter will review the prevalence, diagnostic clinical features, treatment, and prognosis of stress cardiomyopathy. The proposed pathophysiologic mechanisms of this syndrome will be presented, and risk factors that may increase individual susceptibility to SCM will be reviewed.

10.2 A Brief History of the Confusing Taxonomy

The term *stress cardiomyopathy* first appeared in the medical literature in 1980 when Cebelin and Hirsch reported a series of murder victims who had been emotionally and physically traumatized prior to their deaths.[14] None of the victims died from internal injuries, but the majority of them had extensive myocardial contraction band necrosis, a histologic finding frequently observed in states of catecholamine excess. The authors proposed that the cause of death was the deleterious effect of catecholamines on the heart, and they named the condition *human stress cardiomyopathy*.

This term did not reappear in the medical literature until 1997 when Pavin and colleagues used it to describe two women with elevated catecholamine levels and reversible left ventricular dysfunction precipitated by acute emotional stress.[15] A year later, Brandspiegel reported a woman with "a broken heart" who developed transient left ventricular dysfunction following the death of her husband.[16] At the time of these case reports, SCM was an obscure and almost unheard of condition in Western medical literature. In Japan, however, Satoh and colleagues had already described the syndrome as early as 1990 and had named it *takotsubo cardiomyopathy*[11] after the octopus trapping pot with a wide base and narrow neck that they felt resembled the morphologic appearance of the left ventricle of patients with this condition. For the next decade, reports of takotsubo cardiomyopathy appeared exclusively in Japanese medical journals, primarily in the form of case reports and small case series. Ironically, when Japanese authors finally published their experience with this syndrome in an American medical journal in 2001,[13] they chose the name *transient left ventricular apical ballooning syndrome*, a descriptive term they likely felt would be more acceptable to a Western audience.

In February 2005, SCM received worldwide attention when our group at Johns Hopkins and a second group from the Minneapolis Heart Institute reported the clinical and neurohumoral features of the syndrome in two major medical journals.[12,17] The term *stress cardiomyopathy* was formally used in our manuscript, and the nickname *broken heart syndrome* was also introduced and was quickly popularized by the media.[12] In the 5 years since the publication of these manuscripts, the medical literature regarding SCM has increased dramatically. While there is considerable debate over the ideal nomenclature for this condition, we prefer the name *stress cardiomyopathy* because it emphasizes the importance of acute stress, whether emotional or physical, in the pathogenesis of this disorder. Further, it is now clear that the left ventricle in some patients with SCM can assume morphologic appearances that spare the apex,[18,19] making the names *takotsubo* and *transient left ventricular apical ballooning syndrome* both confusing and inaccurate for these subgroups. Until a clear and consistent nomenclature is agreed upon, physicians should be aware that all four names are used interchangeably in the literature to refer to the same clinical condition.

10.3 Prevalence

While SCM was felt to be a rare condition just a few years ago, it is now clear from the rapidly expanding medical literature that the syndrome is far more prevalent than what was originally believed. Retrospective series from countries worldwide have demonstrated that SCM accounts for approximately 2% of patients with a suspected acute coronary syndrome (ACS) (Table 10.1). The prevalence is even higher in women presenting with suspected ACS, with rates ranging from 4.7% to 7.5%.[23,27,33,36] These series likely underestimate the true prevalence of the disorder because they report only those patients undergoing coronary angiography and do not include patients in medical, surgical, and neurologic intensive care units where the syndrome is common but often unrecognized. This idea is supported by one prospective study that reported echocardiographic evidence of left ventricular apical ballooning in 28% of patients admitted to a medical intensive care unit with a noncardiac illness.[39] It will likely require both prospective evaluation and more widespread recognition of this syndrome by physicians in diverse subspecialties before the true prevalence of SCM is fully appreciated.

Table 10.1 Prevalence of stress cardiomyopathy in patients with suspected ACS

Reference	Country	Number of patients	Study period (years)	Population studied	Prevalence in all patients with suspected ACS (%)	Prevalence in women with suspected ACS
Akashi et al.[20]	Japan	637	5	ACS	2.0	NR
Ito et al.[21]	Japan	573	NR	ACS	1.7	NR
Matsuoka et al.[22]	Japan	450	5	ACS	2.2	NR
Wedekind et al.[23]	Germany	215	1	ACS	2.3	7.5%
Haghi et al.[24]	Germany	2,031	3.8	ACS	2.5	NR
Kurowski et al.[25]	Germany	2,944	3	ACS	1.2	NR
Pilliere et al.[26]	France	1,613	5	ACS	0.7	NR
Parodi et al.[27]	Italy	1,811	2.5	STEMI	2.0	6.6%
Azzarelli et al.[28]	Italy	389	1	ACS	2.0	NR
Buja et al.[29]	Italy	1,657	7	STEMI	1.7	NR
Cangella et al.[30]	Italy	1,674	6	ACS	0.4	NR
Spedicato et al.[31]	Italy	728	4.6	ACS	4	NR
Previtali et al.[32]	Italy	1,457	4.3	ACS	1.2	4.9%
Elian et al.[33]	Israel	638	2.7	ACS	2.0	6.0%
Eshtehardi et al.[34]	Switzerland	2,459	3	ACS	1.7	NR
Bybee et al.[35]	United States	727	2	STEMI	2.2	NR
Strunk et al.[36]	United States	409	2.3	ACS	1.7	4.7%
Larson et al.[37]	United States	1,335	3.7	STEMI	1.3	NR

Modified with kind permission from Wittstein[38], Table 1

ACS troponin positive acute coronary syndrome, *NR* not reported, *STEMI ST*-segment elevation myocardial infarction

10.4 Patient Demographics and Clinical Presentation

While initial reports of SCM were exclusively from Japan, the syndrome has now been described in patients with diverse ethnic backgrounds from countries all over the world.[12,13,17,24,26,27,33,40] All series to date have demonstrated a marked age and gender discrepancy, with older postmenopausal women being most commonly affected (Table 10.2). As illustrated by a systematic review of 28 case series, 91% of the reported cases have been women, with mean ages ranging from 62 to 76 years.[50] Coronary risk factors are common, with hypertension being reported in 49% of the cases, hyperlipidemia in 30.5%, diabetes in 10.6%, smoking in 20.7%, and a positive family history of cardiovascular disease in 11.4%. Comorbidities commonly observed in patients with SCM include thyroid disease, chronic obstructive pulmonary disease, and mood disorders such as anxiety and depression.[45,51]

Patients with SCM typically present with symptoms similar to those of an acute myocardial infarction, with chest pain and shortness of breath being the most common (Table 10.2).[50,52] Heart failure and pulmonary edema have been described in 15.9% of the reported cases, with cardiogenic shock and life-threatening arrhythmias occurring in 10.3% and 14.6% of the cases, respectively.[50] In a large Japanese series, 20% of the patients required intra-aortic balloon counterpulsation or pressor support.[13] We have observed that while the majority of patients with SCM are hemodynamically stable at the time of admission, approximately one third present with life-threatening problems that include pulmonary edema, hypotension, cardiogenic shock, and ventricular arrhythmias (unpublished data). Cases of apical thrombus formation, cardioembolic stroke, left ventricular free wall rupture, and pericarditis have also been reported.

10.5 Diagnostic Criteria

There are no uniformly accepted diagnostic criteria for SCM, though guidelines have been proposed.[53,54] The most widely cited criteria were introduced by investigators from the Mayo Clinic in 2004 and were modified in 2008.[55] We have used similar diagnostic criteria with some minor differences (Table 10.3). The following six criteria should be considered when contemplating the diagnosis of SCM and can help to distinguish the syndrome from acute myocardial infarction:

An acute trigger: An acute emotional or physical trigger precipitating SCM can be identified in the vast majority of cases. At our institution, the most common emotional triggers have included grief, often due to the death of a loved one, and fear (e.g., robbed at gunpoint; motor vehicle accident). The syndrome can also be precipitated by a wide variety of physical stressors including respiratory emergencies (e.g., asthma exacerbation, airway compromise, pneumothorax), surgical procedures, metabolic insults (e.g., hypoglycemia), hemodynamic derangements (e.g., hypotensive gastrointestinal bleeding), and various neurologic insults including

Table 10.2 Clinical characteristics of stress cardiomyopathy in some of the larger case series

Reference	Number patients	Age (yrs)	Women (%)	HTN (%)	HLD (%)	DM (%)	TOB (%)	CP (%)	SOB (%)	Syncope (%)	CHF (%)	IABP/ pressors (%)	VT/VF (%)	Trigger identified (%)
Fazio et al.[41]	40	69	85	50	2.5	2.5	NR	68	16	8	NR	NR	5	80
Elesber et al.[42]	42	71	100	64	38	12	12	67	12	12	26	NR	NR	64
Nunez-Gil et al.[43]	62	65	84	71	45	15	27	92	NR	NR	24	NR	NR	47
Parodi et al.[44]	68	74	94	57	38	10	21	NR	40	NR	21	13	NR	72
Regnante et al.[45]	70	67	95	66	49	14	47	77	7	6	NR	9	4	67
Tsuchihashi et al.[13]	88	67	86	48	24	12	NR	67	7	NR	37	20	9	73
Hoyt et al.[46]	97	71	100	68	39	12	19	NR	NR	NR	47	9	NR	NR
Elesber et al.[47]	100	66	95	52	33	5	38	77	8	NR	44	7	2	56
Singh et al.[48]	114	71(A) 64(NA)	93	66	33	8	47	69	18	7	10	7	1	83
Sharkey et al.[49]	136	68	96	43	NR	NR	NR	63	18	3	NR	NR	NR	89

A apical ballooning, *CHF* congestive heart failure on admission, *CP* chest pain on admission, *DM* history of diabetes mellitus, *HLD* history of hyperlipidemia, *HTN* history of hypertension, *IABP* intra-aortic balloon pump, *NA* non-apical ballooning, *NR* not reported, *SOB* shortness of breath on admission, *TOB* current or prior tobacco use, *VF* ventricular fibrillation, *VT* ventricular tachycardia, yrs years

Table 10.3 Proposed criteria for the diagnosis of stress cardiomyopathy

Modified Mayo Clinic criteria[55]	Johns Hopkins criteria
• Transient hypokinesis, akinesis, or dyskinesis of the left ventricular midsegments with or without apical involvement; the regional wall motion abnormalities extend beyond a single epicardial vascular distribution; a stressful trigger is often, but not always present	*Helpful, but not mandatory, criteria* • An acute identifiable trigger (either emotional or physical) • Characteristic electrocardiographic changes that may include some or all of the following:
• Absence of obstructive coronary disease or angiographic evidence of acute plaque rupture	– ST-segment elevation at time of admission (often <2 mm in magnitude, and usually not associated with reciprocal ST-segment depression)
• New electrocardiographic abnormalities (either ST-segment elevation and/or T-wave inversion) or modest elevation in cardiac troponin	– Diffuse deep T-wave inversion (may be present on admission or may evolve during the first several hospital days) – QT interval prolongation (usually maximal by 24–48 h)
• Absence of: Pheochromocytoma and myocarditis	• Mildly elevated cardiac troponin (often appears disproportionately low given the degree of wall motion abnormality) *Mandatory criteria (all 3 criteria must be met)* • Absence of coronary thrombosis or angiographic evidence of acute plaque rupture • Regional ventricular wall motion abnormalities that extend beyond a single epicardial vascular distribution • Complete recovery of regional wall motion abnormalities (recovery is usually within days to weeks)

subarachnoid hemorrhage,[56] seizure,[57] and stroke.[58] The numerous potential triggers of this syndrome have recently been reported in a large single center series.[49] It is important to realize that the triggers of SCM are not always dramatic events and may frequently go unrecognized. In a systematic review of 14 case series, an identifiable trigger was not reported in 34% of the cases,[52] likely reflecting the retrospective nature in which many of these series were collected. In a recent large prospective series, however, an acute precipitant was identified in 89% of the cases,[49] a prevalence similar to what we have observed at our institution. It is our belief that if the diagnosis of SCM is suspected, a thorough history at the time of admission will elucidate the trigger in the majority of cases.

Characteristic electrocardiographic features: While there are no electrocardiographic (ECG) findings that are absolutely diagnostic of SCM, certain characteristic findings should raise suspicion for the diagnosis (Fig. 10.1). Patients with SCM can present with a normal ECG, nonspecific ST-segment and T-wave changes, or ST-segment elevation, typically seen in precordial leads. ST-segment elevation appears to be more common in Japanese patients and has been reported in only 21–49% of cases from the United States.[48,49] Compared to patients with anterior

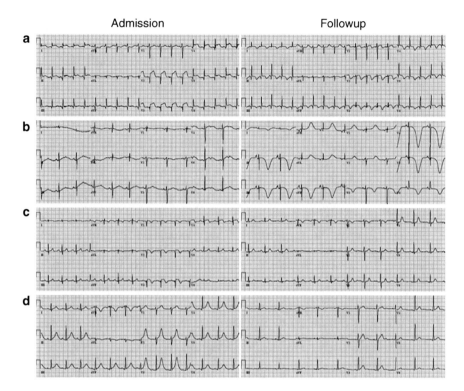

Fig. 10.1 Examples of characteristic ECG findings on admission and at follow-up in four different patients with stress cardiomyopathy. (**a**) Note the marked precordial ST-segment elevation and absence of reciprocal ST-segment depression at the time of admission. Within 24 h, there was diffuse T-wave inversion and QT interval prolongation. (**b**) This patient had nonspecific T-wave abnormalities on admission and developed dramatic diffuse T-wave inversion and QT prolongation within 36 h. (**c**) In addition to ST-segment elevation and T-wave inversion in anteroseptal leads, this patient also had anteroseptal Q waves in leads V1-V3 at the time of admission. These changes had all resolved by follow-up at 3 weeks. (**d**) This patient presented with a non-apical variant of stress cardiomyopathy. In contrast to the apical variant that often has T-wave inversion, note the diffuse broad upright T-waves and QT prolongation on admission that resolved within a few days

ST-segment elevation myocardial infarction (STEMI), patients with SCM tend to have a smaller magnitude of ST-segment elevation[59,60] and are less likely to have reciprocal inferior ST-segment depression at the time of admission.[61]

Within 24–48 h of the initial presentation, patients with SCM typically develop marked QT interval prolongation.[12] The interval is significantly longer than what is seen with acute myocardial infarction.[61] While the QT interval prolongation usually improves over several days, it may take several weeks to completely normalize. The majority of patients with apical ballooning also develop deep diffuse T-wave inversion in both precordial and limb leads. These T-wave abnormalities can persist for days, weeks, or even months.[62] Diffuse T-wave inversion is less commonly observed in patients with mid-ventricular and basal variants of SCM.[63] In contrast, these

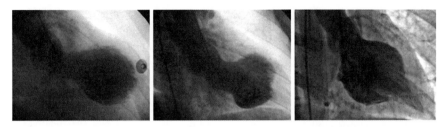

Fig. 10.2 Left ventriculography during systole of the three different variants of stress cardiomyopathy. On the left is the "apical ballooning" variant with apical and mid-ventricular akinesis with sparing of the base. In the middle is the "mid-ventricular ballooning" variant with akinesis of the mid-ventricle but normal contractility of the apex and base. On the right is the "basal ballooning" pattern with basal and mid-ventricular akinesis and normal apical contractility (Reproduced with kind permission from, Wittstein[38], figure 1)

patients often have broad, diffuse, upright T-waves on admission, creating almost a mirror image of the apical variant ECG (Fig. 10.1d).[64] Patients with SCM can also present with pathologic Q waves that are usually seen in precordial leads. Unlike with acute myocardial infarction, these Q waves are transient in most cases and typically resolve within days to weeks of the initial presentation (Fig. 10.1c).[12]

Mild cardiac enzyme elevation: Most patients with SCM have only mildly elevated cardiac enzymes at the time of admission. These enzyme levels can appear paradoxically low given the extensive ventricular wall motion abnormalities that are typical for these patients. Cardiac enzyme levels are much lower in patients with SCM than in patients with acute infarction.[27,61] In addition, the enzyme release kinetics may be different, with troponin levels in SCM peaking earlier after symptom onset than they do with acute infarction.[65] Patients with SCM also have markedly elevated brain natriuretic peptide (BNP) levels at the time of admission, but these levels rapidly decline and do not appear to have prognostic importance.[12]

Absence of coronary thrombosis or acute plaque rupture: Stress cardiomyopathy is characterized by the absence of obstructive coronary disease. While the majority of reported cases have described normal coronary arteries,[50,52] it is now well recognized that many patients with this condition have angiographic evidence of non-obstructive coronary atherosclerosis.[46,66] Because patients typically present with chest pain, dynamic ECG changes, elevated cardiac enzymes, and focal wall motion abnormalities, coronary angiography should be performed unless there is an obvious contraindication to definitively exclude evidence of acute plaque rupture and coronary thrombosis.

Ventricular "ballooning": Perhaps the most defining characteristic of this syndrome is the unusual pattern of left ventricular dysfunction which is typically seen with echocardiography or ventriculography at the time of presentation (Fig. 10.2). In contrast to patients with acute infarction, patients with SCM have left ventricular wall motion abnormalities that extend beyond a single coronary territory. The majority of patients have the well-described "apical ballooning" pattern in which there is akinesis or dense hypokinesis of the apical and mid-ventricular segments with sparing of the base. More recently, variants of this syndrome have been reported in which the apex is not affected.[18,19] Patients with "basal" and "mid-ventricular" ballooning patterns tend to be younger and have less heart failure, but otherwise have many of the same clinical features as patients with apical involvement.[63] While SCM is characterized primarily by left ventricular dysfunction, a third of the patients with left ventricular apical ballooning also have right ventricular dysfunction.[67] Patients with biventricular involvement are more likely to have severe heart failure and hemodynamic instability.

Recovery of left ventricular function: Complete recovery of ventricular systolic function is one of the hallmarks of SCM. Despite extensive wall motion abnormalities at the time of initial presentation, follow-up assessment of ventricular function has demonstrated recovery in all series to date. Most patients demonstrate significant improvement in systolic function within a week of the initial presentation, and complete recovery is often observed by the end of the third week. Cases of very slow left ventricular recovery have been published,[68] and some authors have reported a recovery period of up to 1 year.[49] This tends to be the exception, however, and as a general rule, if systolic function in a patient suspected of having SCM has not completely normalized within 12 weeks, alternative diagnoses should be considered.

10.6   Other Diagnostic Tools

In addition to echocardiography and ventriculography, other imaging modalities have been used to help differentiate SCM from acute infarction.

Cardiac magnetic resonance imaging (MRI): Cardiac MRI has proven itself to be one of the more useful tools for making the diagnosis of SCM.[12,17,69-71] Not only does cardiac MRI provide analysis of regional wall motion abnormalities of both the left and right ventricles, the absence of delayed gadolinium enhancement in the majority of patients with SCM reliably demonstrates myocardial viability and lack of myocardial necrosis, and can be useful at the time of presentation in distinguishing this syndrome from other acute myocardial processes such as infarction and myocarditis (Fig. 10.3).[12,17,69,70]

Positron emission tomography (PET): Several studies have used F-18 fluorodeoxyglucose (FDG) PET to study myocardial metabolic activity in patients with SCM.[72-75] These studies have consistently demonstrated marked metabolic impairment in regions of ventricular akinesis despite normal or only mildly impaired myocardial perfusion. The precise mechanism of this "reversible inverse perfusion/metabolism mismatch" is unknown, but may result either from sympathetically mediated microcirculatory dysfunction or direct catecholamine impairment of myocyte glucose utilization. PET imaging with the norepinephrine analogue ^{11}C hydroxyephedrine has also been used in patients with SCM and has demonstrated increased sympathetic activity in regions of the ventricle with contractile dysfunction.[76]

SCM   **AMI**

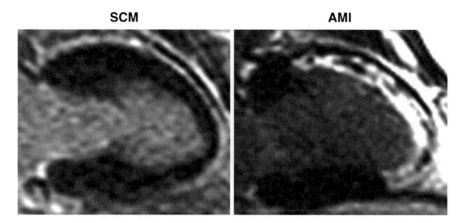

Fig. 10.3 Cardiac MRI in patients with stress cardiomyopathy (*SCM*) and anterior ST-elevation myocardial infarction (*AMI*). Myocardial viability in SCM is suggested by the absence of delayed gadolinium enhancement. In contrast, the left ventricle in AMI demonstrates hyper-enhancement indicative of necrosis and decreased viability (Reproduced with permission, from reference Wittstein et al.[12]. Copyright © 2005 Massachusetts Medical Society. All rights reserved)

123I-metaiodobenzyl-guanidine (*123I-MIBG*) *scintigraphy*: While rarely necessary to make the diagnosis of SCM, 123I-MIBG imaging has helped to elucidate the potential mechanism of this disorder. Studies have shown decreased 123I-MIBG uptake in regions of ventricular akinesis with an increased cardiac washout rate on delayed imaging.[77,78] These findings, which suggest increased cardiac sympathetic activity during the acute phase of the syndrome, typically recover within 6 months of the initial presentation.[73,79]

10.7 Treatment

The treatment of stress cardiomyopathy is primarily supportive. In the acute period, hemodynamically stable patients are frequently treated with diuretics, angiotensin-converting enzyme (ACE) inhibitors, and beta-blockers. Unless there is a clear contraindication, patients with apical akinesis should be anticoagulated until apical contractility improves in order to reduce the risk of thromboembolic events. For hemodynamically unstable patients, reported treatment has included inotropes, vasopressor support, and intra-aortic balloon counterpulsation. There are also some limited reports that patients with hypotension and left ventricular cavity obstruction in the acute period may derive hemodynamic and echocardio-graphic benefit from the administration of intravenous beta-blockade.[80] Because catecholamines may be central to the pathogenesis of SCM and have been associ-ated with ventricular outflow tract obstruction in some patients,[17] we prefer to use intra-aortic balloon counterpulsation for hemodynamically unstable patients and to avoid the administration of exogenous catecholamines whenever possible. Fortunately, even the most unstable patients typically demonstrate rapid clinical improvement and rarely require hemodynamic support for more than a few days.

There is no consensus regarding the long-term management of SCM. While it is reasonable to treat patients with beta-blockers and ACE inhibitors during the period of ventricular recovery, there are currently no data to support that the chronic use of these agents prevents recurrence or improves survival. It has therefore become our practice to stop these medications once left ventricular function has normalized. It is not unreasonable to consider chronic beta-blockade or calcium channel blockade for patients who develop recurrent episodes of SCM, but once again, there are no data to support the efficacy of this treatment strategy. Some patients will continue to have episodic chest discomfort for weeks to months after the initial presentation. Nitrates are often effective in relieving symptoms in these individuals.

While patients with SCM have a high prevalence of anxiety and depression,[51] no studies have examined whether psychological or pharmacologic treatment of these mood disorders improves the long-term outcomes of patients with SCM or helps prevent recurrence. Preliminary data from our institution have revealed an increased mortality in patients with SCM taking antidepressants (unpublished data). While the use of antidepressants may simply identify a group of patients with more severe depression, it is also possible that drugs affecting catecholamine metabolism may have deleterious long-term effects in these patients. Until more data are available, we believe that the routine use of antidepressants in the treatment of SCM should be avoided.

10.8   Prognosis and Recurrence

From the literature reported to date, patients with SCM appear to have a favorable prognosis and a relatively low risk of recurrence. Compared to acute myocardial infarction, patients with SCM have a better long-term survival and fewer major adverse cardiac events.[43] In a systematic review of 28 case series of SCM, the recurrence and in-hospital mortality rates were only 3.1% and 1.7%, respectively.[50] In a large single center retrospective experience from the Mayo Clinic, the recurrence rate of SCM was 11.4% during the 4 years following the initial presentation. The 4-year survival was no different than that observed in an age- and gender-matched population.[47] Sharkey and colleagues recently reported a 15% 5 year mortality rate and a 5% recurrence rate in a large series of patients with SCM.[49] While these patients had reduced survival compared to an age- and sex-matched population, most of the deaths occurred within the first year and were due to noncardiac causes. These mortality and recurrence rates are very similar to what we have observed at our institution.

10.9   Possible Pathophysiologic Mechanisms

While the clinical features of stress cardiomyopathy have become increasingly well recognized, the precise pathophysiologic mechanism of this disorder remains unknown. There is significant clinical evidence to suggest that enhanced sympathetic stimulation may be central to the pathogenesis of SCM. We found that patients with SCM due to emotional stress had markedly elevated plasma catecholamine levels compared to patients with Killip III myocardial infarction,[12] but an elevation in peripheral venous catecholamine levels has been an inconsistent finding.[81] This discrepancy may be due to the fact that sympathetic activation may be differentiated (see also Chap. 3 by Hjemdahl and Esler) and result primarily in local myocardial catecholamine release which can only be detected with coronary sinus sampling.[82] Looking at indices of heart rate variability, Ortak and colleagues have demonstrated sympathetic predominance and a marked depression of cardiac parasympathetic activity during the acute phase of SCM,[83] and parasympathetic blockade with atropine has been shown to exacerbate the signs and symptoms of SCM.[84] Enhanced sympathetic activity has been suggested by the increased washout rate of the norepinephrine analogue ^{123}I-metaiodobenzyl-guanidine (MIBG) using myocardial scintigraphy.[78] Stress cardiomyopathy has also been associated with catecholamine-secreting tumors such as pheochromocytoma and paraganglioma.[85,86] Further, all of the clinical features of SCM, including the various ventricular ballooning patterns, can be precipitated by the intravenous administration of catecholamines and beta-agonists.[64]

Data from animal models also support the central role of adrenergic stimulation in the pathogenesis of SCM. Ueyama was able to precipitate left ventricular apical ballooning which was attenuated by alpha- and beta-blockade in rats subjected to immobilization stress.[87] Izumi and colleagues induced stress cardiomyopathy in monkeys with the infusion of intravenous epinephrine and demonstrated increased myocytolysis in the apical portion of the ventricle.[88] Administration of the beta-blocker metoprolol decreased epinephrine-mediated myocytolysis and resulted in an improvement in left ventricular ejection fraction.

Exactly how increased sympathetic activity might result in the reversible ventricular dysfunction seen with SCM is unclear, but several pathophysiologic mechanisms have been proposed (Fig. 10.4).

Plaque rupture: Catecholamine-mediated plaque rupture with rapid and complete lysis of the ensuing thrombus has been proposed as a possible mechanism of SCM. Despite a normal appearing coronary angiogram in many patients with this condition, some authors have reported eccentric atherosclerotic plaque in the midportion of the left anterior descending (LAD) coronary artery using intravascular ultrasound,[90] but these findings have not been uniformly supported. It has also been proposed that plaque rupture and transient coronary thrombosis must occur in a long wrap-around LAD to explain the apical ballooning pattern.[40] It has now been demonstrated, however, that apical ballooning can occur even in the absence of a wrap-around LAD and that the prevalence of this coronary anatomy is no higher in

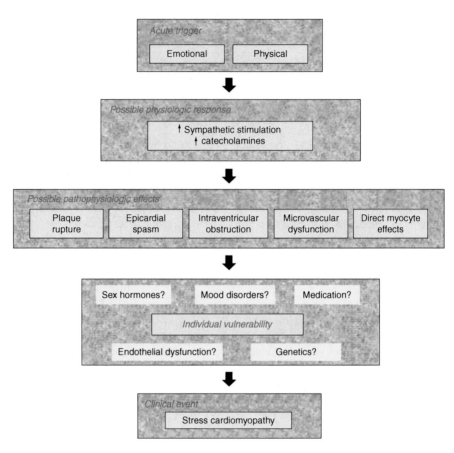

Fig. 10.4 Possible mechanistic link between acute stress and the syndrome of stress cardiomyo-pathy. Evidence suggests that increased sympathetic stimulation is the key physiologic response to acute stress which may mediate myocardial stunning through a variety of possible pathophysio-logic effects. Potential risk factors that may increase individual susceptibility to these physiologic and pathophysiologic responses are also shown (Modified from Bhattacharyya[89], figure 1, copy-right © 2007, with permission from Elsevier)

patients with SCM than it is in a control population.[46] Further, transient thrombosis in a large wrap-around LAD would not explain the basal and mid-ventricular ballooning patterns that have been reported.

Epicardial spasm: Ischemia due to sympathetically mediated coronary spasm could account for the myocardial stunning that characterizes this syndrome, but there are several compelling reasons to challenge this hypothesis. First, while epicardial spasm has been reported in cases of SCM, it is rarely observed during angiography, even when provocative agents such as ergonovine and acetylcholine are administered.[50,91] Second, most patients have only mild cardiac enzyme eleva-tion, and many no evidence of ST-segment elevation on ECG, findings that seem inconsistent with diffuse epicardial spasm. Finally, it is virtually impossible to explain the different "ballooning" patterns based on an epicardial vascular distribution, and even multivessel spasm would not account for the unusual patterns of akinesis that have been reported.

Intraventricular obstruction: An intraventricular pressure gradient can be measured in some patients with SCM during the acute presentation.[13,17] It has been suggested that patients with smaller ventricles and localized mid-ventricular septal thickening may be predisposed to severe mid-cavity obstruction during periods of excessive sympathetic stimulation. This obstruction could result in apical subendocardial ischemia due to a large pressure gradient between the apex and base, resulting in transient apical dysfunction. It is likely, however, that the intraventricular gradient observed in some patients is a consequence rather than the underlying cause of the myocardial dysfunction. Only a small minority of cases reported in the literature have described an intraventricular gradient.[50] In addition, while a large gradient between left ventricular apex and base could theoretically result in apical ischemia and ballooning, it certainly does not provide a very plausible explanation for the basal and mid-ventricular variants or for the right ventricular dysfunction seen in about a third of patients with this syndrome.

Microvascular dysfunction: Sympathetically mediated microcirculatory dysfunction is another potential mechanism of the myocardial stunning seen with SCM. A significant reduction in coronary flow reserve and velocity has been observed using a Doppler flow wire at the time of coronary angiography.[92] Doppler transthoracic echocardiography has also demonstrated abnormal coronary flow reserve in the acute phase of SCM following the infusion of adenosine[93] or dipyridamole.[94] Despite the absence of obstructive coronary disease, patients with SCM have elevated Thrombolysis in Myocardial Infarction (TIMI) frame counts,[35] a well-validated index of coronary blood flow, and abnormal TIMI myocardial perfusion grades.[42] In the majority of these patients, TIMI frame counts are elevated in multiple vessels and perfusion abnormalities involve multiple coronary territories, suggesting that catecholamine-mediated endothelial cell injury could account for the microvascular dysfunction seen with this syndrome. This idea is further supported by a recent study in which patients presenting with SCM were found to have elevated plasma catecholamine levels and evidence from left ventricular endomyocardial biopsy of microvascular endothelial cell apoptosis.[95]

Direct myocyte effects: Myocardial stunning in SCM could alternatively result from the direct effects of catecholamines on cardiac myocytes through adrenergic receptor signaling. Lyon and colleagues have suggested that high levels of circulating epinephrine may cause a switch from G_s to G_i protein signaling in the cardiac myocyte via the β_2-adrenergic receptor.[96] This could result in a negative inotropic effect that is most pronounced at the apex of the heart where the β-receptor density is greatest. While this hypothesis is interesting, it does not readily explain the nonapical variants of SCM that are frequently observed. There is evidence to suggest that catecholamines may affect cardiac function in SCM through alteration of myocyte calcium handling. Catecholamines can decrease myocyte viability through cyclic adenosine monophosphate–mediated calcium overload.[97] This results in contraction band necrosis, a histologic finding known to occur in states of catecholamine excess that has also been observed in the endomyocardial biopsy samples of patients with SCM.[12,98] Recently, Nef and colleagues utilized left ventricular endomyocardial biopsy samples to demonstrate evidence of a disturbed calcium regulatory system in patients with SCM.[99] At the time of presentation, there was significant downregulation of sarcoplasmic Ca^{2+} ATPase (SERCA2a) gene expression, increased ventricular expression of sarcolipin, and dephosphorylation of phospholamban (PLN). The increased PLN/SERCA2a ratio, which could potentially result in myocardial contractile dysfunction through decreased calcium affinity, had normalized when biopsy samples were repeated following ventricular recovery. Data from animal models also support the idea that catecholamine-mediated abnormalities of calcium handling may be central to the pathogenesis of SCM. In a rat model of stress cardiomyopathy, acute beta-adrenergic stimulation resulted in left ventricular dysfunction and myocyte injury through calcium leakage due to hyperphosphorylation of the ryanodine receptor 2 (RyR2).[100]

10.10   Factors That May Increase Susceptibility to Stress Cardiomyopathy

While most individuals are subjected to repeated emotional and physiologic stressors, the fact that only a relatively small number develop SCM suggests that there may be risk factors that increase individual susceptibility to this disorder. These risk factors may influence not only a person's physiologic response to stress but also the pathophysiologic mechanisms that result in myocardial stunning (Fig. 10.4). While it is likely that many such risk factors exist, only a few that are supported by clinical observations and research will be discussed here.

Hormonal influence: A consistent observation in all series reported to date is the striking preponderance of postmenopausal women. Female hormones exert important influences on the sympathetic neurohormonal axis as well as on coronary vasoreactivity and myocyte calcium handling. As women age, cardiac vagal tone, and baroreflex sensitivity decrease significantly,[101] potentially making postmenopausal women more susceptible to the deleterious cardiovascular effects of sympathetic stimulation following an acute stressor. There is clinical evidence that estrogen attenuates catecholamine-mediated vasoconstriction[102] and the catecholamine response to mental stress[103] in postmenopausal women. In an animal model of SCM, Ueyama has demonstrated that estrogen supplementation in ovariectomized rats can attenuate the negative effect of immobilization stress on left ventricular systolic function.[104] While these observations suggest that sex hormones likely have an important influence on stress-related myocardial stunning, there are currently no clinical data to suggest that estrogen replacement can prevent the occurrence or recurrence of SCM. On the contrary, the syndrome has been reported in younger women,[12,49] and 11% of the women with SCM at our institution were taking hormone replacement therapy at the time of presentation.

Mood disorders and antidepressant use: We have previously reported a high prevalence of mood disorders and antidepressant use in patients with SCM.[51] This may have pathogenic importance since patients with depressive disorders have decreased vagal tone and an increased adrenomedullary hormonal response to stressful events,[105] and some patients with depression appear to have very high noradrenaline spillover[106] (see chapter 4 by Esler). Further, the increased use of antidepressants such as selective norepinephrine reuptake inhibitors in this population may facilitate myocardial stunning by increasing local catecholamine levels. Well-designed prospective case control studies will be necessary to determine the true frequency of psychiatric disorders in patients with SCM and to clarify whether antidepressant use increases individual susceptibility to this disorder.

Endothelial dysfunction: Recent data have suggested that patients with SCM may be individuals with inherent endothelial dysfunction and chronic impairment of coronary vasodilatory reserve. In an important study by Barletta and colleagues, subjects who had fully recovered from an episode of SCM were subjected to cold pressor testing (CPT). Peripheral venous catecholamines were measured, and left ventricular function and perfusion were assessed using real-time three-dimensional echocardiography and myocardial contrast 2D echocardiography, respectively.[107] Despite the fact that subjects were 1–3 years out from their initial stress cardiomyopathy episode, CPT resulted in significant catecholamine elevation and transient apical and mid-ventricular wall motion abnormalities, and no increase in coronary blood flow was observed. This contrasted with an age-, sex-, and risk factor–matched control group in which CPT increased coronary flow and resulted in no regional wall motion abnormalities. The results of this study suggest that patients with SCM may be individuals who are particularly susceptible to myocardial stunning during periods of acute stress and catecholamine excess due to intrinsic impairment of coronary flow reserve.

Genetic determinants: SCM has been reported in siblings,[108] but the genetic determinants of this syndrome have yet to be defined. Zaroff and colleagues studied the impact of adrenergic receptor polymorphisms on cardiac dysfunction in patients with neurogenic stunned myocardium, a condition seen commonly after central neurologic injury that almost certainly shares an overlapping pathophysiology with SCM.[109] They demonstrated that following subarachnoid hemorrhage, the risk of cardiac dysfunction and troponin elevation was greatly increased in individuals with specific α- and β-adrenergic receptor polymorphisms. An increased frequency of these same polymorphisms has not been found in patients with SCM.[110] Recently, however, Spinelli and colleagues have demonstrated that compared to a control population, patients with SCM have an increased frequency of the L41Q polymorphism of the G protein–coupled receptor kinase 5 (GRK5).[111] The L41 variant of GRK5 enhances β-adrenergic receptor desensitization and attenuates the receptor's response to catecholamine stimulation. The authors proposed that in the setting of catecholamine stimulation, ventricular ballooning might result from either a negative inotropic effect due to β-receptor uncoupling, or from ischemia resulting from an imbalance between α1-adrenergic coronary vasoconstriction and β-adrenergic vasodilation. While larger genetic studies are warranted, these initial reports suggest the exciting possibility that individual susceptibility to SCM may in part be genetically based.

10.11 Conclusion

In just a few short years, SCM has emerged from relative obscurity and has become a widely recognized and accepted clinical syndrome. It is now clear that SCM occurs fairly commonly and that cardiac contractile abnormalities can be precipitated by a wide variety of emotional and physical triggers. Despite the increasing awareness of this syndrome, the optimal management of patients with SCM remains completely unclear. A variety of both medical and psychological treatments have been proposed, but a significant benefit from any intervention will be difficult to demonstrate with randomized clinical trials given the relatively low recurrence rate, rapid recovery, and good prognosis that are characteristic of this condition. While the precise mechanism of SCM remains unknown, there is increasing evidence that enhanced sympathetic stimulation underlies the pathogenesis of this syndrome. Exciting challenges for the future will include not only elucidating the precise cellular and molecular mechanisms of stress-induced myocardial stunning, but also identifying those risk factors that increase individual susceptibility to this unique disorder.

References

1. Engel GL. Sudden and rapid death during psychological stress. Folklore or folk wisdom? *Ann Intern Med.* 1971;74:771-782.
2. Lecomte D, Fornes P, Nicolas G. Stressful events as a trigger of sudden death: a study of 43 medico-legal autopsy cases. *Forensic Sci Int.* 1996;79:1-10.
3. Leor J, Poole WK, Kloner RA. Sudden cardiac death triggered by an earthquake. *N Engl J Med.* 1996;334:413-419.
4. Meisel SR, Kutz I, Dayan KI, et al. Effect of Iraqi missile war on incidence of acute myocardial infarction and sudden death in Israeli civilians. *Lancet.* 1991;338:660-661.
5. Wilbert-Lampen U, Leistner D, Greven S, et al. Cardiovascular events during World Cup soccer. *N Engl J Med.* 2008;358:475-483.
6. Mittleman MA, Maclure M, Sherwood JB, et al. Triggering of acute myocardial infarction onset by episodes of anger. Determinants of myocardial infarction onset study investigators. *Circulation.* 1995;92:1720-1725.
7. Steptoe A, Strike PC, Perkins-Porras L, McEwan JR, Whitehead DL. Acute depressed mood as a trigger of acute coronary syndromes. *Biol Psychiatry.* 2006;60:837-842.
8. Yeung AC, Vekshtein VI, Krantz DS, et al. The effect of atherosclerosis on the vasomotor response of coronary arteries to mental stress. *N Engl J Med.* 1991;325:1551-1556.
9. Burke AP, Farb A, Malcom GT, Liang Y, Smialek JE, Virmani R. Plaque rupture and sudden death related to exertion in men with coronary artery disease. *JAMA.* 1999;281:921-926.
10. Steinberg JS, Arshad A, Kowalski M, et al. Increased incidence of life-threatening ventricular arrhythmias in implantable defibrillator patients after the world trade center attack. *J Am Coll Cardiol.* 2004;44:1261-1264.

11. Satoh H, Tateishi H, Uchida T, et al. Takotsubo-type cardiomyopathy due to multivessel spasm. In: Kodama K, Haze K, Hon M, eds. *Clinical Aspect of Myocardial Injury, from Ischemia to Heart Failure (in Japanese)*. Tokyo: Kagakuhyouronsya Co; 1990:56-64.

12. Wittstein IS, Thiemann DR, Lima JA, et al. Neurohumoral features of myocardial stunning due to sudden emotional stress. *N Engl J Med*. 2005;352:539-548.

13. Tsuchihashi K, Ueshima K, Uchida T, et al. Transient left ventricular apical ballooning without coronary artery stenosis: a novel heart syndrome mimicking acute myocardial infarction. Angina pectoris-myocardial infarction investigations in Japan. *J Am Coll Cardiol*. 2001;38:11-18.

14. Cebelin MS, Hirsch CS. Human stress cardiomyopathy. Myocardial lesions in victims of homicidal assaults without internal injuries. *Hum Pathol*. 1980;11:123-132.

15. Pavin D, Le Breton H, Daubert C. Human stress cardiomyopathy mimicking acute myocardial syndrome. *Heart*. 1997;78:509-511.

16. Brandspiegel HZ, Marinchak RA, Rials SJ, Kowey PR. A broken heart. *Circulation*. 1998;98:1349.

17. Sharkey SW, Lesser JR, Zenovich AG, et al. Acute and reversible cardiomyopathy provoked by stress in women from the United States. *Circulation*. 2005;111:472-479.

18. Hurst RT, Askew JW, Reuss CS, et al. Transient midventricular ballooning syndrome: a new variant. *J Am Coll Cardiol*. 2006;48:579-583.

19. Reuss CS, Lester SJ, Hurst RT, et al. Isolated left ventricular basal ballooning phenotype of transient cardiomyopathy in young women. *Am J Cardiol*. 2007;99:1451-1453.

20. Akashi YJ, Musha H, Kida K, et al. Reversible ventricular dysfunction takotsubo cardiomyopathy. *Eur J Heart Fail*. 2005;7:1171-1176.

21. Ito K, Sugihara H, Katoh S, Azuma A, Nakagawa M. Assessment of takotsubo (ampulla) cardiomyopathy using 99mTc-tetrofosmin myocardial SPECT – comparison with acute coronary syndrome. *Ann Nucl Med*. 2003;17:115-122.

22. Matsuoka K, Okubo S, Fujii E, et al. Evaluation of the arrhythmogenecity of stress-induced "takotsubo cardiomyopathy" from the time course of the 12-lead surface electrocardiogram. *Am J Cardiol*. 2003;92:230-233.

23. Wedekind H, Moller K, Scholz KH. Tako-tsubo cardiomyopathy. Incidence in patients with acute coronary syndrome. *Herz*. 2006;31:339-346.

24. Haghi D, Athanasiadis A, Papavassiliu T, et al. Right ventricular involvement in takotsubo cardiomyopathy. *Eur Heart J*. 2006;27:2433-2439.

25. Kurowski V, Kaiser A, von Hof K, et al. Apical and midventricular transient left ventricular dysfunction syndrome (tako-tsubo cardiomyopathy): frequency, mechanisms, and prognosis. *Chest*. 2007;132:809-816.

26. Pilliere R, Mansencal N, Digne F, Lacombe P, Joseph T, Dubourg O. Prevalence of tako-tsubo syndrome in a large urban agglomeration. *Am J Cardiol*. 2006;98:662-665.

27. Parodi G, Del Pace S, Carrabba N, et al. Incidence, clinical findings, and outcome of women with left ventricular apical ballooning syndrome. *Am J Cardiol*. 2007;99:182-185.

28. Azzarelli S, Galassi AR, Amico F, et al. Clinical features of transient left ventricular apical ballooning. *Am J Cardiol*. 2006;98:1273-1276.

29. Buja P, Zuin G, Di Pede F, et al. Long-term outcome and sex distribution across ages of left ventricular apical ballooning syndrome. *J Cardiovasc Med*. 2008;9:905-909.

30. Cangella F, Medolla A, De Fazio G, et al. Stress induced cardiomyopathy presenting as acute coronary syndrome: tako-tsubo in Mercogliano, southern Italy. *Cardiovasc Ultrasound*. 2007;5:36.

31. Spedicato L, Zanuttini D, Nucifora G, et al. Transient left ventricular apical ballooning syndrome: a 4-year experience. *J Cardiovasc Med*. 2008;9:916-921.

32. Previtali M, Repetto A, Panigada S, Camporotondo R, Tavazzi L. Left ventricular apical ballooning syndrome: prevalence, clinical characteristics and pathogenetic mechanisms in a European population. *Int J Cardiol*. 2009;134:91-96.

33. Elian D, Osherov A, Matetzky S, et al. Left ventricular apical ballooning: not an uncommon variant of acute myocardial infarction in women. *Clin Cardiol*. 2006;29:9-12.

34. Eshtehardi P, Koestner SC, Adorjan P, et al. Transient apical ballooning syndrome – clinical characteristics, ballooning pattern, and long-term follow-up in a Swiss population. *Int J Cardiol.* 2009;135:370-375.

35. Bybee KA, Prasad A, Barsness GW, et al. Clinical characteristics and thrombolysis in myocardial infarction frame counts in women with transient left ventricular apical ballooning syndrome. *Am J Cardiol.* 2004;94:343-346.

36. Strunk B, Shaw RE, Bull S, et al. High incidence of focal left ventricular wall motion abnormalities and normal coronary arteries in patients with myocardial infarctions presenting to a community hospital. *J Invasive Cardiol.* 2006;18:376-381.

37. Larson DM, Menssen KM, Sharkey SW, et al. "False-positive" cardiac catheterization laboratory activation among patients with suspected ST-segment elevation myocardial infarction. *JAMA.* 2007;298:2754-2760.

38. Wittstein IS. Acute stress cardiomyopathy. *Curr Heart Fail Rep.* 2008;5:61-68.

39. Park JH, Kang SJ, Song JK, et al. Left ventricular apical ballooning due to severe physical stress in patients admitted to the medical ICU. *Chest.* 2005;128:296-302.

40. Ibanez B, Navarro F, Farre J, et al. Tako-tsubo syndrome associated with a long course of the left anterior descending coronary artery along the apical diaphragmatic surface of the left ventricle. *Rev Esp Cardiol.* 2004;57:209-216.

41. Fazio G, Barbaro G, Sutera L, et al. Clinical findings of takotsubo cardiomyopathy: results from a multicenter international study. *J Cardiovasc Med.* 2008;9:239-244.

42. Elesber A, Lerman A, Bybee KA, et al. Myocardial perfusion in apical ballooning syndrome correlate of myocardial injury. *Am Heart J.* 2006;152:469.e9-469.e13.

43. Nunez-Gil IJ, Fernandez-Ortiz A, Perez-Isla L, et al. Clinical and prognostic comparison between left ventricular transient dyskinesia and a first non-ST-segment elevation acute coronary syndrome. *Coron Artery Dis.* 2008;19:449-453.

44. Parodi G, Del Pace S, Salvadori C, Carrabba N, Olivotto I, Gensini GF. Left ventricular apical ballooning syndrome as a novel cause of acute mitral regurgitation. *J Am Coll Cardiol.* 2007;50:647-649.

45. Regnante RA, Zuzek RW, Weinsier SB, et al. Clinical characteristics and four-year outcomes of patients in the Rhode Island Takotsubo Cardiomyopathy Registry. *Am J Cardiol.* 2009;103: 1015-1019.

46. Hoyt J, Lerman A, Lennon RJ, Rihal CS, Prasad A. Left anterior descending artery length and coronary atherosclerosis in apical ballooning syndrome (takotsubo/stress induced cardiomyopathy). *Int J Cardiol.* 2010;145:112-115.

47. Elesber AA, Prasad A, Lennon RJ, Wright RS, Lerman A, Rihal CS. Four-year recurrence rate and prognosis of the apical ballooning syndrome. *J Am Coll Cardiol.* 2007;50:448-452.

48. Singh NK, Rumman S, Mikell FL, Nallamothu N, Rangaswamy C. Stress cardiomyopathy: clinical and ventriculographic characteristics in 107 North American subjects. *Int J Cardiol.* 2010;141:297-303.

49. Sharkey SW, Windenburg DC, Lesser JR, et al. Natural history and expansive clinical profile of stress (tako-tsubo) cardiomyopathy. *J Am Coll Cardiol.* 2010;55:333-341.

50. Pilgrim TM, Wyss TR. Takotsubo cardiomyopathy or transient left ventricular apical ballooning syndrome: a systematic review. *Int J Cardiol.* 2008;124:283-292.

51. Mudd JO, Kapur NK, Champion HC, Schulman SP, Wittstein IS. Patients with stress-induced (takotsubo) cardiomyopathy have an increased prevalence of mood disorders and antidepressant use compared to patients with acute myocardial infarction. *J Card Fail.* 2007;13(suppl 2):S176.

52. Gianni M, Dentali F, Grandi AM, Sumner G, Hiralal R, Lonn E. Apical ballooning syndrome or takotsubo cardiomyopathy: a systematic review. *Eur Heart J.* 2006;27:1523-1529.

53. Kawai S, Kitabatake A, Tomoike H. Guidelines for diagnosis of takotsubo (ampulla) cardiomyopathy. *Circ J.* 2007;71:990-992.

54. Novo S, Akashi Y, Arbustini E, et al. Takotsubo cardiomyopathy: a consensus document. *G Ital Cardiol.* 2008;9:785-797.

55. Prasad A, Lerman A, Rihal CS. Apical ballooning syndrome (tako-tsubo or stress cardiomyopathy): a mimic of acute myocardial infarction. *Am Heart J.* 2008;155:408-417.

56. Otomo S, Sugita M, Shimoda O, Terasaki H. Two cases of transient left ventricular apical ballooning syndrome associated with subarachnoid hemorrhage. *Anesth Analg*. 2006;103: 583-586.
57. Lemke DM, Hussain SI, Wolfe TJ, et al. Takotsubo cardiomyopathy associated with seizures. *Neurocrit Care*. 2008;9:112-117.
58. Yoshimura S, Toyoda K, Ohara T, et al. Takotsubo cardiomyopathy in acute ischemic stroke. *Ann Neurol*. 2008;64:547-554.
59. Sharkey SW, Lesser JR, Menon M, Parpart M, Maron MS, Maron BJ. Spectrum and significance of electrocardiographic patterns, troponin levels, and thrombolysis in myocardial infarction frame count in patients with stress (tako-tsubo) cardiomyopathy and comparison to those in patients with ST-elevation anterior wall myocardial infarction. *Am J Cardiol*. 2008; 101:1723-1728.
60. Bybee KA, Motiei A, Syed IS, et al. Electrocardiography cannot reliably differentiate transient left ventricular apical ballooning syndrome from anterior ST-segment elevation myocardial infarction. *J Electrocardiol*. 2007;40:38.e1-38.e6.
61. Ogura R, Hiasa Y, Takahashi T, et al. Specific findings of the standard 12-lead ECG in patients with 'Takotsubo' cardiomyopathy: comparison with the findings of acute anterior myocardial infarction. *Circ J*. 2003;67:687-690.
62. Mitsuma W, Kodama M, Ito M, et al. Serial electrocardiographic findings in women with takotsubo cardiomyopathy. *Am J Cardiol*. 2007;100:106-109.
63. Hahn JY, Gwon HC, Park SW, et al. The clinical features of transient left ventricular nonapical ballooning syndrome: comparison with apical ballooning syndrome. *Am Heart J*. 2007;154: 1166-1173.
64. Abraham J, Mudd JO, Kapur NK, Klein K, Champion HC, Wittstein IS. Stress cardiomyopathy after intravenous administration of catecholamines and beta-receptor agonists. *J Am Coll Cardiol*. 2009;53:1320-1325.
65. Novaro GM, Almahameed S. Release pattern of cardiac troponin in left ventricular apical ballooning syndrome: insights into the mechanisms of stress cardiomyopathy. *Int J Cardiol*. 2008;131:e31-e32.
66. Winchester DE, Ragosta M, Taylor AM. Concurrence of angiographic coronary artery disease in patients with apical ballooning syndrome (tako-tsubo cardiomyopathy). *Catheter Cardiovasc Interv*. 2008;72:612-616.
67. Elesber AA, Prasad A, Bybee KA, et al. Transient cardiac apical ballooning syndrome: prevalence and clinical implications of right ventricular involvement. *J Am Coll Cardiol*. 2006; 47:1082-1083.
68. Kitaoka T, Ogawa Y, Kato J, et al. Takotsubo-like left ventricular dysfunction with delayed recovery of left ventricular shape: a case report. *J Cardiol*. 2006;47:197-205.
69. Haghi D, Fluechter S, Suselbeck T, Kaden JJ, Borggrefe M, Papavassiliu T. Cardiovascular magnetic resonance findings in typical versus atypical forms of the acute apical ballooning syndrome (takotsubo cardiomyopathy). *Int J Cardiol*. 2007;120:205-211.
70. Eitel I, Behrendt F, Schindler K, et al. Differential diagnosis of suspected apical ballooning syndrome using contrast-enhanced magnetic resonance imaging. *Eur Heart J*. 2008;29: 2651-2659.
71. Leurent G, Larralde A, Boulmier D, et al. Cardiac MRI studies of transient left ventricular apical ballooning syndrome (takotsubo cardiomyopathy): a systematic review. *Int J Cardiol*. 2009;135:146-149.
72. Yoshida T, Hibino T, Kako N, et al. A pathophysiologic study of tako-tsubo cardiomyopathy with F-18 fluorodeoxyglucose positron emission tomography. *Eur Heart J*. 2007;28:2598-2604.
73. Cimarelli S, Sauer F, Morel O, Ohlmann P, Constantinesco A, Imperiale A. Transient left ventricular dysfunction syndrome: patho-physiological bases through nuclear medicine imaging. *Int J Cardiol*. 2010;144:212-218.
74. Feola M, Rosso GL, Casasso F, et al. Reversible inverse mismatch in transient left ventricular apical ballooning: perfusion/metabolism positron emission tomography imaging. *J Nucl Cardiol*. 2006;13:587-590.

75. Bybee KA, Murphy J, Prasad A, et al. Acute impairment of regional myocardial glucose uptake in the apical ballooning (takotsubo) syndrome. *J Nucl Cardiol.* 2006;13:244-250.
76. Prasad A, Madhavan M, Chareonthaitawee P. Cardiac sympathetic activity in stress-induced (takotsubo) cardiomyopathy. *Nat Rev Cardiol.* 2009;6:430-434.
77. Burgdorf C, von Hof K, Schunkert H, Kurowski V. Regional alterations in myocardial sympathetic innervation in patients with transient left-ventricular apical ballooning (tako-tsubo cardiomyopathy). *J Nucl Cardiol.* 2008;15:65-72.
78. Akashi YJ, Nakazawa K, Sakakibara M, Miyake F, Musha H, Sasaka K. 123I-MIBG myocardial scintigraphy in patients with "takotsubo" cardiomyopathy. *J Nucl Med.* 2004;45:1121-1127.
79. Moriya M, Mori H, Suzuki N, Hazama M, Yano K. Six-month follow-up of takotsubo cardiomyopathy with I-123-beta-metyl-iodophenyl pentadecanoic acid and I-123-meta-iodobenzyl-guanidine myocardial scintigraphy. *Intern Med.* 2002;41:829-833.
80. Yoshioka T, Hashimoto A, Tsuchihashi K, et al. Clinical implications of midventricular obstruction and intravenous propranolol use in transient left ventricular apical ballooning (tako-tsubo cardiomyopathy). *Am Heart J.* 2008;155:526-527.
81. Madhavan M, Borlaug BA, Lerman A, Rihal CS, Prasad A. Stress hormone and circulating biomarker profile of apical ballooning syndrome (takotsubo cardiomyopathy): insights into the clinical significance of B-type natriuretic peptide and troponin levels. *Heart.* 2009;95:1436-1441.
82. Kume T, Kawamoto T, Okura H, et al. Local release of catecholamines from the hearts of patients with tako-tsubo-like left ventricular dysfunction. *Circ J.* 2008;72:106-108.
83. Ortak J, Khattab K, Barantke M, et al. Evolution of cardiac autonomic nervous activity indices in patients presenting with transient left ventricular apical ballooning. *Pacing Clin Electrophysiol.* 2009;32(Suppl 1):S21-S25.
84. Sandhu G, Servetnyk Z, Croitor S, Herzog E. Atropine aggravates signs and symptoms of takotsubo cardiomyopathy. *Am J Emerg Med.* 2010;28:258.e5-258.e7.
85. Takizawa M, Kobayakawa N, Uozumi H, et al. A case of transient left ventricular ballooning with pheochromocytoma, supporting pathogenetic role of catecholamines in stress-induced cardiomyopathy or takotsubo cardiomyopathy. *Int J Cardiol.* 2007;114:e15-e17.
86. Van Spall HG, Roberts JD, Sawka AM, Swallow CJ, Mak S. Not a broken heart. *Lancet.* 2007;370:628.
87. Ueyama T, Kasamatsu K, Hano T, Yamamoto K, Tsuruo Y, Nishio I. Emotional stress induces transient left ventricular hypocontraction in the rat via activation of cardiac adrenoceptors: a possible animal model of 'tako-tsubo' cardiomyopathy. *Circ J.* 2002;66:712-713.
88. Izumi Y, Okatani H, Shiota M, et al. Effects of metoprolol on epinephrine-induced takotsubo-like left ventricular dysfunction in non-human primates. *Hypertens Res.* 2009;32:339-346.
89. Bhattacharyya MR, Steptoe A. Emotional triggers of acute coronary syndromes: strength of evidence, biological processes, and clinical implications. *Prog Cardiovasc Dis.* 2007;49:353-365.
90. Ibanez B, Navarro F, Cordoba M, Alberca P, Farre J. Tako-tsubo transient left ventricular apical ballooning: is intravascular ultrasound the key to resolve the enigma? *Heart.* 2005;91:102-104.
91. Martinez-Selles M, Datino T, Pello AM, Fernandez-Aviles F. Ergonovine provocative test in Caucasian patients with left ventricular apical ballooning syndrome. *Int J Cardiol.* 2010;145:89-91.
92. Kume T, Akasaka T, Kawamoto T, et al. Assessment of coronary microcirculation in patients with takotsubo-like left ventricular dysfunction. *Circ J.* 2005;69:934-939.
93. Meimoun P, Malaquin D, Sayah S, et al. The coronary flow reserve is transiently impaired in tako-tsubo cardiomyopathy: a prospective study using serial Doppler transthoracic echocardiography. *J Am Soc Echocardiogr.* 2008;21:72-77.
94. Rigo F, Sicari R, Citro R, Ossena G, Buja P, Picano E. Diffuse, marked, reversible impairment in coronary microcirculation in stress cardiomyopathy: a Doppler transthoracic echo study. *Ann Med.* 2009;41:462-470.

95. Uchida Y, Egami H, Uchida Y, et al. Possible participation of endothelial cell apoptosis of coronary microvessels in the genesis of takotsubo cardiomyopathy. *Clin Cardiol*. 2010;33: 371-377.

96. Lyon AR, Rees PS, Prasad S, Poole-Wilson PA, Harding SE. Stress (takotsubo) cardiomyopathy – a novel pathophysiological hypothesis to explain catecholamine-induced acute myocardial stunning. *Nat Clin Pract Cardiovasc Med*. 2008;5:22-29.

97. Mann DL, Kent RL, Parsons B, Cooper G. Adrenergic effects on the biology of the adult mammalian cardiocyte. *Circulation*. 1992;85:790-804.

98. Nef HM, Mollmann H, Kostin S, et al. Tako-tsubo cardiomyopathy: intraindividual structural analysis in the acute phase and after functional recovery. *Eur Heart J*. 2007;28:2456-2464.

99. Nef HM, Mollmann H, Troidl C, et al. Abnormalities in intracellular Ca2+ regulation contribute to the pathomechanism of tako-tsubo cardiomyopathy. *Eur Heart J*. 2009;30:2155-2164.

100. Ellison GM, Torella D, Karakikes I, et al. Acute beta-adrenergic overload produces myocyte damage through calcium leakage from the ryanodine receptor 2 but spares cardiac stem cells. *J Biol Chem*. 2007;282:11397-11409.

101. Lavi S, Nevo O, Thaler I, et al. Effect of aging on the cardiovascular regulatory systems in healthy women. *Am J Physiol Regul Integr Comp Physiol*. 2007;292:R788-R793.

102. Sung BH, Ching M, Izzo JL Jr, Dandona P, Wilson MF. Estrogen improves abnormal norepinephrine-induced vasoconstriction in postmenopausal women. *J Hypertens*. 1999;17: 523-528.

103. Komesaroff PA, Esler MD, Sudhir K. Estrogen supplementation attenuates glucocorticoid and catecholamine responses to mental stress in perimenopausal women. *J Clin Endocrinol Metab*. 1999;84:606-610.

104. Ueyama T, Ishikura F, Matsuda A, et al. Chronic estrogen supplementation following ovariectomy improves the emotional stress-induced cardiovascular responses by indirect action on the nervous system and by direct action on the heart. *Circ J*. 2007;71:565-573.

105. Cevik C, Nugent K. The role of cardiac autonomic control in the pathogenesis of tako-tsubo cardiomyopathy. *Am Heart J*. 2008;156:e31.

106. Barton DA, Dawood T, Lambert EA, et al. Sympathetic activity in major depressive disorder: identifying those at increased risk? *J Hypertens*. 2007;25:2117-2124.

107. Barletta G, Del Pace S, Boddi M, et al. Abnormal coronary reserve and left ventricular wall motion during cold pressor test in patients with previous left ventricular ballooning syndrome. *Eur Heart J*. 2009;30:3007-3014.

108. Pison L, De Vusser P, Mullens W. Apical ballooning in relatives. *Heart*. 2004;90:e67.

109. Zaroff JG, Pawlikowska L, Miss JC, et al. Adrenoceptor polymorphisms and the risk of cardiac injury and dysfunction after subarachnoid hemorrhage. *Stroke*. 2006;37:1680-1685.

110. Sharkey SW, Maron BJ, Nelson P, Parpart M, Maron MS, Bristow MR. Adrenergic receptor polymorphisms in patients with stress (tako-tsubo) cardiomyopathy. *J Cardiol*. 2009;53: 53-57.

111. Spinelli L, Trimarco V, Di Marino S, Marino M, Iaccarino G, Trimarco B. L41Q polymorphism of the G protein coupled receptor kinase 5 is associated with left ventricular apical ballooning syndrome. *Eur J Heart Fail*. 2010;12:13-16.

Part III
Chronic Stress

Chapter 11
Psychosocial Factors at Work: The Epidemiological Perspective

Mika Kivimäki, Archana Singh-Manoux, G. David Batty, Marianna Virtanen, Jane E. Ferrie, and Jussi Vahtera

Keywords Psychosocial factors • Epidemiological perspective • INTERHEART study • Prospective analysis • Long-term exposure • Iso-strain • Coronary heart disease

11.1 Introduction

The belief that adverse psychosocial work factors or "stresses at work" affect health is widespread in the general public and media. Coronary heart disease (CHD) is a leading cause of mortality and disability in the industrialised world and the health outcome, which has been most commonly related to work stress. Interestingly, however, the status of psychosocial factors at work as a cause of CHD is still a controversial issue, despite evidence accumulated over decades. This is exemplified by the fact that psychosocial stress at work is not included in the list of CHD risk factors in most clinical guidelines,[1-4] although psychosocial factors were mentioned in European guidelines on cardiovascular disease prevention in clinical practice.[5]

In this chapter, we review current evidence on psychosocial stress at work as a risk factor for CHD, highlighting the strengths and limitations in the research. We

M. Kivimäki (✉) • G.D. Batty • J.E. Ferrie
Department of Epidemiology and Public Health, University College London, London, UK
e-mail: m.kivimaki@ucl.ac.uk

A. Singh-Manoux
Centre for Research in Epidemiology & Population Health, Hôpitaux de Paris,
Villejuif Cedex, France

M. Virtanen
Unit of Expertise for Work Organizations, Finnish Institute of Occupational Health,
Helsinki, Finland

J. Vahtera
Department of Public Health, University of Turku and Turku University Hospital, Turku, Finland

P. Hjemdahl et al. (eds.), *Stress and Cardiovascular Disease*,
DOI 10.1007/978-1-84882-419-5_11, © Springer-Verlag London Limited 2012

summarise the data syntheses from the most recent systematic reviews and findings from the seminal studies. To facilitate a balanced evaluation, we also undertake horizontal comparisons, whereby we contrast the existing evidence on psychosocial factors at work with that related to other emerging or established risk factors for CHD. As a prelude we briefly describe the leading theoretical models of psychosocial stress at work.

11.2 The Main Theoretical Models of Psychosocial Factors at Work

What are the most important psychosocial risk factors at work? In general terms, they refer to the aspects of work design, organization, and management and their social and organizational contexts, that have the potential to cause harm to employee health.[6] The main theoretical models aim to describe those psychosocial factors that are likely to elicit harmful stress at work in a significant proportion of employees, but are still specific enough to help design interventions.[7] These factors are conceptualized at a level of generalization that allows for their identification in a wide range of occupations.

The model of psychosocial factors at work most often cited and most widely tested is the two-dimensional job strain model.[8] It proposes that employees who simultaneously have high job demands and low control over work are in a job strain situation which, if prolonged, increases the risk of stress-related diseases. Job control refers to both socially predetermined control over detailed aspects of task performance (e.g., pace, quantity of work, policies and procedures and scheduled hours) and skill discretion (i.e., control over the use of skills by the worker). An expanded version of the job strain model adds social support to the model as a third component. The highest risk of illness is assumed to relate to iso-strain jobs (abbreviation of isolated job strain), characterised by high demands, low job control and low social support.

More recent theoretical models have broadened the view from sole work characteristics to cover aspects of the person and the labour market context. A promising example is the effort–reward imbalance model.[9] This model maintains that the experience of imbalance between high effort spent at work and a perception of low reward received is particularly stressful, as this imbalance violates core expectations about reciprocity and adequate exchange at work. Not only high demands and challenges at work, but also over-commitment and heavy obligations in private life (e.g., large debts) may contribute to a high expenditure of effort. Low rewards can be related to insufficient pay, low esteem (e.g., lack of help or acceptance by supervisors and colleagues) and poor career opportunities (no promotion prospects, poor job security and status inconsistency).

While effort–reward imbalance defines disproportionate costs for an employee in terms of gains received, that is, a distributive injustice condition, the latest research on psychosocial factors at work has also focussed on other aspects of justice. Procedural justice assesses whether decision-making procedures include input from affected parties, are consistently applied, suppress bias, are accurate, are correctable and are ethical. Relational justice refers to treatment of individuals with fairness, politeness and consideration by supervisors. As justice is a fundamental value in social interactions and the organization of society, enduring problems in procedural and relational justice have been hypothesized to form an important source of stress at work, and constitute the organizational injustice model.[10,11]

11.3 The INTERHEART Study

Recent evidence from the INTERHEART study shows that psychosocial factors were associated with acute myocardial infarction in a study on 15,000 cases and controls from 52 countries in Europe, America, Africa, Asia and Australia.[12] The study found that smoking, raised ApoB/ApoA1 ratio, history of hypertension, diabetes, abdominal obesity, low consumption of fruits and vegetables, lack of physical activity and psychosocial factors, including work stress, were all strongly related to acute myocardial infarction. As shown in Fig. 11.1, exposure to psychosocial factors added to risk even after taking into account the combined exposure to smoking, diabetes, hypertension, ApoB/ApoA1 ratio and obesity; the odds ratio

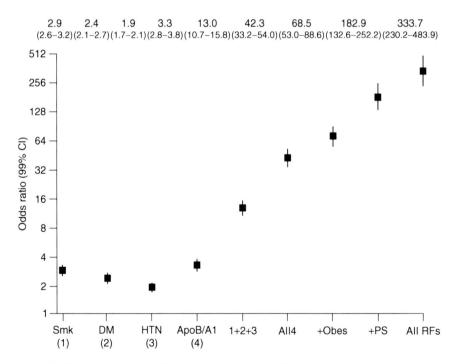

Fig. 11.1 Risk of acute myocardial infarction associated with exposure to multiple risk factors. *Smk* smoking, *DM* diabetes mellitus, *HTN* hypertension, *Obes* abdominal obesity, *PS* psychosocial, *RF* risk factors. (Reproduced with permission from the Yusuf et al.[12])

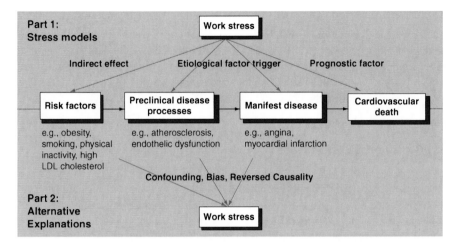

Fig. 11.2 Hypothesized pathways from psychosocial factors to CHD and alternative explanations to this association (Adapted from Kivimaki et al.[13], with permission from the Journal)

increased from 68.5 to 182.9 compared with those free from all these risk factors. These findings were remarkably robust. A similar pattern of associations were found in men and women, old and young, and in all continents of the world.

The INTERHEART study is clearly the largest study in the field. However, given that myocardial infarction is typically preceded by a long subclinical phase of atherosclerosis development, a case–control study, irrespective of its size, is not in a strong position to rule out the possibility that the perception of psychosocial stress is, in fact, a consequence of disease process rather than a cause (Fig. 11.2, Part 2). More specifically, people with advanced atherosclerosis may experience exhaustion more easily than others and therefore attribute their environments as being more demanding than those who are more physically fit. Thus, an important step in the determination of causality is to work out the temporal order of the association between psychosocial factors and CHD using prospective study designs.

11.4 Review of Prospective Evidence

Considering the robust evidence from the INTERHEART study and a number of other studies, there is little doubt about the existence of an association between psychosocial factors and CHD. However, given the problems of information bias in case–control studies – that is, the concern that the assessment of psychosocial factors may be influenced by existing CHD – we limit the following review to prospective cohort studies where this issue is less problematic. Systematic reviews are commonly used to synthesise evidence on relationship. We utilise two recent systematic reviews, and also describe individual high-quality cohort studies that are considered to be key papers in the field.

11.4.1 Meta-analysis

There are several reviews available that have summarised evidence from prospective studies on psychosocial factors at work and CHD.[13-15] Most of these are narrative with only one providing quantitative estimates based on a meta-analysis. The meta-analysis,[13] published in January 2006, includes papers on job strain, effort–reward imbalance and organizational injustice from 14 prospective cohort studies with follow-up periods ranging from 3 years to over 25 years. The findings show that employees exposed to psychosocial risk factors at work (job strain, effort–reward imbalance and organizational injustice) have an average 50% excess risk for CHD compared to those unexposed. An age- and sex-adjusted summary estimate of the relative risk across studies on job strain was 1.5 (95% CI 1.2–1.8) with eight of the ten individual studies reporting either a significant association or an association that was nonsignificant but in the expected direction. In two studies was a nonsignificant inverse association observed (i.e., higher psychosocial risk estimates were associated with lower CHD risk). Multiple adjustments for other risk factors considerably attenuated the overall estimate and it was no longer statistically significant, relative risk $= 1.16$ (95% CI 0.94–1.43, n.s.) (Fig. 11.3). It has been argued that some of the adjusted risk factors were actually mediators of the association between job strain and CHD, leading to overadjustment (see Sect. 11.4.2.4).

Four independent studies were identified for the effort–reward imbalance model.[13] The summary estimate for these studies suggests an age- and sex-adjusted excess risk for employees reporting high effort and low reward (relative risk 1.6; 95% CI 0.8–3.0, n.s.). This overall relative risk was slightly enhanced after multiple adjustments for other CHD risk factors; RR 2.1, 95% CI 1.0–4.3 ($p < 0.05$). The two studies of organizational injustice and CHD reported an age- and sex-adjusted relative risk of 1.6 (95% CI 1.2–2.1), an estimate that remained statistically significant after additional adjustment for other risk factors, including job strain and effort–reward imbalance (1.5, 95% CI 1.2–2.0).

Of particular note in the above figures are the substantial differences in the magnitudes of the associations between studies. This heterogeneity was confirmed statistically for job strain and for effort–reward imbalance, but such a test was not meaningful for organizational injustice due to the low number of studies.[13] Reasons for this heterogeneity remain unclear. One hypothesis is that the excess risk may be dependent on sex, the association being more consistent for men than women. It is also possible that age and measurement of the exposure are important sources of heterogeneity.[16-18] In a Swedish study, for example, including older age individuals in a cohort used to assess job strain attenuated the findings towards the null.[17] Thus, in the 19–55-year age group, participants with job strain had a 1.8 (95% CI 1.1–2.9) times higher age-adjusted risk of incident ischaemic (coronary or cerebrovascular) disease than those free of strain. The impact of job strain was reduced by 70% and was no longer statistically significant after the inclusion of employees older than 55 years in the analysis (hazard ratio 1.2, 95% CI 0.8–2.0).

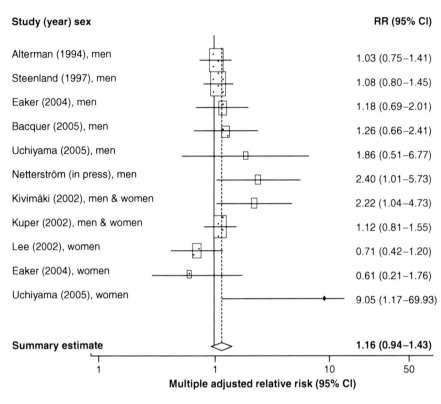

Fig. 11.3 Meta-analysis of prospective studies on job strain: Multivariable adjusted relative risk of incident CHD or cardiovascular events and its summary estimate (*m* male study population, *w* female study population) (Reproduced with permission from the Kivimaki et al.[13])

11.4.2 High-Quality Papers

Variation in methodological quality is recognised as a source of heterogeneity in findings in epidemiological studies. Thus, instead of extracting summary estimates across all studies, selecting the best papers may improve the estimation of true effect size. The most recent systematic review did not include a meta-analysis, but assessed the quality of articles published till 2008 on work-related psychosocial factors and ischaemic heart disease.[15] In that qualitative review, the following issues were evaluated to construct a summary score for study quality (range 0–11 points):

(a) Validity of exposure assessment (0–2 points)
(b) Validity of endpoint assessment (0–2 points)
(c) Ascertainment of CHD-free status at baseline (0 or 1)
(d) Representativeness of working population (0 or 1)
(e) Coverage of full age range (0 or 1)
(f) Follow-up less than 10 years (0 or 1)
(g) Sex-specific analysis (0 or 1)
(h) Adjustment for potential confounding factors (0–2 points)

Of the 33 prospective and case–control studies, only one received the maximum quality score of 11 and three studies reached a score of 9 or 10. The quality score did, however, not take sample size and statistical power (i.e., the possibility to detect differences in outcome) into account. A brief description of these high-quality prospective studies, starting from the one with the best score, follows:

In the Belgian Job Stress Project Cohort, a total of 14,000 middle-aged men from 21 worksites completed the standard Job Content Questionnaire and participated in a clinical examination of standard coronary risk factors (age, body mass index, blood pressure, total and LDL cholesterol and diabetes).[19] Clinical manifest coronary events were ascertained over a 3-year period and they included the occurrence of acute myocardial infarction, unstable angina and hospitalisation for coronary artery bypass grafting or percutaneous transluminal coronary angioplasty. The total number of coronary events in the study was 87, of which 20 cases were fatal myocardial infarctions. Job strain was associated with a 1.5-fold (95% CI 0.9–2.5) age-adjusted risk of incident coronary events. Multiple adjustments slightly attenuated this nonsignificant relative risk, the fully adjusted hazard ratio being 1.4 (95% CI 0.8–2.4), and thus also not statistically significant. The corresponding age-adjusted and fully adjusted figures for iso-strain were 1.9 (95% CI 1.1–3.4) and 1.9 (95% CI 1.1–3.5), respectively. However, the study was underpowered with only 18 events among employees with job strain and 14 events among those with iso-strain.

Two of the remaining "high-quality" studies come from Sweden. The first was on a cohort consisting of 3,000 men and 4,700 women, the Malmö Diet and Cancer (MDC) study.[20] Inclusion criteria for the study of work-related psychosocial factors included continuous employment at the present worksite for 4 years or more (to ensure long-term exposure) and a clear position in the occupational hierarchy (that is, farmers and the self-employed were excluded). The baseline questionnaire included items on job demands, job control and social support, but a standard questionnaire was apparently not used. The almost 8-year follow-up for fatal or nonfatal myocardial infarction was based on record linkage with the National Myocardial Infarction Register. As the unadjusted hazard ratio for job strain was nonsignificant, 1.2 (95% CI 0.7–2.1) for men and 1.3 (0.4–3.9) for women, adjusted estimates were not provided. However, the authors reported a significant association between low social support at work and myocardial infarction among women (unadjusted hazard ratio 2.2, 95% CI 1.2–4.3; age, systolic blood pressure, diabetes and smoking adjusted hazard ratio 2.7, 95% 1.4–5.2). No corresponding association was seen among men and the reason for this sex-specific finding remains unclear.

In the second report from Sweden, data were drawn from the Work, Lipids, Fibrinogen (WOLF) Stockholm Study, a prospective cohort study of employees 19–65 years of age from 40 companies in the Stockholm area.[17] The sample included 3,160 men who participated in the baseline examination and job strain was measured with the Swedish Demand–Control Questionnaire, a widely used self-administered survey measure. To minimize reporting bias, the study was restricted to diagnoses of ischaemic heart disease based on objective criteria (e.g., electrocardiography, enzymes and computed tomography or magnetic resonance imaging). During the mean follow-up of 9.7 years, 93 individuals were diagnosed with ischaemic heart disease. The age-adjusted relative risk for job strain was 1.2 (0.7–2.1) and the study was not powered to show a small effect size with statistical significance.

The last of the four "high-quality" studies comes from Finland, the population-based Kuopio Ischemic Heart Disease Risk Factor Study of 2,300 middle-aged men screened for conventional CHD risk factors.[21] Workplace demands, resources and economic rewards were self-reported using non-validated scales. Acute myocardial infarction was ascertained by linkage to a national acute myocardial infarction register established under the WHO MONICA project. Cardiovascular mortality was assessed by linkage to national death registers. The follow-up periods for these two outcomes were 6 and 8 years respectively. During follow-up, 87 cases of fatal or nonfatal myocardial infarction and 93 cardiovascular deaths occurred. In age-adjusted analyses, a combination of high demands, low resources and low income was associated with a 2.6-fold (95% CI 1.4–4.9) increased risk of myocardial infarction and a 3.1-fold (95% CI 1.5–6.6) risk of cardiovascular death, compared to low demands, high resources and high income. However, after adjustment for behavioural, biological and other psychosocial covariates, the relative hazards were attenuated substantially, 1.6 (95% CI 0.8–3.2) and 1.5 (95% CI 0.7–3.5), respectively.

In sum, most of the "high-quality" studies selected by the authors of the most recent systematic review[15] found a modestly elevated risk of CHD among individuals exposed to adverse psychosocial factors at work, but this risk was rarely significant in the total population due to limited statistical power. The impact of potential confounding was clearly reported only in one study where the effect disappeared after adjustment for other CHD risk factors. Thus, the evidence from the "high-quality" studies seems to be consistent with the conclusions we draw in the meta-analysis published in 2006.

11.4.2.1   The Importance of Long-Term Exposure

The British Whitehall II study [22] is one of the principal studies on psychosocial factors and health. An important contribution of this study has been the use of longitudinal data from the study to demonstrate that poor measurement of long-term exposure to psychosocial factors is a potential source of false null findings.[23,24] As CHD develops over a long time span, long-term rather than short-term levels of adverse psychosocial factors are assumed to impact CHD incidence. Thus, when evaluating the dose–response relation for adverse effects of psychosocial risk factors, it is important to examine not only stimulus strength but also stimulus duration. For employees with stable psychosocial stress, a single measurement may provide an accurate estimate of long-term exposure. However, this is not necessarily the case for others and it is of note that all four "high-quality" studies described above were based on a single measurement of work-related psychosocial factors.

The target population in the Whitehall II study was London-based civil servants aged 35–55 years at baseline.[22] Repeated 5-yearly medical examinations and additional questionnaire surveys between these examinations at 2–3-year intervals included the measurement of job strain and its components. The correlation

Fig. 11.4 Dose–response association between iso-strain and incident CHD in the Whitehall II study of British civil servants. Hazard ratios are adjusted for age, sex, employment grade, hypertension, total cholesterol and smoking history (Source: Chandola et al.[18])

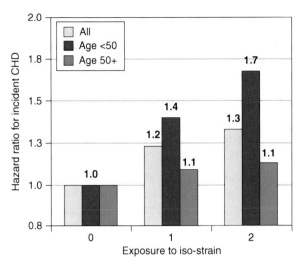

coefficients for the repeated measurements of stress indicators between the first two examinations were moderate, varying between Pearson $r = 0.45$ for job strain and $r = 0.72$ for job control.[23] In addition, short-term repeats, 1–2 months after the examination, were part of the measurement procedure to assess the repeatability of each measure. The regression dilution ratio, based on these short-term repeats, was 0.778 for job strain, 0.800 for work demands and 0.902 for lack of control.[23]

One report from the Whitehall II cohort exploited the short-term repeat data in order to minimize the error caused by instability in exposure measures.[23] In that study, we used Rosner"s formula to create a correction factor. For job strain and work demands, the corrected excess risk for CHD was 30% higher than the uncorrected estimate (the hazard ratio for a one standard deviation increase in job strain was 1.23 before the correction and 1.30 after). This suggests that the use of exposures measured only once may underestimate the importance of job strain as a CHD risk factor.

Further support for the importance of taking into account long-term exposure comes from two more recent Whitehall II reports, one focused on the metabolic syndrome,[24] a risk factor for CHD, and the other on CHD (Fig. 11.4).[18] In the first report, iso-strain was assessed four times. The outcome was presence of the metabolic syndrome, based on the National Cholesterol Education Program definition, measured at the end of the follow-up (a total of 216 cases were identified). A dose–response relation was found between exposure to iso-strain over 14 years and risk of the metabolic syndrome at the end of the follow-up. The age- and socioeconomic status–adjusted odds ratio for developing the metabolic syndrome was 2.3 (95% CI 1.3–3.8) times higher for employees with three or four exposures to iso-strain compared to those with no exposure to iso-strain.

In the CHD study,[18] only the first two study phases were used to define long-term exposure to iso-strain in order to ensure sufficient follow-up and numbers for CHD events. Among participants aged 50 or younger, a total of 174 CHD events occurred during an average follow-up of 12 years. Long-term iso-strain was associated with a 1.7-fold (95% CI 1.2–2.4) increased risk of CHD compared to no exposure to iso-strain. In the 50+ age group with 258 incident CHD events, however, there was no such association (relative risk 1.1, 95% CI 0.7–1.8 with the highest iso-strain level).

11.5   Horizontal Comparison Between Risk Factors

The horizontal review is a method to compare the evidence on diverse risk markers in a unified explicit framework.[25] Comparing evidence horizontally (that is between risk factors) may help to highlight specific deficiencies in the evidence that could be missed in traditional "vertical" reviews focused on only one risk factor and one field of research. Here, we briefly compare the evidence on work-related psychosocial factors with that on C-reactive protein (CRP), a circulating inflammatory marker of uncertain causal status in CHD aetiology, and diabetes, an established causal risk factor for CHD. Summary data for these risk factors are drawn from a horizontal review published in 2009.[25]

Horizontal comparisons reveal that studies have used various methods to define psychosocial factors at work but relatively standardised methods for measurement of CRP and diabetes. In the largest systematic reviews, adjustments for the a priori confounders smoking, blood pressure and cholesterol were found in 11/11 cohort studies for job strain/iso-strain and CHD, and adjustments in the CRP (20/22 studies) and diabetes studies (26/37 studies) were also generally consistent and complete. Summary estimates from meta-analyses for adjusted relative risks of CHD are lower for job strain (1.2, 95% CI 0.9–1.4) than for CRP (the top versus the bottom tertile 1.6 95% CI 1.5–1.7) and diabetes (3.7, 95% CI 2.6–5.2 for women and 2.2, 95% CI 1.8–2.6 for men). There are no randomised controlled trials (RCT) to examine whether removal of psychosocial risk factors at work would reduce CHD. The status of diabetes cannot be randomised and there are no interventions, currently, that specifically target CRP. Consequently, as for psychosocial factors, no RCTs have directly tested the causal importance of CRP and diabetes for CHD.

This horizontal review clearly suggests different evidence "profiles" for the selected risk markers. Compared to CRP and diabetes, the evidence in favour of psychosocial factors was weaker due to (i) the lack of standardised measurements, (ii) the lower number of studies published and (iii) weaker adjusted effects.

11.6   Confounding

Lack of precision in the measurement of long-term exposure to psychosocial factors has been used to explain modest or negative findings. The underlying assumption is that negative findings are false. However, it is equally important to consider the converse assumption, that is, whether the positive findings might be false when the true association is null (Fig. 11.2, Part 2). This is the argument of confounding.

In observational epidemiological studies, confounding by imprecisely or unmeasured third factors is an alternative explanation for observed associations between exposure and outcome. CHD has an extended induction period, often taking decades to develop, and it is associated with a large variety of risk factors in adulthood and from the pre-employment period in childhood and adolescence. The possibility of confounding arises when these risk factors additionally predict psychosocial factors at work. Only randomised controlled trials can rule out confounding, but such trials are currently not available and it has been argued that they would be impractical, unfeasible and unethical. However, we believe that one unproblematic intervention approach would be to start with people at very high risk for future cardiac events, such as people with existing CHD. Based on observational evidence,[26] reduction of job strain should prevent recurrent cardiac events in this group.

In observational studies, one potential confounder for the psychosocial factors–CHD relation is material disadvantage, that is, individuals with adverse psychosocial environment may also experience socioeconomic adversity characterised by an increased exposure to infectious agents and passive smoking, poorer diets and fewer opportunities for physical activity and high-quality health care. A study of 27 workplaces in Scotland between 1970 and 1973 provides an interesting setting to examine this issue.[27] In that study, perceived psychological stress (used as a proxy measure for psychosocial factors) was, in contrast with most other studies, associated with material advantage rather than material disadvantage. Cardiovascular deaths over a period of 21 years were followed up by linkage to the UK's National Health Service central mortality register; 785 of the 5,388 men died from cardiovascular disease. Surprisingly, higher psychological stress was associated with *lower* age-adjusted cardiovascular mortality (relative risk for high versus low perceived stress 0.84, 95% CI 0.67–1.05 and for moderate versus low stress 0.83, 95% CI 0.71–0.97) and thus seemed to have a protective effect. The authors concluded that material circumstances may confound the association between psychosocial factors and health, but that in their study, this was largely avoided because of the exceptional association between psychological stress and material advantage in that population.

The findings from Scottish men have not been replicated in other cohorts or with data based on validated measures of psychosocial factors at work. However, the issue of residual confounding has also been raised by the authors of a study of Swedish men aged 40–53 years.[28] It reported a 1.6-fold increased risk of CHD among employees who worked in occupations that on average had low job control. Supporting the confounding hypothesis, this excess risk was attenuated and no longer reached statistical significance after controlling for pre-employment risk factors (e.g., socioeconomic position of the father and low education) and health behaviours. In other studies, however, the association of directly measured psychosocial factors with intima-media thickness in the carotid artery (a structural indicator of preclinical atherosclerosis) and incident CHD remained after adjustment for a range of indicators of adulthood and early life material conditions,[29,30] suggesting that the association may not be confounded.

11.7 Plausible Mechanisms Linking Psychosocial Factors with Coronary Heart Disease

Plausibility is an important consideration in examining causality. Several plausible mechanisms have been proposed through which psychosocial factors may have an adverse impact[16] (Fig. 11.2, Part 1). First, they may influence CHD risk indirectly by increasing health risk behaviours and reducing help-seeking and compliance with medical treatment. For example, the Finnish Public Sector study of over 50,000 participants – one of the largest cohort studies in the field – found little difference in smoking status between those reporting an adverse psychosocial work environment compared to those with a more favourable environment.[31] However, among current smokers, adverse psychosocial factors were associated with significantly greater smoking intensity: Smokers who reported job strain or effort–reward imbalance were 50% more likely to smoke over 20 cigarettes per day than those free of these conditions. The first group was also less likely to quit smoking.

Second, in addition to indirect effects, psychosocial factors may relate to biological changes directly involved in CHD aetiology and prognosis. These mechanisms include prolonged overactivation and dysregulation of the autonomic nervous system and the hypothalamus-pituitary-adrenal cortex (HPA) axis[32]; both are assumed to increase disease risk, accelerate existing disease processes, act as triggers of acute events, such as heart attack, and worsen prognosis. Psychosocial risk factors are also hypothesized to increase risk of the metabolic syndrome: insulin resistance, lipoprotein disturbances, reduced fibrolysis and central obesity, in susceptible individuals.

The Whitehall II study has probably reported the most comprehensive test of different potential mediating mechanisms for the association between psychosocial factors at work and CHD.[18] In that study, long-term iso-strain was associated with low physical activity, unhealthy diet, the metabolic syndrome, lower heart rate variability and a higher morning rise in cortisol.[18] Approximately 16% of the association with CHD was explained by health behaviours and another 16% by the metabolic syndrome (which is also a consequence of health behaviours), a total of 32%. These findings suggest that both direct and indirect mechanisms may be operating. However, given that only one third of the association was explained, much of the pathways linking psychosocial factors and CHD remained unknown.

11.8 Conclusions and Future Challenges

During the discovery phase, it is reasonable to have a higher tolerance for false-positive findings as the aim is not to abandon a potentially important risk marker prematurely. For the hypothesis of psychosocial factors as a cause of CHD, this phase has probably been passed and now strong evidence is necessary to make an influence on public health policy.

We have sought to provide a balanced review of the evidence on psychosocial factors at work and CHD as well as to highlight potential drawbacks that could explain why causality still remains a controversial issue. The following arguments can be made to support the status of psychosocial factors as a causal risk factor for CHD:

- There is strong evidence of cross-sectional associations between psychosocial factors and CHD across different populations.
- Prospective cohort studies showing that psychosocial factors at work predict future CHD in employees free from CHD at study inception have established that the temporal order fits a causal association.
- A dose–response association has been shown in the British Whitehall II study: The longer exposure to psychosocial risk factors at work, the greater risk of the metabolic syndrome and, among those younger than 50, incident CHD.

However, we also found that the current evidence is not strong enough to exclude the possibility of confounding and bias as an explanation for observed associations. This is because:

- There is large heterogeneity in the magnitude of effect estimates between prospective studies and the reasons for these differences remain unclear.
- Risk estimates adjusted for conventional risk factors tend to be substantially lower than the age- and sex-adjusted estimates. This may indicate confounding, but also indirect, effects where psychosocial factors additionally alter conventional risk factor levels.
- Studies are prone to information biases with multiple instruments used to determine exposure to psychosocial factors at work and absence of a widely agreed standardised instrument.
- In most studies, psychosocial factors at work have a relatively small effect on CHD; even the age- and sex-adjusted associations failed to reach conventional levels of statistical significance in 3 of the 4 "best-quality" studies listed in a recent review. The studies were generally underpowered to show these modest effect sizes.
- There is no evidence of reversibility, i.e., that elimination of psychosocial risk factors at work would lead to a reduction in CHD risk among employees.

Regarding the next steps in the psychosocial research field, we believe there is a fundamental need to reach wider agreement on how to define and assess exposure to adverse psychosocial factors at work in a standard way, taking into account the need to capture long-term exposure. Increased specificity of the study questions (i.e., to whom and under what circumstances are psychosocial factors likely to increase the risk of CHD) is also of considerable importance, because this may help identify reasons for the heterogeneity in findings. Of equal importance, to tackle confounding and the role of selection into psychosocially unfavourable work environments, are longitudinal analyses, covering both the pre-employment and employment periods. Finally, developing standard interventions and testing them in randomised controlled trials should be the ultimate goal, both as a scientific test of causality and a way to inform policy and guidelines.

References

1. De Backer G, Ambrosioni E, Borch-Johnsen K, et al. European guidelines on cardiovascular disease prevention in clinical practice. Third joint task force of European and other societies on cardiovascular disease prevention in clinical practice. *Eur Heart J.* 2003;24(17): 1601-1610.
2. Pearson TA, Blair SN, Daniels SR, et al. AHA guidelines for primary prevention of cardiovascular disease and stroke: 2002 update: consensus panel guide to comprehensive risk reduction for adult patients without coronary or other atherosclerotic vascular diseases. American Heart Association Science Advisory and Coordinating Committee. *Circulation.* 2002;106(3): 388-391.
3. Redberg RF, Benjamin EJ, Bittner V, et al. ACCF/AHA 2009 performance measures for primary prevention of cardiovascular disease in adults: a report of the American College of Cardiology Foundation/American Heart Association task force on performance measures (writing committee to develop performance measures for primary prevention of cardiovascular disease): developed in collaboration with the American Academy of Family Physicians; American Association of Cardiovascular and Pulmonary Rehabilitation; and Preventive Cardiovascular Nurses Association: endorsed by the American College of Preventive Medicine, American College of Sports Medicine, and Society for Women's Health Research. *Circulation.* 2009;120(13):1296-1336.
4. Nathan DM, Buse JB, Davidson MB, et al. Management of hyperglycemia in type 2 diabetes: a consensus algorithm for the initiation and adjustment of therapy: a consensus statement from the American Diabetes Association and the European Association for the study of diabetes. *Diabetes Care.* 2006;29(8):1963-1972.
5. Graham I, Atar D, Borch-Johnsen K, Boysen G, et al. European guidelines on cardiovascular disease prevention in clinical practice: full text. Fourth Joint Task Force of the European Society of Cardiology and other societies on cardiovascular disease prevention in clinical practice (constituted by representatives of nine societies and by invited experts). *Eur J Cardiovasc Prev Rehabil.* 2007;14(Suppl 2):S1-S113.
6. Cox T, Griffiths A. Assessment of psychosocial hazards at work. In: Schabracq MJ, Winnubst JAM, Cooper CL, eds. *Handbook of Work and Health Psychology.* Chichester: Wiley; 1996: 127-146.
7. Kivimäki M, Lindström K. Psychosocial approach to occupational health. In: Salvendy G, ed. *Handbook of Human Factors and Ergonomics.* 3rd ed. New York: Wiley; 2006:801-817.
8. Karasek R, Theorell T. *Healthy Work: Stress, Productivity, and the Reconstruction of Working Life.* New York: Basic Books; 1990.
9. Siegrist J. Adverse health effects of high-effort/low-reward conditions. *J Occup Health Psychol.* 1996;1(1):27-41.
10. Elovainio M, Kivimaki M, Vahtera J. Organizational justice: evidence of a new psychosocial predictor of health. *Am J Public Health.* 2002;92(1):105-108.
11. Kivimäki M, Ferrie JE, Brunner E, et al. Justice at work and reduced risk of coronary heart disease among employees: the Whitehall II study. *Arch Intern Med.* 2005;165(19):2245-2251.
12. Yusuf S, Hawken S, Ounpuu S, et al. Effect of potentially modifiable risk factors associated with myocardial infarction in 52 countries (the INTERHEART study): case-control study. *Lancet.* 2004;364(9438):937-952.
13. Kivimaki M, Virtanen M, Elovainio M, Kouvonen A, Vaananen A, Vahtera J. Work stress in the etiology of coronary heart disease – a meta-analysis. *Scand J Work Environ Health.* 2006; 32(6):431-442.
14. Belkic KL, Landsbergis PA, Schnall PL, Baker D. Is job strain a major source of cardiovascular disease risk? *Scand J Work Environ Health.* 2004;30(2):85-128.
15. Eller NH, Netterstrom B, Gyntelberg F, et al. Work-related psychosocial factors and the development of ischemic heart disease: a systematic review. *Cardiol Rev.* 2009;17(2):83-97.

16. Theorell T, Perski A, Orth-Gomer K, Hamsten A, de Faire U. The effects of the strain of returning to work on the risk of cardiac death after a first myocardial infarction before the age of 45. *Int J Cardiol.* 1991;30(1):61-67.
17. Kivimaki M, Theorell T, Westerlund H, Vahtera J, Alfredsson L. Job strain and ischaemic disease: does the inclusion of older employees in the cohort dilute the association? The WOLF Stockholm study. *J Epidemiol Community Health.* 2008;62(4):372-374.
18. Chandola T, Britton A, Brunner E, et al. Work stress and coronary heart disease: what are the mechanisms? *Eur Heart J.* 2008;29(5):640-648.
19. De Bacquer D, Pelfrene E, Clays E, et al. Perceived job stress and incidence of coronary events: 3-year follow-up of the Belgian Job Stress Project cohort. *Am J Epidemiol.* 2005;161(5):434-441.
20. Andre-Petersson L, Engstrom G, Hedblad B, Janzon L, Rosvall M. Social support at work and the risk of myocardial infarction and stroke in women and men. *Soc Sci Med.* 2007;64(4): 830-841.
21. Lynch J, Krause N, Kaplan GA, Tuomilehto J, Salonen JT. Workplace conditions, socioeconomic status, and the risk of mortality and acute myocardial infarction: the Kuopio Ischemic Heart Disease Risk Factor study. *Am J Public Health.* 1997;87(4):617-622.
22. Marmot MG, Davey Smith G, Stansfeld S, et al. Health inequalities among British civil servants: the Whitehall II study. *Lancet.* 1991;337(8754):1387-1393.
23. Kivimaki M, Head J, Ferrie JE, et al. Why is evidence on job strain and coronary heart disease mixed? An illustration of measurement challenges in the Whitehall II study. *Psychosom Med.* 2006;68(3):398-401.
24. Chandola T, Brunner E, Marmot M. Chronic stress at work and the metabolic syndrome: prospective study. *BMJ.* 2006;332:521-525.
25. Kuper H, Nicholson A, Kivimäki M, et al. Evaluating the causal relevance of diverse risk markers: a horizontal systematic review. *BMJ.* 2009;339:b4265.
26. Aboa-Eboule C, Brisson C, Maunsell E, et al. Job strain and risk of acute recurrent coronary heart disease events. *JAMA.* 2007;298(14):1652-1660.
27. Macleod J, Davey Smith G, Heslop P, Metcalfe C, Carroll D, Hart C. Are the effects of psychosocial exposures attributable to confounding? Evidence from a prospective observational study on psychological stress and mortality. *J Epidemiol Community Health.* 2001;55(12): 878-884.
28. Hemmingsson T, Lundberg I. Is the association between low job control and coronary heart disease confounded by risk factors measured in childhood and adolescence among Swedish males 40–53 years of age? *Int J Epidemiol.* 2006;35(3):616-622.
29. Kivimaki M, Hintsanen M, Keltikangas-Jarvinen L, et al. Early risk factors, job strain, and atherosclerosis among men in their 30s: the Cardiovascular Risk in Young Finns study. *Am J Public Health.* 2007;97(3):450-452.
30. Hintsa T, Shipley MJ, Gimeno D, et al. Do pre-employment influences explain the association between psychosocial factors at work and coronary heart disease? The Whitehall II study. *Occup Environ Med.* 2010;67(5):330-334.
31. Kouvonen A, Kivimäki M, Virtanen M, Pentti J, Vahtera J. Work stress, smoking status, and smoking intensity: an observational study of 46,190 employees. *J Epidemiol Community Health.* 2005;59(1):63-69.
32. McEwen BS. Protective and damaging effects of stress mediators. *N Engl J Med.* 1998; 338(3):171-179.

Chapter 12
Depression and Cardiovascular Disease Progression: Epidemiology, Mechanisms, and Treatment

Petra Hoen, Nina Kupper, and Peter de Jonge

Keywords Depression • Cardiovascular disease progression • Epidemiology • Mechanisms • Treatment • Inflammation • Platelet function • Serotonin metabolism • Screening

12.1 Background

Depression and coronary heart disease (CHD) are the two strongest contributors to the global burden of disease.[1] Both disorders are common, and while cardiovascular disease is an important factor directly contributing to mortality, depression is primarily associated with decreased health-related quality of life,[2] and imposes a significant economic burden on society.[3] However, there are also signs that depression may contribute to higher mortality rates, perhaps due to its association with somatic disease, and in particular CHD.

The term depression can refer both to the presence of depressive symptoms, including low mood and fatigue, and to the presence of depressive disorder, referring to a psychiatric diagnosis. Among the mood disorders defined in the Diagnostic and Statistical Manual of Mental Disorders, Fourth Edition (DSM-IV), major depressive disorder (MDD) is the most important single disorder in terms of prevalence and severity. MDD is characterized by one or more episodes of depressed mood and loss of interest and is defined in DSM-IV as follows (Box 12.1).

P. Hoen (✉) • P. de Jonge (✉)
Department of Interdisciplinary Center for Psychiatric Epidemiology,
University Medical Center Groningen, Groningen, The Netherlands
e-mail: p.w.hoen@med.umcg.nl; peter.de.jonge@med.umcg.nl

N. Kupper
Department of Medical Psychology, Center of Research on Psychology in Somatic Diseases,
Tilburg University, Tilburg, The Netherlands

P. Hjemdahl et al. (eds.), *Stress and Cardiovascular Disease*,
DOI 10.1007/978-1-84882-419-5_12, © Springer-Verlag London Limited 2012

Box 12.1. Diagnostic Criteria DSM-IV

Category 1
- Depressed mood
- Lack of interest

Category 2
- Change in appetite or weight
- Insomnia or hypersomnia
- Psychomotor agitation or retardation
- Fatigue or loss of energy
- Feelings of worthlessness and guilt
- Concentration problems
- Suicidal ideation

To be diagnosed with MDD, individuals have to experience at least one of the symptoms from Category 1 and at least three or more symptoms from Category 2, for a total of at least five out of nine symptoms. These symptoms must be present for most of the day, nearly every day, for at least 2 weeks. MDD is thus operationalized as a syndrome, of which the appearance may vary among individuals.

12.1.1   Depression and Cardiovascular Disease

Patients with cardiovascular disease have a high risk of developing depression.[4] Approximately one out of five patients is affected by depression following CHD,[5-7] which contrasts with the prevalence of MDD of approximately 7% in the US general population over the last 12 months.[8] Since Carney et al.[9] identified MDD as a risk factor for cardiac events in patients with stable coronary heart disease and Frasure-Smith et al.[10] showed an increased risk of mortality in post-myocardial infarction (MI) depressive patients, the association between clinical depression and CHD raised much attention. Currently, a large body of literature has confirmed that healthy patients with MDD are at risk of developing incident CHD[11,12] and that depressive patients with established heart disease have an increased risk of suffering adverse cardiovascular outcomes.[13,14] Specifically, this second line of research has developed exponentially and its results have by now been summarized in several systematic reviews and meta-analyses[6,13-15] (Table 12.1).

From these meta-analyses, a consistent picture emerges in which depression is a risk factor for cardiac disease progression. The association between post-MI depression and prognosis was not influenced by the way depression was assessed (i.e., depressive symptoms vs. depressive disorder).[14] Although the first studies on the association between post-MI depression and cardiac prognosis may have been too optimistic, suggesting increased odds of 6–11.[10,16] More recent studies tend to report

Table 12.1 Depression and coronary heart disease: meta-analyses

	Publication year	Number of studies	Patients	Outcomes	Result
Van Melle et al.[14]	2004	22 prospective studies of 16 different cohorts	6,367 MI patients	All-cause mortality, cardiovascular mortality, cardiovascular events	All-cause mortality: OR 2.38 cardiovascular mortality: OR 2.59 cardiovascular events: OR 1.95
Barth et al.[13]	2004	29 prospective studies of 20 different cohorts	11,018 CHD patients	All-cause mortality, cardiovascular mortality	Mortality: OR 2.24 (short term, unadjusted) and OR 1.76 (long term, adjusted)
Nicholson et al.[15]	2006	21 etiological studies and 34 prognostic studies	146,538 CHD patients	Etiological: Fatal CHD and incident MI. Prognostic: Fatal CHD and all-cause mortality	Etiological: future CHD OR 1.81. Prognostic: OR 1.80. Adjusting for LVEF: OR from 2.18 to 1.53
Rutledge et al.[6]	2006	36 studies	149,847 CHD patients	Mortality, hospitalization, clinical events, health care costs, health care use	Mortality and secondary events: RR 2.1

CHD coronary heart disease, *CHF* chronic heart failure, *MI* myocardial infarction

lower odds ratios for mortality attributed to depression,[17] while a minority of studies even failed to confirm an impact of post-MI depression on cardiac prognosis.[18,19]

12.1.2   Confounding by Cardiac Disease Severity and Overlap Between Psychosocial Factors

Despite the growth and relative consistency of results in this area of research, debates on the interpretation of findings have continued,[20-22] focusing on the extent to which the association can be interpreted as causal.[14,15,23,24] Two issues are central in this discussion: confounding by disease severity and overlap between psychosocial factors.

There is substantial disagreement on the possible confounding of the apparent cardiotoxic effects of depression by MI severity and its consequences.[20,21,25] As a first sign of potential confounding, the previous observation that MDD is present in 20–25% of post-MI patients, while the prevalence of depression over the past 12 months in the general population is only 7%, should be kept in mind. However, this could also be due to the fact that MI, for many individuals, can be a significant psychological stressor and trigger depression in persons already at increased risk.[26]

Evidence for the possibility of confounding can be seen in the association between left ventricular ejection fraction (LVEF) and post-MI depression. LVEF is an important determinant of cardiac disease severity in the post-MI setting, and reflects the adequacy of pump function of the heart. In a sample of about 2,000 MI patients, Van Melle et al. observed a dose-response like association between LVEF at the time of MI and subsequent risk of depression during the post-MI year.[25] The authors also summarized the existing studies on this association, and found significantly higher proportions of depression in MI patients with more LVEF dysfunction, although some heterogeneity in findings was observed.[20,21] (Table 12.2). Confounding may also occur by complaints attributable to the MI, such as pain or physical limitations, or by somatic comorbidities such as heart failure, diabetes, or arthritis.[31] For instance, Watkins et al. showed that in post-MI patients the Beck Depression Inventory (BDI) score was correlated with the Charlson comorbidity index, in which the number of somatic diseases is counted. Of interest, the authors found that the somatic symptoms of depression, such as fatigue, sleeping difficulties, and working difficulties, were mainly associated. Also, the underlying process that has led to the occurrence of the MI, atherosclerosis, may be related directly to the occurrence of depression. This will be discussed in the context of mechanisms.

An association between disease severity factors and depression does not automatically imply that the association between depression and cardiac prognosis is confounded. Confounding implies that, when cardiac disease severity is added to a prediction model for cardiac prognosis, the association between depression and prognosis is attenuated.[20] Several of the prognostic studies included have therefore added such an analysis. In their meta-analysis, Van Melle et al. found that of the five

Table 12.2 Studies presenting the prevalence of depression in post-MI patients according to LVEF

First author	Sample size (n)	LVEF cut-off value (%)	Prevalence of depression (%)		
			Below cut-off	Above cut-off	P-value
Frasure-Smith[16]	222	35	35	29	0.43
Frasure-Smith[27]	896	35	39	30	0.03
Bush[28]	285[a]	35	34	19	0.07
Strik[29]	318[b]	50	48	47	0.90
Strik[30]	206[c]	50	39	26	0.06[d]
Carney[20]	766[e]	40	49	46	0.58[d]
Total	2,693	35–50	42	35	<0.01

Van Melle et al.[25]. By permission of Oxford University Press
[a] MI patients ≥ 65 years
[b] Male patients with first MI
[c] Patients with first MI
[d] Computed from data as presented in article (χ^2 test)
[e] Controls free of depression and social isolation

studies that adjusted for LVEF, the association between depression and prognosis was substantially attenuated in one study, while in two of the studies the odds ratios were not even significant anymore. Nicholson and colleagues even concluded that almost half of the variance in the association was explained away when LVEF was added to the prediction models.[15] Thus, LVEF appears to be an important source of possible confounding.[32]

A second factor that needs to be discussed is the presence of competing psychosocial factors, since observed associations between depression and cardiac prognosis may be related to other psychosocial factor(s) also related to, or underlying, depression.[33] Researchers have tended to evaluate the effects of putative psychological risk factors for physical disease by analyzing or measuring only a single psychological construct at a time.[33] However, the increased risk of cardiac events may extend to patients with symptoms of negative affect other than depression. In the field of psychological and cardiological research, several candidates of such psychosocial risk factors have been investigated, although rarely simultaneously.[34]

Anxiety may be an interesting factor in this respect, as depression and anxiety are highly comorbid disorders,[35] and symptoms of depression and anxiety frequently co-occur in post-MI patients.[36] Some studies have reported symptoms of anxiety to be predictive of subsequent cardiac events and mortality post-MI, independently of established biomedical risk factors,[29,34] while others found no association.[18] In a recent meta-analysis on the prognostic association between post-MI anxiety and cardiac prognosis, it was found that overall anxious MI patients had 36% increased risk of adverse cardiac events.[37] The extent to which these findings are attributable to depression, or conversely, the extent to which the results with respect to depression are attributable to anxiety, is not known to date.

A second possibly competing risk factor is Type D personality,[38,39] which differs from depression in that it includes social inhibition apart from negative affectivity, and is conceptualized as a trait rather than a state. Type D personality has been associated with vulnerability to emotional distress[40] and an increased risk for adverse clinical events in CHD patients.[38] Consequently, personality may comprise a general disposition that acts as an underlying variable promoting both depression and CHD risk.

A third psychosocial factor is social isolation.[41-43] Social factors that may influence a patient's psychological status include social networks, social relationships, and social support. These factors may lead to social isolation. Research has shown that social isolation is associated with adverse cardiac outcome, and the impact seems to be greatest in those patients who are most isolated. However, mixed findings have been reported.[44]

As a fourth potential factor, vital exhaustion is a related construct to depression. It is characterized by feelings of fatigue, irritability, and demoralization, and may also be associated with adverse clinical outcome.[45,46]

Other psychosocial factors that have been studied are anger and hostility. These factors are associated with more mixed findings and a recent meta-analysis suggests small effect sizes in CHD patients (1.24; 95% CI 1.08–1.42).[47] Given this level of risk, hostility and anger do not seem to be major cardiac risk factors. Further research is needed to identify psychological risk indicators in patients with heart disease, as well as how they operate in concert. For a more detailed discussion on this topic, see Suls and Bunde.[33]

12.2   Mechanisms

Several physiological as well as behavioral mechanisms have been proposed to explain how depression may lead to cardiac events (Table 12.3).[61-64]

12.2.1   Heart Rate Variability

Among the suggested mechanisms linking depression and cardiac events, an often studied candidate is altered autonomic nervous system (ANS) activity,[61] characterized by sympathetic overactivity and/or parasympathetic withdrawal. Heart rate variability (HRV) is a noninvasive marker of ANS activation of the heart, with reduced HRV being an important independent risk factor for cardiac mortality.[65] Some,[48,66,67] but not all studies[68-70] have associated depression with reduced HRV in CHD patients. In the ENRICHD patient group, in which depression was associated with low HRV, more specifically very low frequency (VLF) HRV, it was shown that VLF HRV partially mediated the effect of depression on survival

Table 12.3 Mechanisms through which depression may lead to cardiac events

Biological mechanisms	Behavioral mechanisms
Lower heart rate variability (HRV) reflecting altered cardiac autonomic tone[48]	Cigarette smoking and hypertension[49,50]
Inflammatory processes[51]	Nonadherence to cardiac prevention and treatment regimens[52]
Increased platelet aggregation[53]	Dietary factors[52]
Enhanced activity of the hypothalamic pituitary axis[54]	Lack of exercise[55]
Increased whole blood serotonin[56]	Poor social support[57]
Lower omega-3 fatty acid levels[58]	
Antidepressant cardiotoxicity[59]	
Increased catecholamine levels[60]	

after acute MI.[71] Conversely, the Heart and Soul study, in which low HRV was not associated with depression, showed that VLF HRV did not predict adverse cardiac events, nor did it mediate the effect of depression on adverse cardiac events when adjusting for the appropriate clinical confounders.[72] However, when the authors evaluated the differential association of somatic and cognitive depressive symptoms with HRV, they found that somatic depressive symptoms were associated with lower HRV, while cognitive depressive symptoms were not.[73] These results suggest that individual symptoms of depression may have a differential association with HRV.

12.2.2 Inflammation

Higher levels of inflammatory markers, including C-reactive protein (CRP), interleukin (IL)-6, and tumor necrosis factor (TNF)-alpha have been found in CHD patients. These elevations impose an increased risk of adverse cardiac outcome.[74] On the other hand, depression has also been associated with increased levels of inflammation (i.e., CRP and IL-6) in CHD patients.[75] Whether the effects of depression are mediated by inflammation has only been examined in the Heart and Soul study, in which it was found that the increased risk of adverse cardiac events could only be partly explained by increased levels of inflammatory markers.[72] Of interest, this proposed mechanism is also linked to the vascular depression hypothesis,[76] which suggests that cerebrovascular lesions due to prolonged atherosclerosis play a role in the etiology of late-life depression. As atherosclerosis is also associated with MI, it may account for the supposed cardiotoxicity of depression. Furthermore, a pro-inflammatory state is accompanied by "sickness-behavior," in which somatic, flu-like symptoms of depression such as fatigue, decreased appetite, and psychomotor retardation become dominant.[51] This provides an additional potential explanation for the relation between depression and inflammation.

12.2.3   Platelet Function

Platelets are involved in thrombus formation and play an important role in MI, unstable angina, and in atherogenesis.[77] A recent systematic review suggests that depressed cardiac patients experience increased platelet aggregation.[78] It is suggested that platelet aggregation may contribute to the process of atherogenesis as well as to the increased risk of cardiac events in depressed patients. Further, serotonin reuptake inhibitors are potentially able to normalize platelet activity. However, findings in this area are far from conclusive, as there are mixed findings for platelet activation markers and platelet aggregability.[78] This suggests the need for larger and better-designed studies. See also the Chap. 6 by Hjemdahl and von Känel.

12.2.4   Hypothalamus-Pituitary-Adrenal Axis

The hypothalamus-pituitary-adrenal axis (HPA) axis is involved in the human stress response (see also the Chap. 5 by Chrousos). In individuals with depression, or as a consequence of continued exposure to stress, the HPA axis may become deregulated, resulting in either hyperactivity or hypoactivity. HPA axis dysregulation has also been associated with several CHD risk factors (e.g., abdominal obesity, hypercholesterolemia, hypertension), and HPA axis dysfunction is implicated in the pathogenesis of CHD.[79] CHD patients with depression have been characterized by an impaired feedback control of the HPA axis, and consequently elevated levels of cortisol due to HPA axis hyperactivity.[80] However, studies also report flattened cortisol day profiles with lower morning values and higher evening values,[81] or even report null-findings.[82] Therefore, although some research findings hint at a mediatory role for HPA axis dysregulation, more research is necessary. Along with the mediating role of cortisol, genetic studies indicate that cortisol might be a shared risk factor for depression and CHD.[83]

12.2.5   Serotonin Metabolism

Serotonin has a wide variety of cardiovascular effects (e.g., brady- and tachycardia, vasoconstriction and vasodilatation), and long-term exposure can lead to endothelial dysfunction and thickening of the cardiac valves. Serotonin dysfunction is considered to be one of the main pathophysiological factors leading to depression.[84] Genetic studies support the role of serotonin in the association between depression and CHD. A twin study reported a substantial genetic contribution to the covariance between CHD and depression,[85] and an association study reported the association between post-MI depression and specific variants of the serotonin transporter genes.[86] Nonetheless, these findings should be viewed as preliminary, and could benefit from replication in larger samples using prospective designs when examining

CHD prognosis. Of note, to date serotonin has not been investigated as a risk marker of worsening prognosis in CAD.

Besides biological mechanisms, several behavioral mechanisms have been proposed as well, though remarkably fewer studies have evaluated these pathways than the physiological ones.[87]

12.2.6 Medication Adherence and Other Forms of Health Behavior

Poor adherence to medication regimens is a common problem and can cause substantial worsening of the disease and its prognosis.[88] Roughly, 50% of patients with chronic conditions are not compliant with their treatment regimen. Adherence rates to medication are higher in short-term treatment regimens in comparison with the longer medication usage in chronic conditions,[89] and post-MI patients are usually put on long-term medication regimens. Thereby, it has been found that depressed patients are less adherent to medication treatment than nondepressed patients.[90] Given that poor adherence is a risk factor for poor cardiac outcome[91] and the association between depression and poor adherence, poor adherence may be a possible behavioral mediator.

An important part of the medical treatment regimen is cardiac rehabilitation, which has been found to reduce mortality in post-MI patients.[92] However, only a minority of eligible patients seem to attend, due to several possible factors: sociodemographic factors such as low income, living alone, and living far away from rehabilitation facilities; lifestyle factors, such as lack of regular exercise habits; and clinical factors, such as more severe illness and lack of active physician endorsement.[93] Mental factors are also important, as illustrated by the finding that depression is a predictor of not attending and completing cardiac rehabilitation.[94]

Also supporting the role of health behavior in explaining the association between depression and cardiac prognosis is the finding from several large cohort studies that cardiac patients with mental disorders receive less cardiac aftercare. In a cohort study of over 100,000 MI patients aged 65 years and older, the patients with a documented ICD-9 mental disorder at the time of the MI had lower rates of subsequent revascularization procedures (i.e., percutaneous coronary intervention (PCI) and coronary artery bypass graft (CABG)).[95] One of the strongest associations found was for depression, with 49% lower rates of PCI use and 37% lower rates of CABG use. These findings were replicated in other cohort studies, including a study performed in Canada, in which over 300,000 patients younger than 65 were included.[96] A limitation of these studies is that these are registry studies in which only diagnosed depression cases have been evaluated. This has likely resulted in a vast underrepresentation of true depression cases. Therefore, it is necessary for future research to consider whether CHD patients with depression are receiving adequate cardiac intervention procedures, based on a depression assessment of all patients in the cohort.

12.2.7 Inability to Modify Lifestyle

Lifestyle modification is an important means of secondary prevention in patients with established CHD, and the two most important examples include smoking cessation and promoting physical exercise. Smoking is an independent major risk factor for CHD,[97] and patients who continue to smoke have an increased mortality risk and poorer cardiovascular prognosis.[98] Patients with mental health problems smoke more, are more often nicotine dependent, and suffer from greater morbidity and mortality from smoking-related illnesses than the general population.[99] Thus, smoking or failure to quit smoking can be a possible explanation for the poorer cardiovascular prognosis in depressed post-MI patients.[100]

Lifestyle modification may also involve increasing one's amount of exercise. In a study focused on the association between health behavior, depressive symptoms, and new cardiovascular events, it was concluded that the association between depressive symptoms and adverse cardiovascular events was largely explained by lack of physical activity.[72] In depression treatment, exercise is used as an alternative approach, and a recent meta-analysis found that the effect of exercise on depressive symptoms was not significantly different from that of cognitive therapy in terms of effectiveness.[101] Therefore, lack of exercise is considered as a possibly important mediator between depression and cardiac disease prognosis, and one that is potentially amenable.

12.2.8 General Discussion

The extent to which these proposed biological and behavioral mechanisms explain the increased risk of cardiovascular events in depressed patients is unknown. This is due to several factors. First, to date, the design of relevant studies has often been ineffective in testing for mediation. Mediation testing can be done following the Baron and Kenny model, in which the initial variable is correlated with the outcome variable and mediator variable. The mediator must affect the outcome variable and, for complete mediation, the effect of the initial variable on the outcome variable must be zero while controlling for the mediator variable.[102] Studies conducted so far are mainly cross-sectional, while longitudinal studies are necessary for adequate mediation testing.[103] Second, most of the proposed mechanisms have been studied in isolation, while in reality they are interrelated.[104] It is unlikely that a single psychophysiological or behavioral mechanism will fully explain the prospective association between depression and cardiac outcome. Rather, the bidirectional association between mood disorders and heart disease is multifaceted, involving an integration of several central and peripheral processes.[104] Several recent studies testify to the presence of a network of effects between depression and cardiac outcome, as studies have linked measures of HRV to pro-inflammatory cytokine IL-6[68,105,106] and fibrinogen.[105]

In one of the exceptional studies, in which several physiological and behavioral mechanisms were studied in concert, it was found that the increased risk of adverse cardiovascular events associated with depression was largely explained by behavioral factors, notably lack of physical exercise.[72] However, it should be noted that, in this study, depression and proposed mechanisms were still assessed at the same time point so that a strong mediation test could not be performed.

In sum, much of the role of biological and behavioral factors in explaining the association between depression and CHD remains unclear to date, as the literature is hampered by imperfect study designs. Using longitudinal designs, more attention should be directed to the identification of the underlying pathophysiological and behavioral processes by which depression contributes to cardiovascular prognosis.

12.3 Treatment

The treatment of depression in CHD patients has drawn a lot of attention, especially because it has the potential to evaluate the extent to which the association between depression and cardiovascular prognosis is causal. In the general population, the most popular forms of treatment are psychotherapy, antidepressant drugs, and combinations of the two. A large body of evidence has demonstrated that both forms of treatment are moderately effective in terms of reducing depressive symptomatology, although recently it has been argued that the efficacy of antidepressive drugs has been over-estimated due to publication bias.[107,108] The evaluation of treatment forms for depressed CHD patients has been done in two phases.

12.3.1 Phase 1: Psychological Treatments with Rather Poor Study Design

Many studies have evaluated the effectiveness of various forms of psychological treatment in CHD patients, such as relaxation therapy, structured health education, and stress management. The results have been summarized in several meta-analyses.[109-111] Rees et al. examined nonspecific psychological interventions in CHD patients in general.[111] This Cochrane review indicated small reductions in depression, but no significant effects of psychological interventions on all-cause or cardiac mortality. Linden et al. examined various forms of psychological treatment of cardiac patients,[110] and found mortality benefits due to psychotherapy in men only. However, there were several problems associated with the studies included in these meta-analyses. Notably, there was significant heterogeneity in terms of the nature of the interventions, for example, stress management versus meditation, versus cognitive-behavioral therapy, and individual versus group therapy. Similarly, some trials evaluated psychological treatment as a single intervention, while others evaluated the treatment as part of a comprehensive cardiac rehabilitation program. Another source of heterogeneity was the patient type. Some patients received the intervention post-MI while others received it postsurgery, and some studies also included patients with chronic CHD and angina. Also, several studies did not evaluate the effects of depression-specific treatment in the population of CHD patients with comorbid depressive disorder. Rather, they evaluated the effects in the population of CHD patients with comorbid anxiety, depression, composite psychological outcomes, and others (stress and type A behavior). Overall, we feel that, although suggesting efficacy in terms of psychological and cardiac outcomes, this evaluation phase has not produced definitive evidence for or against the effects of depression treatment.

12.3.2 Phase 2: Depression Treatment and the Effect on Depression and Cardiac Outcome

Despite the prevalence of depression and its association with negative cardiac prognosis, only a limited number of pharmacological and behavioral randomized controlled trials has been performed in CHD patients with comorbid depressive disorder. Overall, treating depressive patients has served three goals: studying the safety of antidepressive treatments, evaluating the effects on depression per se (as well as quality of life), and studying the effects of depression treatment on cardiovascular outcomes.

First of all, it is important to know whether treatment is safe. The Sertraline Heart Attack Randomized Trial (SADHART) was designed as a safety trial, and is, to date, the largest RCT evaluating antidepressant medication use for depressed patients with unstable ischemic heart disease[112] ($N=369$). The primary safety outcome measure was change from baseline in left ventricular ejection fraction. The authors reported that sertraline is a "safe" treatment for depression in patients with recent MI or unstable angina and without other life-threatening medical conditions. Second, the Canadian Cardiac Randomized Evaluation of Antidepressant and Psychotherapy Efficacy Trial (CREATE) evaluated whether depression treatment improved depression scores in CHD patients. CREATE compared citalopram to placebo, and compared short-term interpersonal psychotherapy combined with clinical management to clinical management alone in patients with coronary artery disease[113] ($N=284$). The authors reported a statistically significant effect of citalopram in comparison with placebo in depressed CHD patients. There was no demonstrable benefit of psychotherapeutic intervention over clinical management alone.

The MIND-IT study was designed to evaluate whether antidepressive treatment for post-MI depression improves long-term depression status and cardiovascular prognosis.[114,115] The MIND-IT study was an effectiveness study rather than an efficacy study, and compared the effects of an active treatment strategy with usual care. In this multicenter randomized clinical trial, patients with a post-MI depressive episode were randomized to intervention (i.e., antidepressive treatment; $N=209$) or care as usual (CAU; $N=122$). First-choice treatment consisted of placebo-controlled treatment with mirtazapine. In case of refusal or nonresponse, alternative open treatment with citolapram was offered. In the CAU arm the patient was not informed about the research diagnosis. Psychiatric treatment outside the study was recorded, but no treatment was offered. Both arms were followed for endpoints. Cardiac events included cardiac death or hospital admission for documented nonfatal myocardial infarction, myocardial infarction, coronary revascularization, heart failure, or ventricular tachycardia. Forty-two cardiac events occurred in the time between randomization and 18 months post-myocardial infarction. Antidepressive treatment was significantly more effective than placebo after 8 weeks of treatment,[114] but no differences in depression status or cardiac event rates were found between patients in the intervention arm of the study and the care-as-usual arm at 18 months post-infarction.[115] However, the study was not well powered to evaluate treatment effects on coronary events.

The Enhancing Recovery in Coronary Heart Disease (ENRICHD) determined whether treating depression would alter CHD outcomes. ENRICHD was a randomized trial comparing cognitive behavioral therapy (CBT), plus sertraline in case of insufficient response, with usual care following MI[116] ($N = 2,481$). Overall, this study found that CBT improved depression, although only modestly. However, this study was unable to demonstrate that CBT, in comparison to usual care, reduced the composite endpoint of all-cause mortality and nonfatal-MI over 2 years.

Some researchers have suggested cardiac benefits for patients receiving antidepressive treatment in secondary analyses. In the ENRICHD trial, it was found that the prescription of serotonin reuptake inhibitors was associated with 40% reductions in both recurrent MI and death.[117] In addition, several studies suggest that unsuccessful treatment of depression identifies a subgroup of patients with high cardiac risk, and that response to antidepressive treatment is associated with less subsequent cardiac events[118,119] (see also Chap. 19 by Talbot Ellis and Linden). However, both of these findings must be interpreted with caution as they do not represent randomized comparisons.

A recent systematic review evaluated the effect of depression treatment on depressive symptoms and cardiac outcome. Overall, the authors found that depression treatment in CHD patients had only minor effects in terms of reducing depressive symptoms (effect size: 0.20–0.38; r^2: 1–4%), and that these effects did not lead to enhanced survival.[120]

12.4   Differential Effects of Intervention in Subtypes of Depression

12.4.1   Subtypes of Depression

Because randomized comparisons have found that depression treatment does not affect cardiac prognosis (albeit with reservations about statistical inadequacies), it may be reasonable to think that depression does not have a causal effect on cardiac events. However, depression is a heterogeneous condition, and it is possible that some types are cardiotoxic while others are not, and some types may respond to treatment while others do not. It is therefore important to identify patients who are at the highest risk for adverse cardiac outcome. Several subtypes of depression may be of importance in this respect. Recently, several studies have reported interesting subgroup analyses and re-analyses of existing epidemiologic studies and clinical trials.

The first observation concerns reports that there are prognostic differences between various depressive symptoms and/or symptom clusters. There seems to be a relevant distinction between somatic and cognitive depressive symptoms. Evidence indicates that self-reported somatic/affective, but not cognitive/affective symptoms of depression are highly prevalent in cardiac patients.[121] Furthermore, these symptoms are predictive of cardiovascular mortality and cardiac events, even after somatic health status has been controlled for.[122,123] Recently, these findings were replicated in two independent samples of post-MI patients,[124,125] and in patients with chronic heart failure.[126]

The second observation concerns reports that the increased cardiac risk in post-MI depression appears to be restricted to first-ever (incident) depressions in individuals who have not had depression before; however, this evidence is inconsistent.[127-132]

Third, the role of depression severity has been considered.[100,132] Fourth and most recently, the importance of depression persistence and treatment resistance has been evaluated with regard to prediction of cardiac events.[132-134]

So far, there is no consensus on which of these distinctions is clinically relevant, but additional research is needed. The identification of certain cardiotoxic aspects of depression could be an important step in the development of interventions. In this context, the distinction between somatic and cognitive depressive symptoms seems to be important as this distinction may contribute to finding an intervention to alleviate the depression-associated risk of cardiovascular events.

12.5   Discussion

The bidirectional relationship between CHD and depression represents a major challenge in health care. The field of depression and CHD has expanded enormously over the last two decades, but continues to be faced with several unresolved issues.

12.5.1   Screening

An important unresolved issue is whether patients with heart disease should be routinely screened for depression in clinical practice. There is an ongoing debate considering the benefits of depression screening in patients with cardiovascular disease. Recently, the American Heart Association science advisory recommended screening all post-MI patients for depression at regular intervals during the post-MI period, including during hospitalization, using a standardized depression symptoms checklist, and treat identified depression aggressively to improve not only the depression but also cardiac prognosis.[135] The recommendation was based on the high prevalence of depression in CHD and on the association of depression with poor cardiovascular prognosis, but a careful review of benefits and harms of routine depression screening was not performed.[136] In a careful systematic review, routine screening was discouraged at this time, because there is a lack of evidence that depression screening in patients with cardiovascular disease produces better outcomes.[120] So far, no study has actually evaluated whether screening for depression in patients with CHD improves access to depression care and thereby cardiac outcomes.

12.5.2   Mechanisms

In this chapter, we have proposed several possible mechanisms by which depression may lead to cardiac events. However, the role of factors that might explain the association between depression and CHD remains largely unclear. Clarifying how depression may lead to adverse cardiac outcome will be achieved, to some extent, by prospective research designs that simultaneously and carefully monitor depression, possible mediators and CHD outcomes. Additionally, such studies should include a variety of measures of plausible behavioral and physiological pathways through which the CHD effects of depression may be carried forward. Such research will help to pinpoint the mechanistic pathways that link depression to CHD progression.

12.5.3   Future Trials

Further research regarding the association between depression and CHD should be aimed at identifying or developing effective interventions. It is important that promising interventions are properly tested in new RCTs. Perhaps a more individualized form of treatment for depressed patients, based on their cardiac risks or markers of cardiac pathophysiology, is needed. We also need to know more about factors contributing to noncompliance with treatment.

For future trials, several (combinations of) pharmacological and behavioral interventions could be considered. There is strong evidence from the Heart and Soul study that lifestyle and physical exercise represent important pathways between depression and CHD outcomes in stable CHD patients. Physical exercise could therefore be an important and effective component of rehabilitation programs in future trials.[137,138]

Health care–related behavior may be a relevant target for intervention in depressed MI-patients.[52] Interventions focused on health care–related behavior could be implemented in collaborative care models for depressed patients. Collaborative care is based on the principle of structured care involving a greater role of nonmedical specialists to augment primary care. According to a recent meta-analysis, collaborative care is more effective than standard care in improving depression outcomes in the short and long terms.[139] Perhaps in depressed CHD patients, collaborative care can serve two goals: treatment of depression and enhancement of cardiac aftercare.

12.6 Conclusion

In a recent review, Frasure-Smith and Lespérance portrayed the present status and future directions of research regarding depression and cardiac risk, making a comparison between depression and Type A.[140] In 1981, a review stated that Type A behavior was associated with an increased risk of CHD.[141] However, soon after this statement, contradictory evidence began to appear, and today Type A research is scarce. Frasure-Smith and Lespérance concluded that, "only time will tell whether depression will follow in the footsteps of Type A behavior, or whether the efforts at isolating and treating its most cardiotoxic elements or behavioral and pathophysiological pathways will succeed." Future research will hopefully help to pinpoint the precise nature of the harmful aspects of depression, as well as the mechanistic pathways that link depression to CHD progression.

In this context, the distinction between somatic and cognitive depressive symptoms seems to be the most promising. Several studies showed that there is a consistent association between adverse cardiac outcome and somatic/affective, but not cognitive/affective symptoms of depression.[122-125] It is possible that depression treatment trials in CHD patients have primarily targeted the cognitive symptoms of depression, and that their inability to demonstrate reductions in cardiovascular morbidity and mortality may be partly attributable to under-treatment of the somatic features of depression. Although treating cognitive depressive symptoms is of importance, it may not result in improved cardiovascular outcome. The results from studies focusing on somatic and cognitive depressive symptoms indicate the need for future research directed at identifying the underlying pathophysiological processes by which somatic depressive symptoms contribute to prognosis in CHD patients. In addition, various interventions must be tested in order to alleviate the associated risk.

Depression and CHD are the two strongest contributors to the global burden of disease. Despite some efforts, several issues remain unresolved, with regard to the precise nature of the harmful CHD effects, the mechanistic pathways that link depression to CHD, the implementation of depression screening in CHD patients, and the best treatment for CHD patients with depression. Clarification of these issues in future research is important in order to identify depression treatments that have the potential to reduce both depressive symptoms and adverse cardiovascular outcomes.

References

1. Mathers CD, Loncar D. Projections of global mortality and burden of disease from 2002 to 2030. *PLoS Med.* 2006;3(11):e442.
2. Rumsfeld JS. Health status and clinical practice: when will they meet? *Circulation.* 2002;106(1):5-7.
3. Zellweger MJ, Osterwalder RH, Langewitz W, Pfisterer ME. Coronary artery disease and depression. *Eur Heart J.* 2004;25(1):3-9.
4. Schleifer SJ, ari-Hinson MM, Coyle DA, et al. The nature and course of depression following myocardial infarction. *Arch Intern Med.* 1989;149(8):1785-1789.
5. Rudisch B, Nemeroff CB. Epidemiology of comorbid coronary artery disease and depression. *Biol Psychiatry.* 2003;54(3):227-240.
6. Rutledge T, Reis VA, Linke SE, Greenberg BH, Mills PJ. Depression in heart failure a meta-analytic review of prevalence, intervention effects, and associations with clinical outcomes. *J Am Coll Cardiol.* 2006;48(8):1527-1537.
7. Thombs BD, Bass EB, Ford DE, et al. Prevalence of depression in survivors of acute myocardial infarction. *J Gen Intern Med.* 2006;21(1):30-38.
8. Kessler RC, Merikangas KR, Wang PS. Prevalence, comorbidity, and service utilization for mood disorders in the United States at the beginning of the twenty-first century. *Annu Rev Clin Psychol.* 2007;3:137-158.
9. Carney RM, Rich MW, Freedland KE, et al. Major depressive disorder predicts cardiac events in patients with coronary artery disease. *Psychosom Med.* 1988;50(6):627-633.
10. Frasure-Smith N, Lesperance F, Talajic M. Depression following myocardial infarction. Impact on 6-month survival. *JAMA.* 1993;270(15):1819-1825.
11. Lett HS, Blumenthal JA, Babyak MA, et al. Depression as a risk factor for coronary artery disease: evidence, mechanisms, and treatment. *Psychosom Med.* 2004;66(3):305-315.
12. Van der Kooy K, van Hout H, Marwijk H, Marten H, Stehouwer C, Beekman A. Depression and the risk for cardiovascular diseases: systematic review and meta analysis. *Int J Geriatr Psychiatry.* 2007;22(7):613-626.
13. Barth J, Schumacher M, Herrmann-Lingen C. Depression as a risk factor for mortality in patients with coronary heart disease: a meta-analysis. *Psychosom Med.* 2004;66(6):802-813.
14. Van Melle JP, de Jonge P, Spijkerman TA, et al. Prognostic association of depression following myocardial infarction with mortality and cardiovascular events: a meta-analysis. *Psychosom Med.* 2004;66(6):814-822.
15. Nicholson A, Kuper H, Hemingway H. Depression as an aetiologic and prognostic factor in coronary heart disease: a meta-analysis of 6362 events among 146,538 participants in 54 observational studies. *Eur Heart J.* 2006;27(23):2763-2774.
16. Frasure-Smith N, Lesperance F, Talajic M. Depression and 18-month prognosis after myocardial infarction. *Circulation.* 1995;91(4):999-1005.
17. Spijkerman TA, van den Brink RH, May JF, et al. Decreased impact of post-myocardial infarction depression on cardiac prognosis? *J Psychosom Res.* 2006;61(4):493-499.
18. Lane D, Carroll D, Ring C, Beevers DG, Lip GY. Mortality and quality of life 12 months after myocardial infarction: effects of depression and anxiety. *Psychosom Med.* 2001;63(2):221-230.
19. Mayou RA, Gill D, Thompson DR, et al. Depression and anxiety as predictors of outcome after myocardial infarction. *Psychosom Med.* 2000;62(2):212-219.
20. Carney RM, Blumenthal JA, Catellier D, et al. Depression as a risk factor for mortality after acute myocardial infarction. *Am J Cardiol.* 2003;92(11):1277-1281.
21. Lane D, Carroll D, Lip GY. Anxiety, depression, and prognosis after myocardial infarction: is there a causal association? *J Am Coll Cardiol.* 2003;42(10):1808-1810.
22. Pickering TG, Davidson K, Shimbo D. Is depression a risk factor for coronary heart disease? *J Am Coll Cardiol.* 2004;44(2):472-473.
23. Kuper H, Nicholson A, Kivimaki M, et al. Evaluating the causal relevance of diverse risk markers: horizontal systematic review. *BMJ.* 2009;339:b4265.

24. Sorensenf C, Friis-Hasche E, Haghfelt T, Bech P. Postmyocardial infarction mortality in relation to depression: a systematic critical review. *Psychother Psychosom.* 2005;74(2): 69-80.

25. Van Melle JP, de Jonge P, Ormel J, et al. Relationship between left ventricular dysfunction and depression following myocardial infarction: data from the MIND-IT. *Eur Heart J.* 2005;26(24):2650-2656.

26. Brown GW, Harris TO, Hepworth C. Life events and endogenous depression. A puzzle reexamined. *Arch Gen Psychiatry.* 1994;51(7):525-534.

27. Frasure-Smith N, Lesperance F, Juneau M, Talajic M, Bourassa MG. Gender, depression, and one-year prognosis after myocardial infarction. *Psychosom Med.* 1999;61(1):26-37.

28. Bush DE, Ziegelstein RC, Tayback M, et al. Even minimal symptoms of depression increase mortality risk after acute myocardial infarction. *Am J Cardiol.* 2001;88(4):337-341.

29. Strik JJ, Denollet J, Lousberg R, Honig A. Comparing symptoms of depression and anxiety as predictors of cardiac events and increased health care consumption after myocardial infarction. *J Am Coll Cardiol.* 2003;42(10):1801-1807.

30. Strik JJ, Lousberg R, Cheriex EC, Honig A. One year cumulative incidence of depression following myocardial infarction and impact on cardiac outcome. *J Psychosom Res.* 2004;56(1): 59-66.

31. Moussavi S, Chatterji S, Verdes E, Tandon A, Patel V, Ustun B. Depression, chronic diseases, and decrements in health: results from the World Health Surveys. *Lancet.* 2007;370(9590): 851-858.

32. Kronish IM, Rieckmann N, Schwartz JE, Schwartz DR, Davidson KW. Is depression after an acute coronary syndrome simply a marker of known prognostic factors for mortality? *Psychosom Med.* 2009;71(7):697-703.

33. Suls J, Bunde J. Anger, anxiety, and depression as risk factors for cardiovascular disease: the problems and implications of overlapping affective dispositions. *Psychol Bull.* 2005;131(2): 260-300.

34. Frasure-Smith N, Lesperance F, Talajic M. The impact of negative emotions on prognosis following myocardial infarction: is it more than depression? *Health Psychol.* 1995;14(5): 388-398.

35. Zimmerman M, McDermut W, Mattia JI. Frequency of anxiety disorders in psychiatric outpatients with major depressive disorder. *Am J Psychiatry.* 2000;157(8):1337-1340.

36. Denollet J, Strik JJ, Lousberg R, Honig A. Recognizing increased risk of depressive comorbidity after myocardial infarction: looking for 4 symptoms of anxiety-depression. *Psychother Psychosom.* 2006;75(6):346-352.

37. Roest AM, Martens EJ, Denollet J, de Jonge P. Prognostic association of anxiety post myocardial infarction with mortality and new cardiac events: a meta-analysis. *Psychosom Med.* 2010;72(6):563-569. Epub 2010 Apr 21.

38. Denollet J, Sys SU, Stroobant N, Rombouts H, Gillebert TC, Brutsaert DL. Personality as independent predictor of long-term mortality in patients with coronary heart disease. *Lancet.* 1996;347(8999):417-421.

39. Denollet J, Type D. Personality. A potential risk factor refined. *J Psychosom Res.* 2000;49(4):255-266.

40. Denollet J. Personality and coronary heart disease: the type-D scale-16 (DS16). *Ann Behav Med.* 1998;20(3):209-215.

41. Berkman LF, Leo-Summers L, Horwitz RI. Emotional support and survival after myocardial infarction. A prospective, population-based study of the elderly. *Ann Intern Med.* 1992;117(12): 1003-1009.

42. Kawachi I, Colditz GA, Ascherio A, et al. A prospective study of social networks in relation to total mortality and cardiovascular disease in men in the USA. *J Epidemiol Community Health.* 1996;50(3):245-251.

43. Williams RB, Barefoot JC, Califf RM, et al. Prognostic importance of social and economic resources among medically treated patients with angiographically documented coronary artery disease. *JAMA.* 1992;267(4):520-524.

44. Mookadam F, Arthur HM. Social support and its relationship to morbidity and mortality after acute myocardial infarction: systematic overview. *Arch Intern Med.* 2004;164(14):1514-1518.
45. Appels A, Kop W, Bar F, de Swart H, Mendes de Leon C. Vital exhaustion, extent of atherosclerosis, and the clinical course after successful percutaneous transluminal coronary angioplasty. *Eur Heart J.* 1995;16(12):1880-1885.
46. Kop WJ, Appels AP, de Leon CF Mendes, de Swart HB, Bar FW. Vital exhaustion predicts new cardiac events after successful coronary angioplasty. *Psychosom Med.* 1994;56(4):281-287.
47. Chida Y, Steptoe A. The association of anger and hostility with future coronary heart disease: a meta-analytic review of prospective evidence. *J Am Coll Cardiol.* 2009;53(11):936-946.
48. Carney RM, Blumenthal JA, Stein PK, et al. Depression, heart rate variability, and acute myocardial infarction. *Circulation.* 2001;104(17):2024-2028.
49. Glassman AH, Helzer JE, Covey LS, et al. Smoking, smoking cessation, and major depression. *JAMA.* 1990;264(12):1546-1549.
50. Pfohl B, Rederer M, Coryell W, Stangl D. Association between post-dexamethasone cortisol level and blood pressure in depressed inpatients. *J Nerv Ment Dis.* 1991;179(1):44-47.
51. Dantzer R, O'Connor JC, Freund GG, Johnson RW, Kelley KW. From inflammation to sickness and depression: when the immune system subjugates the brain. *Nat Rev Neurosci.* 2008;9(1):46-56.
52. Ziegelstein RC, Fauerbach JA, Stevens SS, Romanelli J, Richter DP, Bush DE. Patients with depression are less likely to follow recommendations to reduce cardiac risk during recovery from a myocardial infarction. *Arch Intern Med.* 2000;160(12):1818-1823.
53. Musselman DL, Tomer A, Manatunga AK, et al. Exaggerated platelet reactivity in major depression. *Am J Psychiatry.* 1996;153(10):1313-1317.
54. Otte C, Marmar CR, Pipkin SS, Moos R, Browner WS, Whooley MA. Depression and 24-hour urinary cortisol in medical outpatients with coronary heart disease: the Heart and Soul Study. *Biol Psychiatry.* 2004;56(4):241-247.
55. Ruo B, Rumsfeld JS, Pipkin S, Whooley MA. Relation between depressive symptoms and treadmill exercise capacity in the Heart and Soul Study. *Am J Cardiol.* 2004;94(1):96-99.
56. Schins A, Hamulyak K, Scharpe S, et al. Whole blood serotonin and platelet activation in depressed post-myocardial infarction patients. *Life Sci.* 2004;76(6):637-650.
57. Barefoot JC, Burg MM, Carney RM, et al. Aspects of social support associated with depression at hospitalization and follow-up assessment among cardiac patients. *J Cardiopulm Rehabil.* 2003;23(6):404-412.
58. Frasure-Smith N, Lesperance F, Julien P. Major depression is associated with lower omega-3 fatty acid levels in patients with recent acute coronary syndromes. *Biol Psychiatry.* 2004;55(9):891-896.
59. Cohen HW, Gibson G, Alderman MH. Excess risk of myocardial infarction in patients treated with antidepressant medications: association with use of tricyclic agents. *Am J Med.* 2000;108(1):2-8.
60. Otte C, Neylan TC, Pipkin SS, Browner WS, Whooley MA. Depressive symptoms and 24-hour urinary norepinephrine excretion levels in patients with coronary disease: findings from the Heart and Soul Study. *Am J Psychiatry.* 2005;162(11):2139-2145.
61. Carney RM, Freedland KE, Miller GE, Jaffe AS. Depression as a risk factor for cardiac mortality and morbidity: a review of potential mechanisms. *J Psychosom Res.* 2002;53(4):897-902.
62. De Jonge P, Rosmalen JG, Kema IP, et al. Psychophysiological biomarkers explaining the association between depression and prognosis in coronary artery patients: a critical review of the literature. *Neurosci Biobehav Rev.* 2010;35(1):84-90. Epub 2009 Dec 3.
63. Joynt KE, Whellan DJ, O'Connor CM. Why is depression bad for the failing heart? a review of the mechanistic relationship between depression and heart failure. *J Card Fail.* 2004;10(3):258-271.
64. Whooley MA. Depression and cardiovascular disease: healing the broken-hearted. *JAMA.* 2006;295(24):2874-2881.
65. Grippo AJ, Johnson AK. Biological mechanisms in the relationship between depression and heart disease. *Neurosci Biobehav Rev.* 2002;26(8):941-962.

66. Krittayaphong R, Cascio WE, Light KC, et al. Heart rate variability in patients with coronary artery disease: differences in patients with higher and lower depression scores. *Psychosom Med.* 1997;59(3):231-235.
67. Stein PK, Carney RM, Freedland KE, et al. Severe depression is associated with markedly reduced heart rate variability in patients with stable coronary heart disease. *J Psychosom Res.* 2000;48(4–5):493-500.
68. Frasure-Smith N, Lesperance F, Irwin MR, Talajic M, Pollock BG. The relationships among heart rate variability, inflammatory markers and depression in coronary heart disease patients. *Brain Behav Immun.* 2009;23(8):1140-1147.
69. Gehi A, Mangano D, Pipkin S, Browner WS, Whooley MA. Depression and heart rate variability in patients with stable coronary heart disease: findings from the Heart and Soul Study. *Arch Gen Psychiatry.* 2005;62(6):661-666.
70. Martens EJ, Nyklicek I, Szabo BM, Kupper N. Depression and anxiety as predictors of heart rate variability after myocardial infarction. *Psychol Med.* 2008;38(3):375-383.
71. Carney RM, Blumenthal JA, Freedland KE, et al. Low heart rate variability and the effect of depression on post-myocardial infarction mortality. *Arch Intern Med.* 2005;165(13): 1486-1491.
72. Whooley MA, de Jonge P, Vittinghoff E, et al. Depressive symptoms, health behaviors, and risk of cardiovascular events in patients with coronary heart disease. *JAMA.* 2008;300(20): 2379-2388.
73. De Jonge P, Mangano D, Whooley MA. Differential association of cognitive and somatic depressive symptoms with heart rate variability in patients with stable coronary heart disease: findings from the Heart and Soul Study. *Psychosom Med.* 2007;69(8):735-739.
74. Sukhija R, Fahdi I, Garza L, et al. Inflammatory markers, angiographic severity of coronary artery disease, and patient outcome. *Am J Cardiol.* 2007;99(7):879-884.
75. Howren MB, Lamkin DM, Suls J. Associations of depression with C-reactive protein, IL-1, and IL-6: a meta-analysis. *Psychosom Med.* 2009;71(2):171-186.
76. Alexopoulos GS, Meyers BS, Young RC, Campbell S, Silbersweig D, Charlson M. 'Vascular depression' hypothesis. *Arch Gen Psychiatry.* 1997;54(10):915-922.
77. Nemeroff CB, Musselman DL. Are platelets the link between depression and ischemic heart disease? *Am Heart J.* 2000;140(4 suppl):57-62.
78. Von Kanel R. Platelet hyperactivity in clinical depression and the beneficial effect of antidepressant drug treatment: how strong is the evidence? *Acta Psychiatr Scand.* 2004;110(3): 163-177.
79. Nijm J, Jonasson L. Inflammation and cortisol response in coronary artery disease. *Ann Med.* 2009;41(3):224-233.
80. Rosmond R, Bjorntorp P. The hypothalamic-pituitary-adrenal axis activity as a predictor of cardiovascular disease, type 2 diabetes and stroke. *J Intern Med.* 2000;247(2):188-197.
81. Bhattacharyya MR, Molloy GJ, Steptoe A. Depression is associated with flatter cortisol rhythms in patients with coronary artery disease. *J Psychosom Res.* 2008;65(2):107-113.
82. Whitehead DL, Perkins-Porras L, Strike PC, Magid K, Steptoe A. Cortisol awakening response is elevated in acute coronary syndrome patients with type-D personality. *J Psychosom Res.* 2007;62(4):419-425.
83. Koeijvoets KC, van der Net JB, van Rossum EF, et al. Two common haplotypes of the glucocorticoid receptor gene are associated with increased susceptibility to cardiovascular disease in men with familial hypercholesterolemia. *J Clin Endocrinol Metab.* 2008;93(12):4902-4908.
84. Bach-Mizrachi H, Underwood MD, Tin A, Ellis SP, Mann JJ, Arango V. Elevated expression of tryptophan hydroxylase-2 mRNA at the neuronal level in the dorsal and median raphe nuclei of depressed suicides. *Mol Psychiatry.* 2008;13(5):507-513, 465.
85. McCaffery JM, Frasure-Smith N, Dube MP, et al. Common genetic vulnerability to depressive symptoms and coronary artery disease: a review and development of candidate genes related to inflammation and serotonin. *Psychosom Med.* 2006;68(2):187-200.
86. Nakatani D, Sato H, Sakata Y, et al. Influence of serotonin transporter gene polymorphism on depressive symptoms and new cardiac events after acute myocardial infarction. *Am Heart J.* 2005;150(4):652-658.

87. Skala JA, Freedland KE, Carney RM. Coronary heart disease and depression: a review of recent mechanistic research. *Can J Psychiatry*. 2006;51(12):738-745.
88. Osterberg L, Blaschke T. Adherence to medication. *N Engl J Med*. 2005;353(5):487-497.
89. Haynes RB, McDonald HP, Garg AX. Helping patients follow prescribed treatment: clinical applications. *JAMA*. 2002;288(22):2880-2883.
90. DiMatteo MR, Lepper HS, Croghan TW. Depression is a risk factor for noncompliance with medical treatment: meta-analysis of the effects of anxiety and depression on patient adherence. *Arch Intern Med*. 2000;160(14):2101-2107.
91. Gehi AK, Ali S, Na B, Whooley MA. Self-reported medication adherence and cardiovascular events in patients with stable coronary heart disease: the heart and soul study. *Arch Intern Med*. 2007;167(16):1798-1803.
92. Jolliffe JA, Rees K, Taylor RS, Thompson D, Oldridge N, Ebrahim S. Exercise-based rehabilitation for coronary heart disease. *Cochrane Database Syst Rev*. 2001;(1):CD001800.
93. Lane D, Carroll D, Ring C, Beevers DG, Lip GY. Predictors of attendance at cardiac rehabilitation after myocardial infarction. *J Psychosom Res*. 2001;51(3):497-501.
94. Casey E, Hughes JW, Waechter D, Josephson R, Rosneck J. Depression predicts failure to complete phase-II cardiac rehabilitation. *J Behav Med*. 2008;31(5):421-431.
95. Druss BG, Bradford DW, Rosenheck RA, Radford MJ, Krumholz HM. Mental disorders and use of cardiovascular procedures after myocardial infarction. *JAMA*. 2000;283(4):506-511.
96. Kisely S, Smith M, Lawrence D, Cox M, Campbell LA, Maaten S. Inequitable access for mentally ill patients to some medically necessary procedures. *CMAJ*. 2007;176(6):779-784.
97. Jee SH, Suh I, Kim IS, Appel LJ. Smoking and atherosclerotic cardiovascular disease in men with low levels of serum cholesterol: the Korea Medical Insurance Corporation Study. *JAMA*. 1999;282(22):2149-2155.
98. Goldenberg I, Jonas M, Tenenbaum A, et al. Current smoking, smoking cessation, and the risk of sudden cardiac death in patients with coronary artery disease. *Arch Intern Med*. 2003; 163(19):2301-2305.
99. Siru R, Hulse GK, Tait RJ. Assessing motivation to quit smoking in people with mental illness: a review. *Addiction*. 2009;104(5):719-733.
100. Carney RM, Freedland KE, Steinmeyer B, et al. Depression and five year survival following acute myocardial infarction: a prospective study. *J Affect Disord*. 2008;109(1–2):133-138.
101. Mead GE, Morley W, Campbell P, Greig CA, McMurdo M, Lawlor DA. Exercise for depression. *Cochrane Database Syst Rev*. 2009;(3):CD004366.
102. Baron RM, Kenny DA. The moderator-mediator variable distinction in social psychological research: conceptual, strategic, and statistical considerations. *J Pers Soc Psychol*. 1986;51(6): 1173-1182.
103. Kraemer HC, Kiernan M, Essex M, Kupfer DJ. How and why criteria defining moderators and mediators differ between the Baron & Kenny and MacArthur approaches. *Health Psychol*. 2008;27(2 suppl):S101-S108.
104. Grippo AJ, Johnson AK. Stress, depression and cardiovascular dysregulation: a review of neurobiological mechanisms and the integration of research from preclinical disease models. *Stress*. 2009;12(1):1-21.
105. Carney RM, Freedland KE, Stein PK, et al. Heart rate variability and markers of inflammation and coagulation in depressed patients with coronary heart disease. *J Psychosom Res*. 2007;62(4):463-467.
106. Janszky I, Ericson M, Lekander M, et al. Inflammatory markers and heart rate variability in women with coronary heart disease. *J Intern Med*. 2004;256(5):421-428.
107. Melander H, Ahlqvist-Rastad J, Meijer G, Beermann B. Evidence b(i)ased medicine–selective reporting from studies sponsored by pharmaceutical industry: review of studies in new drug applications. *BMJ*. 2003;326(7400):1171-1173.
108. Turner EH, Matthews AM, Linardatos E, Tell RA, Rosenthal R. Selective publication of antidepressant trials and its influence on apparent efficacy. *N Engl J Med*. 2008;358(3): 252-260.
109. Dusseldorp E, van Elderen T, Maes S, Meulman J, Kraaij V. A meta-analysis of psychoeducational programs for coronary heart disease patients. *Health Psychol*. 1999;18(5):506-519.

110. Linden W, Phillips MJ, Leclerc J. Psychological treatment of cardiac patients: a meta-analysis. *Eur Heart J*. 2007;28(24):2972-2984.

111. Rees K, Bennett P, West R, Davey SG, Ebrahim S. Psychological interventions for coronary heart disease. *Cochrane Database Syst Rev*. 2004;(2):CD002902.

112. Glassman AH, O'Connor CM, Califf RM, et al. Sertraline treatment of major depression in patients with acute MI or unstable angina. *JAMA*. 2002;288(6):701-709.

113. Lesperance F, Frasure-Smith N, Koszycki D, et al. Effects of citalopram and interpersonal psychotherapy on depression in patients with coronary artery disease: the Canadian Cardiac Randomized Evaluation of Antidepressant and Psychotherapy Efficacy (CREATE) trial. *JAMA*. 2007;297(4):367-379.

114. Honig A, Kuyper AM, Schene AH, et al. Treatment of post-myocardial infarction depressive disorder: a randomized, placebo-controlled trial with mirtazapine. *Psychosom Med*. 2007; 69(7):606-613.

115. Van Melle JP, de Jonge P, Honig A, et al. Effects of antidepressant treatment following myocardial infarction. *Br J Psychiatry*. 2007;190:460-466.

116. Berkman LF, Blumenthal J, Burg M, et al. Effects of treating depression and low perceived social support on clinical events after myocardial infarction: the Enhancing Recovery in Coronary Heart Disease Patients (ENRICHD) randomized trial. *JAMA*. 2003;289(23): 3106-3116.

117. Taylor CB, Youngblood ME, Catellier D, et al. Effects of antidepressant medication on morbidity and mortality in depressed patients after myocardial infarction. *Arch Gen Psychiatry*. 2005;62(7):792-798.

118. Carney RM, Blumenthal JA, Freedland KE, et al. Depression and late mortality after myocardial infarction in the Enhancing Recovery in Coronary Heart Disease (ENRICHD) study. *Psychosom Med*. 2004;66(4):466-474.

119. De Jonge P, Honig A, van Melle JP, et al. Nonresponse to treatment for depression following myocardial infarction: association with subsequent cardiac events. *Am J Psychiatry*. 2007; 164(9):1371-1378.

120. Thombs BD, de Jonge P, Coyne JC, et al. Depression screening and patient outcomes in cardiovascular care: a systematic review. *JAMA*. 2008;300(18):2161-2171.

121. Martens EJ, Denollet J, Pedersen SS, et al. Relative lack of depressive cognitions in post-myocardial infarction depression. *J Affect Disord*. 2006;94(1–3):231-237.

122. De Jonge P, Ormel J, van den Brink RH, et al. Symptom dimensions of depression following myocardial infarction and their relationship with somatic health status and cardiovascular prognosis. *Am J Psychiatry*. 2006;163(1):138-144.

123. Linke SE, Rutledge T, Johnson BD, et al. Depressive symptom dimensions and cardiovascular prognosis among women with suspected myocardial ischemia: a report from the National Heart, Lung, and Blood Institute-sponsored Women's Ischemia Syndrome Evaluation. *Arch Gen Psychiatry*. 2009;66(5):499-507.

124. Martens EJ, Hoen PW, Mittelhaeuser M, de Jonge P, Denollet J. Symptom dimensions of post-myocardial infarction depression, disease severity and cardiac prognosis. *Psychol Med*. 2009;20:1-8.

125. Smolderen KG, Spertus JA, Reid KJ, et al. The association of cognitive and somatic depressive symptoms with depression recognition and outcomes after myocardial infarction. *Circ Cardiovasc Qual Outcomes*. 2009;2(4):328-337.

126. Schiffer AA, Pelle AJ, Smith OR, Widdershoven JW, Hendriks EH, Pedersen SS. Somatic versus cognitive symptoms of depression as predictors of all-cause mortality and health status in chronic heart failure. *J Clin Psychiatry*. 2009;70(12):1667-1673. Epub 2009 Jul 28.

127. Carney RM, Freedland KE, Steinmeyer B, et al. History of depression and survival after acute myocardial infarction. *Psychosom Med*. 2009;71(3):253-259.

128. De Jonge P, van den Brink RH, Spijkerman TA, Ormel J. Only incident depressive episodes after myocardial infarction are associated with new cardiovascular events. *J Am Coll Cardiol*. 2006;48(11):2204-2208.

129. Grace SL, Abbey SE, Kapral MK, Fang J, Nolan RP, Stewart DE. Effect of depression on five-year mortality after an acute coronary syndrome. *Am J Cardiol.* 2005;96(9):1179-1185.
130. Parker GB, Hilton TM, Walsh WF, et al. Timing is everything: the onset of depression and acute coronary syndrome outcome. *Biol Psychiatry.* 2008;64(8):660-666.
131. Lesperance F, Frasure-Smith N, Talajic M. Major depression before and after myocardial infarction: its nature and consequences. *Psychosom Med.* 1996;58(2):99-110.
132. Glassman AH, Bigger JT Jr, Gaffney M. Psychiatric characteristics associated with long-term mortality among 361 patients having an acute coronary syndrome and major depression: seven-year follow-up of SADHART participants. *Arch Gen Psychiatry.* 2009;66(9):1022-1029.
133. Carney RM, Freedland KE. Treatment-resistant depression and mortality after acute coronary syndrome. *Am J Psychiatry.* 2009;166(4):410-417.
134. Kaptein KI, de Jonge P, van den Brink RH, Korf J. Course of depressive symptoms after myocardial infarction and cardiac prognosis: a latent class analysis. *Psychosom Med.* 2006;68(5):662-668.
135. Lichtman JH, Bigger JT Jr, Blumenthal JA, et al. Depression and coronary heart disease: recommendations for screening, referral, and treatment: a science advisory from the American Heart Association Prevention Committee of the Council on Cardiovascular Nursing, Council on Clinical Cardiology, Council on Epidemiology and Prevention, and Interdisciplinary Council on Quality of Care and Outcomes Research: endorsed by the American Psychiatric Association. *Circulation.* 2008;118(17):1768-1775.
136. Thombs BD, Jewett LR, Knafo R, Coyne JC, Ziegelstein RC. Learning from history: a commentary on the American Heart Association Science Advisory on depression screening. *Am Heart J.* 2009;158(4):503-505.
137. Blumenthal JA, Babyak MA, Doraiswamy PM, et al. Exercise and pharmacotherapy in the treatment of major depressive disorder. *Psychosom Med.* 2007;69(7):587-596.
138. Blumenthal JA. Depression and coronary heart disease: association and implications for treatment. *Cleve Clin J Med.* 2008;75(suppl 2):S48-S53.
139. Gilbody S, Bower P, Fletcher J, Richards D, Sutton AJ. Collaborative care for depression: a cumulative meta-analysis and review of longer-term outcomes. *Arch Intern Med.* 2006; 166(21):2314-2321.
140. Frasure-Smith N, Lesperance F. Depression and cardiac risk: present status and future directions. *Heart.* 2010;96(3):173-176.
141. Coronary-prone behavior and coronary heart disease: a critical review. The review panel on coronary-prone behavior and coronary heart disease. *Circulation.* 1981;63(6):1199-1215.

Chapter 13
Post-traumatic Stress Disorder: Emerging Risk Factor and Mechanisms

Roland von Känel and Marie-Louise Gander Ferrari

Keywords Clinical management • Emerging risk factor • Mechanisms • Pathophysiologic links • Post-traumatic stress disorder • Predictors • Prevalence • Therapeutic approach

13.1 Introduction

The psychological impact of man-made and natural disaster-related traumatic experiences is well known. For instance, in former prisoners of war as well as in survivors of terrorist attacks and earthquakes, trauma-related distress and psychiatric diseases such as post-traumatic stress disorder (PTSD), anxiety disorder, and major depressive disorders are prevalent.[1-3] In addition to the more traditional causes of a psychological trauma, it is now acknowledged that medical diagnoses and procedures such as multiple physical trauma, severe burns, cancer, and heart diseases can also be experienced as emotionally painful, distressful, and shocking.[4-7]

Moreover, recent research shows that psychological traumas may not only result in lasting mental but also in physical effects setting the stage for the development of somatic diseases. For instance, there was a graded relationship between the severity of adverse childhood experiences, including psychological, physical, or

R. von Känel (✉) • M.-L.G. Ferrari
Department of General Internal Medicine, Division of Psychosomatic Medicine,
Inselspital, Bern University Hospital, CH-3010, Bern, Switzerland
e-mail: roland.vonkaenel@insel.ch; marie-louise.gander@insel.ch

P. Hjemdahl et al. (eds.), *Stress and Cardiovascular Disease*,
DOI 10.1007/978-1-84882-419-5_13, © Springer-Verlag London Limited 2012

sexual abuse, and the presence of adult diseases including coronary heart disease (CHD), cancer, chronic lung disease, and liver disease.[8] Many decades after having served in Vietnam, traumatized combat veterans showed an increased prevalence of common autoimmune diseases, including rheumatoid arthritis and insulin-dependent diabetes, as well as musculoskeletal, respiratory, and cardiovascular diseases (CVD).[9,10] Taken together, there is emerging evidence to suggest that both man-made and non-man-made (i.e., disaster- or disease-related) psychological traumas may profoundly impact physical health.

This chapter summarizes the current knowledge about the possible role of post-traumatic stress and PTSD for the manifestation and course of CVD, particularly myocardial infarction (MI). Epidemiological, behavioral, psychophysiologic, and therapeutic aspects of this still nascent field of research will be discussed.

13.2   Definition of Post-traumatic Stress Disorder

Table 13.1 shows the diagnostic criteria for PTSD according to the fourth edition of the Diagnostic and Statistical Manual of Mental Diseases (DSM-IV).[11] Post-traumatic stress disorder is a debilitating form of chronic psychological stress, which develops after exposure to a traumatic event to which a person responded with fear, helplessness, or horror (criterion A). Patients with PTSD have three distinct clusters of symptoms consisting of reexperiencing of the event (criterion B), avoidance of reminders of the event (criterion C), and hyperarousal (criterion D) for at least 1 month. As an example, we saw a patient who reported to have experienced intense fear of dying during the MI, recollected intrusive thoughts in her dreams about being referred to the hospital in the ambulance with sounding siren, and avoided visiting relatives in the hospital to prevent being reminded of her own heart attack.

Several subtypes of PTSD can be distinguished based on the severity and time course of the disorder. Full (i.e., syndromal) PTSD meets criteria B, C, and D, and subthreshold (i.e., subsyndromal) PTSD meets criterion B plus either criterion C or D.[12] Acute PTSD refers to symptoms that last less than 3 months, whereas chronic PTSD refers to symptoms that last 3 months or longer. Delayed-onset PTSD refers to symptoms that begin at least 6 months after the trauma.[13]

Several self-rated post-traumatic symptom questionnaires such as the Post-traumatic Diagnostic Scale[14] and the Impact of Event Scale[15] are available for the assessment of PTSD symptom levels and case definitions of PTSD based on established cut-off points. Importantly, a standardized interview is required to make a clinical diagnosis of DSM-IV PTSD. For instance, own work cited in this chapter applied the widely used semi-structured Clinician-Administered PTSD Scale (CAPS) interview.[16] The CAPS quantifies the frequency and intensity of each of 17 PTSD symptoms. Overall severity of PTSD is obtained by adding up symptom scores of criteria B, C, and D.

Table 13.1 Diagnostic criteria for post-traumatic stress disorder

(A) A person must have been exposed to a traumatic event.
   – The event involved a perceived or actual threat to the person's own life or physical integrity or that of another, such as a physical or sexual assault, rape, a serious accident, a natural disaster, combat, being taken hostage, torture, displacement as a refugee, sudden unexpected death of a loved one, and witnessing a traumatic event.
   – The person's response to the event involved fear, helplessness, or horror.
(B) The person persistently reexperiences the event in at least one of several ways:
   – The person has intrusive recollections of the event.
   – The person has nightmares.
   – The person has flashbacks, which are particularly vivid memories that occur while he or she is awake and make him or her act or feel as though the event was recurring.
   – The person has intense psychological distress in response to reminders of the traumatic event.
   – The person has intense physiological reactions in response to reminders of the event (including palpitations, sweating, difficulty breathing, and other panic responses).
(C) The person avoids reminders of the event and has generalized numbness of feeling, as indicated by the presence of at least three of the following:
   – The person actively avoids pursuits, people, and places that remind him or her of the event.
   – The person avoids thinking of or talking about the event.
   – The person is unable to recall aspects of the event.
   – The person has lost interest in or participates less in activities.
   – The person has felt detached or estranged from other people since the event.
   – The person has a restricted range of emotions or a feeling of numbness.
   – The person feels as though his or her life has been foreshortened or as though there is no need to plan for the future, with respect to his or her career, getting married, or having children.
(D) The person has symptoms of increased arousal, as evidenced by the presence of at least two of the following:
   – The person has difficulty falling or staying asleep (sometimes related to fear of having nightmares).
   – The person is irritable and has feelings of outbursts of anger.
   – The person has difficulty concentrating.
   – The person has become more vigilant and concerned about safety.
   – The person has exaggerated startle reactions in response to sounds or movements.
Three types of symptoms (B–D) must be present together for at least 1 month.
The disorder must cause clinically significant distress or impairment in social, occupational, or other areas of functioning.

Adapted from American Psychiatric Association[11]

13.3   Prevalence of Post-traumatic Stress Disorder

Depending upon the type of trauma and country in which population-based studies were performed, the life-time prevalence of PTSD varies widely, from less than 1% to about 10%.[17] In the USA, the estimated lifetime prevalence of PTSD is almost 8%, whereby combat exposure and being a witness to combat exposure among men and sexual assaults among women are the most common traumas associated with PTSD.[18] More than one third of people with an index episode of PTSD fail to recover even after many years.

The prevalence of PTSD caused by experiencing a potentially life-threatening cardiac disease and heart-related procedures has most often been studied in post-MI patients and seems at least as high as in man-made and disaster-related trauma.[6] In our previous review of 13 published studies (mainly from European countries) we found that the prevalence of PTSD caused by MI was approximately 10% when based on clinical interviews, whereas questionnaire-based surveys yielded prevalence rates of about 15%.[19] For comparison, the prevalence of major depression in patients who have had MI is about 20%. In a consecutively recruited sample of 951 patients who had had a verified MI, we found 10.4% of respondents to have either a full or subthreshold diagnosis of PTSD.[20] Two thirds of the patients with PTSD who consented to a follow-up interview 1–3 years after their index MI still qualified for a PTSD diagnosis.[21] In another study, post-traumatic stress symptoms persisted at least 3 years after an acute cardiac event.[22] Therefore, PTSD caused by MI is a frequently persistent condition. PTSD has also been attributed to the traumatic experiences of surviving a sudden cardiac arrest, cardiac surgery, and heart transplantation with prevalence rates comparable to those observed in relation to MI or even higher.[6] The psychological response to experiencing cumulative shocks in patients with an implantable cardioverter-defibrillator (ICD) may also comprise PTSD.[23]

13.4 Predictors of Post-traumatic Stress After Myocardial Infarction

Several potential predictors ("risk factors") for the development of PTSD symptomatology and diagnostic PTSD in post-MI patients have been described. As shown in Table 13.2, these risk factors relate to demographic and personality characteristics, prior mental and cardiac history, coping strategies, the subjective experience of the index MI, and acute stress disorder (ASD).[20,22,24-36] With regard to the latter, clinicians are aware and studies show that the majority of patients experience moderate to intense distress during the acute phase of MI.[37] Within the first month after an acute MI, post-traumatic stress symptomatology may reach a level that qualifies for DSM-IV ASD in about 4% of the patients.[38] Unlike PTSD, ASD is characterized by dissociative symptoms, meaning that a patient with ASD may for instance feel detached from his or her body and experiences the world as unreal or dreamlike.[11] Notably, the subjective perception of the MI as life- threatening and leaving one helpless reliably predicts PTSD development, whereas objective markers of myocardial damage such as cardiac enzymes and left ventricular ejection fraction do not.[20,30] Conversely, positive affect at the time of hospitalization because of MI predicted a lower risk of developing MI-related PTSD symptoms.[26] The use of sedation and analgesia during or after cardiac arrest in resuscitated patients was unrelated to the risk of developing PTSD.[39]

Table 13.2 Risk factors of PTSD in the aftermath of myocardial infarction

Risk factor	Source
Sociodemographic factors	
Ethnic origin/minority	Wikman et al.[22], Kutz et al.[24]
Younger age	Bennett and Brooke[25]
Prior history	
Prior myocardial infarction	Kutz et al.[24]
Prior cardiac hospitalization	Kutz et al.[24]
Recurrence of cardiac symptoms	Wikman et al.[22]
Recurrent medical intervention	Chung et al.[26]
Previous traumatization, PTSD	Kutz et al.[24]
Life events	Ginzburg[27]
Aspects related to myocardial infarction	
Anticipation of disability	Kutz et al.[24]
Awareness of event as infarct	Bennett and Brooke[25]
Perceived threat and helplessness	Guler et al.[20], Bennett et al.[28], Ginzburg et al.[29], Wiedemar et al.[30]
Dissociation at the time of infarct	Bennett et al.[28], Ginzburg et al.[31]
Acute stress disorder	Ginzburg et al.[29], Ginzburg et al.[31,32]
Negative effect, incl. depression	Wikman et al.[22], Bennett et al.[28], Pedersen et al.[33], Whitehead et al.[34], Chung et al.[35]
Somatic problems/complaints	Ginzburg et al.[32], Chung et al.[35]
Pain during infarct	Wiedemar et al.[30], Whitehead et al.[34]
Personality characteristics	
Type D personality	Pedersen and Denollet [36]
Neuroticism	Chung et al.[35], Pedersen and Denollet[36]
Agreeableness	Chung et al.[35]
Non-repressive coping style	Ginzburg et al.[29,32]
Alexithymia	Bennett and Brooke[25]
Social support	
Lack of social support	Bennett and Brooke[25]
Social deprivation	Wikman et al.[22]
Social dysfunction	Chung et al.[35]

13.5   Post-traumatic Stress Disorder as a Risk Factor for Cardiovascular Disease

Table 13.3 summarizes studies in which PTSD symptomatology and PTSD diagnosis have been associated with an increased risk of different cardiovascular endpoints. Whereas most of these studies are cross-sectional,[9,40-47] there is emerging evidence to suggest that PTSD adversely impacts cardiovascular health several decades down the line in individuals who were initially free of CVD.[48-51] In particular, various case definitions of PTSD predicted the risk of suffering nonfatal MI and fatal CHD combined[49] and mortality from cardiac disease[50] in male veterans. In the latter study, there was also a graded relationship between the level of PTSD symptoms, and

Table 13.3 Association of post-traumatic stress disorder with cardiovascular endpoints

Source	Diagnostic tools	Type of trauma	Subjects	Control for cardiovascular risk factors	Cardiovascular endpoints
Boscarino[9]	DIS (DMS-III)	Combat exposure or noncombat-related trauma	1,399 male veterans, 24% with PTSD	Age, income, race, education, smoking	Higher rates of self-reported circulatory diseases in PTSD patients
Shalev et al.[40]	Clinical interview for PTSD (DMS-III), PTSD scale	Combat exposure	98 male veterans, 1.2% with PTSD	Alcohol, smoking	Lower effort tolerance and performance on ergometer and more self-reported cardiovascular symptoms in PTSD patients
Falger et al.[41]	SCID (DSM-III-revised)	Combat exposure	147 male veterans, 56% with PTSD	None	Higher rate of self-reported angina pectoris in PTSD patients
McFarlane et al.[42]	DIS (DMS-III), IES	Bushfire disaster	140 fire-fighters, 50% PTSD	None	Higher rate of self-reported cardiovascular symptoms in PTSD patients
Cwikel et al.[43]	IES	Nuclear accident	520 immigrants, 58 exposed to trauma	None	More PTSD symptoms correlate with higher rate of self-reported heart disease
Boscarino and Chang[44]	DIS (DMS-III)	Combat exposure or any other trauma	4,462 male veterans, 51% with PTSD	Age, race, body mass index, alcohol, cigarette smoking, education	More electrocardiographic signs of atrioventricular conduction defects and infarctions in PTSD patients
Schnurr et al.[45]	SCID (DSM-III-revised) Mississippi Scale for combat-related PTSD	Combat exposure	605 male veterans, 1% with PTSD	Age, smoking regular alcohol, body mass index	PTSD symptoms correlate with higher rate of physician-diagnosed arterial disease (ICDA-8)

Dobie et al.[46]	PTSD Checklist – civilian version	Not specified	1,259 female veterans, 21% with PTSD	Age	Higher rates of stroke but not of MI or CAD in PTSD patients
Sawchuk et al.[47]	WHO diagnostic interview (DSM-IV)	Natural disaster, physical abuse, serious accident, witnessing traumatic events	1,414 American Indians, 15% with PTSD	Sex, age, education, smoking, self-reported diabetes and high blood pressure, alcohol	High rates of self-reported cardiovascular disease (i.e., heart disease or stroke) in PTSD patients
Boscarino[48]	DIS (DSM-III), Research Triangle Institute PTSD scale	Combat exposure or any other trauma	7,924 male veterans, 11% PTSD	Age, race	Higher cardiovascular mortality in PTSD patients 30 years after military service
Kubzansky et al.[49]	Mississippi Scale for combat-related PTSD or Keane PTSD scale	Veterans from the NAS (Normative Aging Study); men served in military	1,002 (MSCR-PTSD): 944 (K-PTSD); very few with PTSD, therefore PTSD symptoms	Depressive symptoms Age, BMI, cholesterol, smoking, blood pressure, family history, alcohol, education	PTSD increased age-adjusted risk for nonfatal MI and fatal CHD combined and for all of the CHD outcomes combined (nonfatal MI, fatal CHD, and angina)
Boscarino[50]	DSM-III measure (D-PTSD) and Keane measure (K-PTSD)	Vietnam Veterans	4,328 men; 10% PTSD in theater veterans (service in Vietnam) and 3% PTSD in era veterans (service elsewhere)	Lifetime depression and combat exposure, age, race, intelligence, family history of HD, obesity, smoking, alcohol abuse, antisocial personality	D-PTSD doubled the risk for early age heart disease mortality and approached significance for K-PTSD
Kubzansky et al.[51]	NIMH DIS (DMS-III)	Different type of trauma: sexual and physical assault, serious accidents/injuries, natural disaster	1,059 women of the community, 28 (2.6%) with PTSD, PTSD symptom counts: low (0), moderate (1–4), high (>5)	Standard coronary risk factors, depression, trait anxiety	Women with >5 symptoms 3x higher risk of incident CHD

(continued)

Table 13.3 (continued)

Source	Diagnostic tools	Type of trauma	Subjects	Control for cardiovascular risk factors	Cardiovascular endpoints
Shemesh et al.[52]	IES	Myocardial infarction	65 male and female post-MI patients; 20% with PTSD	None	Higher rate of cardiovascular readmissions (composite index of reinfarction, unstable angina, hypertensive complications, indications of heart failure) in PTSD patients and with more PTSD symptoms
Ladwig et al.[53]	IES-revised	Cardiac disease and treatment with an implantable cardioverter-defibrillator	147 (125 men and 22 women), 38 Pat (=26%) with PTSD	Age, sex, diabetes mellitus, left ventricular ejection fraction, beta-blocker, prior resuscitation, ICD shocks received, depression, anxiety	PTSD group with increased mortality risk

CAD coronary artery disease, *CHD* coronary heart disease, *MI* myocardial infarction, *PTSD* post-traumatic stress disorder, *SCID* structured clinical interview for DSM-III and IV revised, *ICDA-8* eighth revision of the International Classification of Diseases, adapted, *IES* impact of event scale, *DIS* diagnostic interview schedule, *DSM* diagnostic and statistical manual of mental disorders, *WHO* World Health Organization

CHD risk suggesting that individuals with the highest level of trauma-related psychological distress run the greatest risk of developing CHD. After a 14-year follow-up, middle-aged civilian women with increased PTSD symptoms showed an increased risk of incident CHD.[51]

Few studies have investigated the prognostic role of PTSD in patients with established cardiac diseases. One study was performed in 65 post-MI patients of whom 20% had above-threshold PTSD symptoms. In addition to age >55 years, a history of coronary artery bypass surgery before the index MI and nonadherence to aspirin, PTSD increased the risk of hospital readmissions owing to a combined endpoint of CVD events that also included recurrent MI and unstable angina during the first year after MI (OR 2.8, 95% CI 1.2–8.8).[52] A second study investigated the predictive value of post-traumatic symptoms attributable to cardiac arrest or acute MI for the prognosis in patients with an ICD.[53] After a mean follow-up of 5 years, patients with a PTSD case definition showed higher adjusted relative mortality risk (HR 3.5, 95% CI 1.6–7.6).

13.6   Pathways and Mechanisms Underlying the Link Between Post-traumatic Stress Disorder and Cardiovascular Disease

Current evidence suggests that PTSD exerts its cardiotoxic effects via several pathways and mechanisms. First, there might be a common genetic background that interacts with toxic environmental exposures to determine the development of both PTSD and CVD. For instance, the S allele of the serotonin transporter gene-linked polymorphic region increased the risk of PTSD in a high-risk environment characterized by high crime and low employment rates on the one hand[54] and of new cardiac events in patients with a previous MI on the other.[55] Second, PTSD clusters with psychosocial risk factors for CHD, including low social support and type D personality.[36] Third, PTSD is strongly comorbid with other lifetime psychiatric disorders, especially anxiety and depression[18], which have been shown to predict CHD in their own right.[56] Fourth, established cardiovascular risk factors such as smoking, dyslipidemia, elevated blood pressure, obesity, diabetes, and low physical activity have all been found to be more prevalent in individuals with PTSD than in those without.[19] In particular, a number of studies found elevated levels of total cholesterol, low-density lipoprotein cholesterol, and triglycerides on one hand and decreased levels of high-density lipoprotein cholesterol on the other; reduced levels of high-density lipoprotein cholesterol were also found in patients with PTSD caused by MI after adjusting for statin therapy.[57] Of note, several large studies found PTSD symptomatology to predict future CHD, even when controlling for classic cardiovascular risk factors and symptoms of depression and anxiety.[49-51] Fifth, adherence to cardiac therapy is relatively poor in PTSD as, for instance, these patients may skip regular intake of cardiac medications in order to avoid being reminded of their heart attack.[58] Sixth, there is an increasing literature on direct pathophysiologic links between PTSD and CHD as discussed in the following paragraph.

13.7 Pathophysiologic Links Between Post-traumatic Stress Disorder and Coronary Heart Disease

In agreement with a conceptual model that prolonged stress reactions ultimately lead to atherosclerosis and cardiovascular system damage,[56,59] elevated circulating levels of several biomarkers of atherothrombotic risk-related to inflammation, coagulation, and endothelial dysfunction have been shown in patients with PTSD. Most of this research has been performed on individuals with post-traumatic symptoms and PTSD who did not have CHD.[19] Previous research mainly investigated circulating markers of inflammation as summarized in Table 13.4.[60-75] Although there is some inconsistency across study findings, the notion is that PTSD might confer a low-grade inflammatory state that is characterized by increased and decreased levels, respectively, of proinflammatory (e.g., interleukin-1β) and anti-inflammatory (e.g., interleukin-4) cytokines.

We compared several biomarkers between non-medicated individuals with PTSD, in most cases attributable to an accident, and carefully matched trauma-exposed non-PTSD controls. We corroborated associations between PTSD symptomatology or PTSD with the inflammatory markers tumor necrosis factor-α, interleukin-1β, and interleukin-4.[71] Additionally, associations were observed for soluble tissue factor, von Willebrand factor antigen, clotting factor VIII, and fibrinogen.[69,73] In the hitherto sole study on inflammatory markers in patients with PTSD and CHD, we found that PTSD caused by MI was associated with higher plasma levels of interleukin-6 and of cellular adhesion molecules relative to post-MI patients with no PTSD.[74,75] Controlling for anxiety and depressive symptoms partially accounted for the relationship between PTSD and biomarkers in our studies (Table 13.4).

Perturbations in circulating levels of biomarkers could be explained by altered hypothalamic-pituitary adrenal axis and autonomic function found in PTSD.[76] These alterations are thought to mediate a dysfunctional peripheral stress response. They involve a range of immunological and other changes with the associated wear and tear of the cardiovascular system and give raise to clinical manifestation of chronic CHD and acute atherothrombotic events such as MI.[19,77] In PTSD there is evidence for hypocortisolemia and peripheral noradrenergic hyperactivity under basal conditions.[78,79] We also found lowered resting plasma cortisol levels in post-MI patients with PTSD, but only when taking comorbid depressive symptoms into account.[80] In response to trauma- and non-trauma-specific stimuli, individuals with PTSD also showed increased sympathetic nervous system activation.[13,79] Similarly, in response to a trauma-specific interview, soluble cellular adhesion molecules increased in patients with PTSD caused by MI relative to post-MI patients with no PTSD.[75]

Table 13.4 Changes in circulating biomarkers of atherothrombotic risk in post-traumatic stress disorder

Source	Diagnostic tools	Type of trauma	Subjects	Biomarker
Spivak et al.[60]	SCID (DMS-III-revised)	Combat exposure	19 men with PTSD, 19 age and sex-matched healthy volunteers	IL-1β: higher in PTSD patients than in controls sIL-2R: no group difference
Maes et al.[61]	CIDI (DMS-III-revised)	Hotel fire or multiple collision car crash	13 men and women with PTSD, 32 healthy volunteers of same age and rate of sex	IL-6: higher in PTSD patients than in controls sIL-6R: higher in PTSD patients than in controls IL-1R antagonist: no group difference
Baker et al.[62]	SCID (DMS-III-revised)	Combat exposure	11 male veterans with PTSD, 8 healthy volunteers of same age and rate of smokers	IL-6: no group difference; if adjusted for age, IL-6 higher in PTSD patients than in controls during daytime
Kawamura et al.[63]	DIS (DSM-IV)	Motor vehicle accident, bullying, witnessing a cruel death, violence, fire, death in the family, and flood	12 men with PTSD, 48 men matched for age and smoking habits without PTSD	IL-4: lower in PTSD patients than in controls
Miller et al.[64]	ICD-10, DTS, RIES	Motor vehicle or work-related accident, victims of an assault or fall, witnessing an upsetting event	15 Trauma patients with PTSD, 8 trauma controls without PTSD	CRP: direct association with intrusive symptoms sIL-6R: direct association with intrusive symptoms IL-6: no group difference
Rohleder et al.[65]	Interview (DSM-IV)	Bosnian war refugees	12 men and women with PTSD, 13 healthy controls	LPS-stimulated cytokine production in whole blood: IL-6 production greater in PTSD patients than in controls; no group difference in TNF-α

(continued)

Table 13.4 (continued)

Source	Diagnostic tools	Type of trauma	Subjects	Biomarker
Sondergaard et al.[66]	CAPS interview (DSM-IV)	Flight from war zone	25 men and women with PTSD, 38 without PTSD	High-sensitive CRP: lower in PTSD patients than in controls
Tucker et al.[67]	SCID and CAPS interview (DMS-IV)	Sexual or physical violence, witnessing violent death, tornado, combat, motor vehicle accident, terrorist bomb, nuclear bomb exposure, life-threatening event	58 men and women with PTSD, 21 traumatized controls without PTSD	IL-1β: higher in PTSD patients than in controls Serum sIL-2R: lower in PTSD patients than in controls
Woods et al.[68]	DTS (Davidson Trauma Scale)	Intimate Partner Violence	62 abused women, 39 nonabused women	LPS-stimulated INF-γ production in whole blood: higher in abused women and in women with recurrent PTSD symptoms
von Känel et al.[69]	CAPS interview (DSM-IV)	Different types of accidents	14 PTSD patients, 14 age- and gender-matched non-PTSD controls	Coagulation factors FVII:C, FVIII:C, FXII:C, fibrinogen, D-dimer: no group difference FVIII:C: direct association with total PTSD symptoms in all subjects Fibrinogen: direct association with total PTSD symptoms in PTSD patients
Song et al.[70]	CIDI (DMS-IV)	Earthquake survivors	34 with PTSD, 30 without PTSD and 34 controls	IL-8: lower in PTSD patients than in other groups IL-2: lower in earthquake survivors (with or without PTSD) than in controls

von Känel et al.[71]	CAPS interview (DSM-IV)	Different types of accidents	14 PTSD patients, 14 age- and gender-matched non-PTSD controls	TNF-α: higher in PTSD patients than in controls (n.s. if adjusted for blood pressure and time since trauma) IL-4: lower in PTSD patients than in controls if adjusted for blood pressure and smoking High-sensitive CRP, IL-1β, IL-10: no group difference
Gill et al.[72]	CAPS interview (DMS-IV)	Insured women: child sex abuse, unexpected death of a family member, rape, sexual assault, child physical abuse, intimate partner violence, witnessing physical assault or murder	26 with PTSD, 24 traumatized non-PTSD controls, 21 non-traumatized controls	LPS-stimulated cytokine production in whole blood: IL-6 and TNF-α production greater in PTSD patients than in other groups; no group difference in IL-1β
von Känel et al.[73]	CAPS interview (DSM-IV)	Different types of accidents	14 PTSD patients, 14 age- and gender-matched non-PTSD controls	Soluble tissue factor: higher in PTSD patients than in controls (n.s. if adjusted for symptoms of anxiety and depression) von Willebrand factor: no group difference; direct association with total PTSD symptoms in all subjects Soluble ICAM-1: no group difference

(continued)

Table 13.4 (continued)

Source	Diagnostic tools	Type of trauma	Subjects	Biomarker
von Känel et al.[74]	CAPS interview (DSM-IV)	Myocardial Infarction	15 post-MI with PTSD, 29 post-MI patients with no PTSD	IL-6: higher in PTSD patients than in controls if adjusted for smoking and depressive symptoms
				Leptin: higher in PTSD patients than in controls if adjusted for medication and sex (n.s. if also adjusted for depressive symptoms)
				High-sensitive CRP: lower in PTSD patients than in controls if adjusted for medication, physical activity, and depressive symptoms
				Soluble CD40 ligand: lower in PTSD patients than in controls if adjusted for depressive symptoms
von Känel et al.[75]	CAPS interview (DSM-IV)	Myocardial Infarction	15 post-MI with PTSD, 7 post-MI patients with remitted PTSD, 22 post-MI patients with no PTSD	Soluble ICAM-1 and VCAM-1: Higher in PTSD patients and in patients with remitted PTSD than in patients with no PTSD; no difference between patients with PTSD and patients with remitted PTSD
				Soluble P-selectin: no group difference

CAPS clinician-administered PTSD scale, *CIDI* composite international diagnostic interview, *CRP* C-reactive protein, *DIS* diagnostic interview schedule, *DSM* diagnostic and statistical manual of mental disorders, *DTS* Davidson trauma scale, *ICAM-1* inter-cellular adhesion molecule-1, *ICD-10* tenth revision of the International Classification of Diseases, *IL* interleukin, *MI* myocardial infarction, *n.s.* nonsignificant, *RIES* revised impact of events scale, *LPS* lipopolysaccharide, *SCID* structured clinical interview for DSM-IV, *sIL-2R* soluble IL-2 receptor, *TNF* tumor necrosis factor, *VCAM-1* vascular cellular adhesion molecule-1

A relative lack in endogenous cortisol might fail to curtail inflammatory processes. Sympathetic overactivity with elevated norepinephrine levels might kindle proinflammatory and procoagulant changes, which all contribute to low-grade inflammation and coagulation in PTSD.[19,81,82] Moreover, there is low vagal tone in PTSD.[83] This finding is intriguing regarding the inflammatory state in PTSD because the vagus nerve exerts tonic inhibition of proinflammatory cytokine production by immune cells.[84] More precisely, experimental models have shown that acetylcholine release from the vagus nerve modulates immune responses at least in part via alpha 7 nicotinic receptors that inhibit NF kappa B and thus cytokine synthesis and release from tissue macrophages.[85]

It should be noted that the above-discussed mechanisms are notoriously difficult to disentangle as behavioral and pathophysiological stress responses intertwine to some extent.[86] For instance, how much of the variance in the PTSD-related CHD risk is attributable to smoking-triggered inflammation, and how much is accounted for by a direct autonomic effect on inflammation? The current lack of sophisticated statistical and conceptual models precludes strong inferences about whether these mechanisms are best conceptualized as confounders, mediators, or moderators of the link between PTSD and CHD. On the one hand, smoking could directly affect (i.e., confound) inflammation and coagulation activity in PTSD. On the other hand, PTSD could also prompt subjects to smoke as a means of stress relief. In the latter instance, smoking would mediate the effect of PTSD on the low-grade inflammatory and procoagulant state.

13.8 Clinical Management

Being aware that PTSD is frequent and persistent, it is important that cardiologists are able to recognize and manage post-traumatic distress in practice.[87] Factors which emerged as predictors for the development of PTSD (Table 13.2) might help cardiologists to draw their attention to at-risk patients. More specifically, an adapted Primary Care PTSD Screen instrument comprises four questions and may help identify patients with significant post-traumatic distress related to cardiac disease (Table 13.5). Poor adherence to cardiac therapy and reluctance to participate in cardiac rehabilitation programs due to avoidance behavior needs particular attention. If three items are answered with yes, the screen shows a sensitivity of 78% and specificity of 87% for PTSD.[88] To our knowledge, the screen has not been validated in cardiac patients with PTSD. However, our clinical experience is that cardiac patients might endorse relevant levels of post-traumatic distress even when confirming less than three items.

Whereas we do not know yet whether alleviating post-traumatic distress benefits cardiovascular outcome, improvements in quality of life and daily functioning of the cardiac patients with PTSD might be predicted. The treatment provided to the cardiac patient with PTSD by the cardiologists and the time of referral to a mental health care provider depends on several issues. These include the severity of post-

Table 13.5 Primary care PTSD screen adapted for cardiac patients

Have you experienced your heart disease (e.g., myocardial infarction) so frightening, horrible, or upsetting that, in the past month, you

1. Have had nightmares about it or thought about it when you did not want to?
2. Tried hard not to think about it or went out of your way to avoid situations that reminded you of it?
3. Were constantly on guard, watchful, or easily startled?
4. Felt numb or detached from others, activities, or your surroundings?

Screen is positive if patient answers "yes" to any three items

traumatic distress, the presence of comorbid psychosocial and psychiatric problems, as well as the therapeutic skills and experience with the psychological needs of traumatized individuals of the individual cardiologist. Cardiology departments in many countries now routinely work together with behavioral cardiologists, psychocardiologists and psychiatric and psychosomatic consultation-liaison services. These are particularly familiar with the psychological sequelae of living with a heart disease and the appropriate diagnostic and therapeutic procedures.[56]

An important question to investigate is whether PTSD could be prevented early on after a cardiac event. Staff of coronary care units might play a crucial role in employing such preventive strategies. Interventions might aim at reducing dramatic referrals and statements by staff, helplessness, pain, and fear of dying, particularly in populations at risk (e.g., younger patients and those with low social support). Means to achieve this task are providing a secure place, reducing the exposure to further stress, taking care of physiological needs, providing information and orientation, recruiting social support, and emphasizing the expectation of returning to normal (e.g., by assuring that the patient shows a normal psychological response to the abnormal situation of a heart attack and that he or she will do fine).[89] Importantly, compulsory psychological debriefing of traumatized patients should no longer be used as it may increase the risk of developing PTSD.[90]

13.9 Therapeutic Approach

The most effective psychotherapies for PTSD are trauma focused and include individual and cognitive-behavioral therapy, eye movement desensitization and reprocessing, and stress management.[91] Trauma-related erroneous automatic thoughts and beliefs associated with PTSD are corrected and restructured, and intolerable traumatic memories are extinguished by repetitive exposure through imaginal or actual reexperience of the traumatic event.[92] Selective serotonin reuptake inhibitors (SSRIs) and venlafaxine, a serotonin norepinephrine reuptake inhibitor (SNRI), are appropriate first-line agents in the pharmacotherapy of PTSD. Second-generation antipsychotics and other agents may be useful for treatment-resistant cases.[93] The SSRIs appear to ameliorate all three symptom clusters of PTSD as well as associated depression and disability. Notably, most randomized trials have tested only a particular monotherapy for PTSD. However, most patients receive two or more treatments concurrently, including different forms of psychotherapy plus one or more medications; partial improvement often prevails over remission.[92]

In cardiac patients with PTSD, randomized controlled trials on the efficacy of pharmacological and psychotherapeutic interventions are currently lacking. As yet, there is only one intervention study available on 14 patients with PTSD attributable to MI who received five group sessions of psychotherapy. At 6-month follow-up, the group that received trauma-focused cognitive behavioral therapy combined with education had greater improvement in post-traumatic stress symptoms and in some traditional cardiovascular risk factors compared to the group that received education only. Importantly, adherence to cardiac medication improved in both groups.[94]

In terms of psychopharmacotherapy of cardiac patients with PTSD, it should be remembered that venlafaxine may increase systolic blood pressure and that many second-generation antipsychotics may have cardiac and metabolic side effects. However, the two SSRIs sertraline and citalopram proved to be safe in patients with CHD.[95,96] Except in very extreme stress reactions, benzodiazepines are best avoided for the treatment of acute stress symptoms in traumatized individuals because these medications may actually increase the risk of developing PTSD.[89] Although this has not been investigated in cardiac patients, propranolol, a nonselective and lipophilic beta blocker, when applied shortly after a trauma, mitigated the development of PTSD likely by preventing the storage of traumatic memories.[97] Beta-blockers may also ameliorate the vicious circle of anxiety caused by elevated heart rates and contractility.

13.10 Summary and Future Directions

Post-traumatic stress disorder occurs in about 10–15% of the patients after MI and seems similarly prevalent in other cardiac diseases. Post-traumatic stress disorder may adversely impact the prognosis of patients with established CHD although studies on this issue are scarce. In contrast, in patients free of CHD, PTSD has emerged as a reliable risk factor for future cardiovascular events, particularly incident CHD. Although PTSD is associated with virtually all established cardiovascular risk factors and also with some psychosocial risk factors of CHD, including depression, these may not fully account for the link between PTSD and CHD. The psychophysiologic mechanisms underlying the link between PTSD and atherosclerosis initiation and progression as well as atherothrombotic events are plausible. Current evidence implicates a low-grade inflammatory state that seems to be accompanied by endothelial dysfunction and hypercoagulability. Due to the lack of systematic trials, recommendations for the clinical management and therapy of cardiac patients with PTSD must largely be inferred from the PTSD literature at large. Before appropriate treatments like trauma-focused cognitive behavioral therapy and SSRIs can be considered, PTSD must be recognized. Therefore, cardiologists are encouraged to screen for significant PTSD symptomatology by asking a few questions as part of their clinical routine.

More research is needed in terms of the prognostic impact of PTSD in patients with established CHD and on effective behavioral interventions to treat and prevent PTSD in cardiac patients. Specifically, we lack studies about the appropriate counseling of patients and staff on acute coronary care units to mitigate the development of PTSD. We also lack studies on interventions specifically tailored for the needs of patients with PTSD caused by MI and other cardiac diseases as compared to PTSD caused by other trauma. Whether tailored interventions will improve compliance, the cardiovascular risk factor profile, and the psychophysiologic disturbances is important to know. Favorable changes in the intermediate pathways leading from PTSD to the initiation and progression of atherosclerosis, thrombotic complications, and ultimately clinical manifestation of atherothrombotic events might help reduce cardiovascular morbidity and mortality in patients with PTSD.

Funding/Support Own work cited in this chapter was supported by an unrestricted grant of Pfizer AG Switzerland and by a research grant of the University of Bern, Switzerland.

References

1. Engdahl B, Dikel TN, Eberly R, Blank A Jr. Comorbidity and course of psychiatric disorders in a community sample of former prisoners of war. *Am J Psychiatry.* 1998;155:1740-1745.
2. Silver RC, Holman EA, McIntosh DN, Poulin M, Gil-Rivas V. Nationwide longitudinal study of psychological responses to September 11. *JAMA.* 2002;288:1235-1244.
3. Lai TJ, Chang CM, Connor KM, Lee LC, Davidson JR. Full and partial PTSD among earthquake survivors in rural Taiwan. *J Psychiatr Res.* 2004;38:313-322.
4. Gurevich M, Devins GM, Rodin GM. Stress response syndromes and cancer: conceptual and assessment issues. *Psychosomatics.* 2002;43:259-281.
5. Tedstone JE, Tarrier N. Posttraumatic stress disorder following medical illness and treatment. *Clin Psychol Rev.* 2003;23:409-448.
6. Spindler H, Pedersen SS. Posttraumatic stress disorder in the wake of heart disease: prevalence, risk factors, and future research directions. *Psychosom Med.* 2005;67:715-723.
7. Schelling G. Post-traumatic stress disorder in somatic disease: lessons from critically ill patients. *Prog Brain Res.* 2008;167:229-237.
8. Felitti VJ, Anda RF, Nordenberg D, et al. Relationship of childhood abuse and household dysfunction to many of the leading causes of death in adults. The Adverse Childhood Experiences (ACE) Study. *Am J Prev Med.* 1998;14:245-258.
9. Boscarino JA. Diseases among men 20 years after exposure to severe stress: implications for clinical research and medical care. *Psychosom Med.* 1997;59:605-614.
10. Boscarino JA. Posttraumatic stress disorder and physical illness: results from clinical and epidemiologic studies. *Ann N Y Acad Sci.* 2004;1032:141-153.
11. American Psychiatric Association. *Diagnostic and Statistical Manual of Mental Disorders.* 4th ed. Washington DC: APA; 1994.
12. Schnyder U, Moergeli H, Trentz O, Klaghofer R, Buddeberg C. Prediction of psychiatric morbidity in severely injured accident victims at one-year follow-up. *Am J Respir Crit Care Med.* 2001;164:653-656.
13. Yehuda R. Post-traumatic stress disorder. *N Engl J Med.* 2002;346:108-114.
14. Foa EB, Cashman L, Jaycox L, Perry K. Validation of a self-report measure of posttraumatic stress disorder: the Posttraumatic Diagnostic Scale. *Psychol Assess.* 1997;9:445-451.
15. Horowitz M, Wilner N, Alvarez W. Impact of event scale: a measure of subjective stress. *Psychosom Med.* 1979;41:209-218.

16. Blake DD, Weathers FW, Nagy LM, et al. The development of a Clinician-Administered PTSD Scale. *J Trauma Stress*. 1995;8:75-90.
17. Hepp U, Gamma A, Milos G, et al. Prevalence of exposure to potentially traumatic events and PTSD. The Zurich Cohort Study. *Eur Arch Psychiatry Clin Neurosci*. 2006;256:151-158.
18. Kessler RC, Sonnega A, Bromet E, Hughes M, Nelson CB. Posttraumatic stress disorder in the National Comorbidity Survey. *Arch Gen Psychiatry*. 1995;52:1048-1060.
19. Gander ML, von Känel R. Myocardial infarction and post-traumatic stress disorder: frequency, outcome, and atherosclerotic mechanisms. *Eur J Cardiovasc Prev Rehabil*. 2006;13:165-172.
20. Guler E, Schmid JP, Wiedemar L, Saner H, Schnyder U, von Känel R. Clinical diagnosis of posttraumatic stress disorder after myocardial infarction. *Clin Cardiol*. 2009;32:125-129.
21. Abbas CC, Schmid JP, Guler E, et al. Trajectory of posttraumatic stress disorder caused by myocardial infarction: a two-year follow-up study. *Int J Psychiatry Med*. 2009;39:359-376.
22. Wikman A, Bhattacharyya M, Perkins-Porras L, Steptoe A. Persistence of posttraumatic stress symptoms 12 and 36 months after acute coronary syndrome. *Psychosom Med*. 2008;70: 764-772.
23. Sears SF Jr, Conti JB. Quality of life and psychological functioning of ICD patients. *Heart*. 2002;87:488-493.
24. Kutz I, Shabtai H, Solomon Z, Neumann M, David D. Post-traumatic stress disorder in myocardial infarction patients: prevalence study. *Isr J Psychiatry Relat Sci*. 1994;31:48-56.
25. Bennett P, Brooke S. Intrusive memories, post-traumatic stress disorder and myocardial infarction. *Br J Clin Psychol*. 1999;38:411-416.
26. Chung MC, Berger Z, Rudd H. Coping with posttraumatic stress disorder and comorbidity after myocardial infarction. *Compr Psychiatry*. 2008;49:55-64.
27. Ginzburg K. Life events and adjustment following myocardial infarction: a longitudinal study. *Soc Psychiatry Psychiatr Epidemiol*. 2006;41:825-831.
28. Bennett P, Conway M, Clatworthy J, Brooke S, Owen R. Predicting post-traumatic symptoms in cardiac patients. *Heart Lung*. 2001;30:458-465.
29. Ginzburg K, Solomon Z, Bleich A. Repressive coping style, acute stress disorder, and posttraumatic stress disorder after myocardial infarction. *Psychosom Med*. 2002;64:748-757.
30. Wiedemar L, Schmid JP, Müller J, et al. Prevalence and predictors of posttraumatic stress disorder in patients with acute myocardial infarction. *Heart Lung*. 2008;37:113-121.
31. Ginzburg K, Solomon Z, Dekel R, Bleich A. Longitudinal study of acute stress disorder, posttraumatic stress disorder and dissociation following myocardial infarction. *J Nerv Ment Dis*. 2006;194:945-950.
32. Ginzburg K, Solomon Z, Koifman B, et al. Trajectories of posttraumatic stress disorder following myocardial infarction: a prospective study. *J Clin Psychiatry*. 2003;64:1217-1223.
33. Pedersen SS, Middel B, Larsen ML. Posttraumatic stress disorder in first-time myocardial infarction patients. *Heart Lung*. 2003;32:300-307.
34. Whitehead DL, Perkins-Porras L, Strike PC, Steptoe A. Post-traumatic stress disorder in patients with cardiac disease: predicting vulnerability from emotional responses during admission for acute coronary syndromes. *Heart*. 2006;92:1225-1229.
35. Chung MC, Berger Z, Rudd H. Comorbidity and personality traits in patients with different levels of posttraumatic stress disorder following myocardial infarction. *Psychiatry Res*. 2007; 152:243-252.
36. Pedersen SS, Denollet J. Validity of the type D personality construct in Danish post-MI patients and healthy controls. *J Psychosom Res*. 2004;57:265-272.
37. Whitehead DL, Strike P, Perkins-Porras L, Steptoe A. Frequency of distress and fear of dying during acute coronary syndromes and consequences for adaptation. *Am J Cardiol*. 2005;96: 1512-1516.
38. Roberge MA, Dupuis G, Marchand A. Acute stress disorder after myocardial infarction: prevalence and associated factors. *Psychosom Med*. 2008;70:1028-1034.
39. Gamper G, Willeit M, Sterz F, et al. Life after death: posttraumatic stress disorder in survivors of cardiac arrest–prevalence, associated factors, and the influence of sedation and analgesia. *Crit Care Med*. 2004;32:378-383.

40. Shalev A, Bleich A, Ursano RJ. Posttraumatic stress disorder: somatic comorbidity and effort tolerance. *Psychosomatics.* 1990;31:197-203.

41. Falger PR, Op den Velde W, Hovens JE, Schouten EG, De Groen JH, Van Duijn H. Current posttraumatic stress disorder and cardiovascular disease risk factors in Dutch Resistance veterans from World War II. *Psychother Psychosom.* 1992;57:164-171.

42. McFarlane AC, Atchison M, Rafalowicz E, Papay P. Physical symptoms in post-traumatic stress disorder. *J Psychosom Res.* 1994;38:715-726.

43. Cwikel J, Abdelgani A, Goldsmith JR, Quastel M, Yevelson II. Two-year follow up study of stress-related disorders among immigrants to Israel from the Chernobyl area. *Environ Health Perspect.* 1997;105(suppl 6):1545-1550.

44. Boscarino JA, Chang J. Electrocardiogram abnormalities among men with stress-related psychiatric disorders: implications for coronary heart disease and clinical research. *Ann Behav Med.* 1999;21:227-234.

45. Schnurr PP, Spiro A 3rd, Paris AH. Physician-diagnosed medical disorders in relation to PTSD symptoms in older male military veterans. *Health Psychol.* 2000;19:91-97.

46. Dobie DJ, Kivlahan DR, Maynard C, Bush KR, Davis TM, Bradley KA. Posttraumatic stress disorder in female veterans: association with self-reported health problems and functional impairment. *Arch Intern Med.* 2004;164:394-400.

47. Sawchuk CN, Roy-Byrne P, Goldberg J, et al. The relationship between post-traumatic stress disorder, depression and cardiovascular disease in an American Indian tribe. *Psychol Med.* 2005;35:1785-1794.

48. Boscarino JA. Posttraumatic stress disorder and mortality among U.S. Army Veterans 30 years after military service. *Ann Epidemiol.* 2006;16:248-256.

49. Kubzansky LD, Koenen KC, Spiro A 3rd, Vokonas PS, Sparrow D. Prospective study of posttraumatic stress disorder symptoms and coronary heart disease in the Normative Aging Study. *Arch Gen Psychiatry.* 2007;64:109-116.

50. Boscarino JA. A prospective study of PTSD and early-age heart disease mortality among Vietnam veterans: implications for surveillance and prevention. *Psychosom Med.* 2008;70:668-676.

51. Kubzansky LD, Koenen KC, Jones C, Eaton WW. A prospective study of posttraumatic stress disorder symptoms and coronary heart disease in women. *Health Psychol.* 2009;28:125-130.

52. Shemesh E, Yehuda R, Milo O, et al. Posttraumatic stress, nonadherence, and adverse outcome in survivors of a myocardial infarction. *Psychosom Med.* 2004;66:521-526.

53. Ladwig KH, Baumert J, Marten-Mittag B, Kolb C, Zrenner B, Schmitt C. Posttraumatic stress symptoms and predicted mortality in patients with implantable cardioverter defibrillators: results from the prospective living with an implanted cardioverter defibrillator study. *Arch Gen Psychiatry.* 2008;65:1324-1330.

54. Koenen KC, Aiello AE, Bakshis E, et al. Modification of the association between serotonin transporter genotype and risk of posttraumatic stress disorder in adults by county-level social environment. *Am J Epidemiol.* 2009;169:704-711.

55. Nakatani D, Sato H, Sakata Y, et al. Influence of serotonin transporter gene polymorphism on depressive symptoms and new cardiac events after acute myocardial infarction. *Am Heart J.* 2005;150:652-658.

56. Rozanski A, Blumenthal JA, Davidson KW, Saab PG, Kubzansky L. The epidemiology, pathophysiology, and management of psychosocial risk factors in cardiac practice: the emerging field of behavioral cardiology. *J Am Coll Cardiol.* 2005;45:637-651.

57. von Känel R, Kraemer B, Saner H, Schmid JP, Abbas CC, Begré S. Posttraumatic stress disorder and dyslipidemia: previous research and novel findings from patients with PTSD caused by myocardial infarction. *World J Biol Psychiatry.* 2010;11:141-147.

58. Shemesh E, Rudnick A, Kaluski E, et al. A prospective study of posttraumatic stress symptoms and nonadherence in survivors of a myocardial infarction (MI). *Gen Hosp Psychiatry.* 2001;23:215-222.

59. Matthews KA, Zhu S, Tucker DC, Whooley MA. Blood pressure reactivity to psychological stress and coronary calcification in the Coronary Artery Risk Development in Young Adults Study. *Hypertension*. 2006;47:391-395.
60. Spivak B, Shohat B, Mester R, et al. Elevated levels of serum interleukin-1 beta in combat-related posttraumatic stress disorder. *Biol Psychiatry*. 1997;42:345-348.
61. Maes M, Lin AH, Delmeire L, et al. Elevated serum interleukin-6 (IL-6) and IL-6 receptor concentrations in posttraumatic stress disorder following accidental man-made traumatic events. *Biol Psychiatry*. 1999;45:833-839.
62. Baker DG, Ekhator NN, Kasckow JW, et al. Plasma and cerebrospinal fluid interleukin-6 concentrations in posttraumatic stress disorder. *Neuroimmunomodulation*. 2001;9:209-217.
63. Kawamura N, Kim Y, Asukai N. Suppression of cellular immunity in men with a past history of posttraumatic stress disorder. *Am J Psychiatry*. 2001;158:484-486.
64. Miller RJ, Sutherland AG, Hutchison JD, Alexander DA. C-reactive protein and interleukin-6 receptor in post-traumatic stress disorder: a pilot study. *Cytokine*. 2001;13:253-255.
65. Rohleder N, Joksimovic L, Wolf JM, Kirschbaum C. Hypocortisolism and increased glucocorticoid sensitivity of pro-inflammatory cytokine production in Bosnian war refugees with posttraumatic stress disorder. *Biol Psychiatry*. 2004;55:745-751.
66. Sondergaard HP, Hansson LO, Theorell T. The inflammatory markers C-reactive protein and serum amyloid A in refugees with and without posttraumatic stress disorder. *Clin Chim Acta*. 2004;342:93-98.
67. Tucker P, Ruwe WD, Masters B, et al. Neuroimmune and cortisol changes in selective serotonin reuptake inhibitor and placebo treatment of chronic posttraumatic stress disorder. *Biol Psychiatry*. 2004;56:121-128.
68. Woods AB, Page GG, O'Campo P, Pugh LC, Ford D, Campbell JC. The mediation effect of posttraumatic stress disorder symptoms on the relationship of intimate partner violence and IFN-gamma levels. *Am J Community Psychol*. 2005;36:159-175.
69. von Känel R, Hepp U, Buddeberg C, et al. Altered blood coagulation in patients with posttraumatic stress disorder. *Psychosom Med*. 2006;68:598-604.
70. Song Y, Zhou D, Guan Z, Wang X. Disturbance of serum interleukin-2 and interleukin-8 levels in posttraumatic and non-posttraumatic stress disorder earthquake survivors in northern China. *Neuroimmunomodulation*. 2007;14:248-254.
71. von Känel R, Hepp U, Kraemer B, et al. Evidence for low-grade systemic proinflammatory activity in patients with posttraumatic stress disorder. *J Psychiatr Res*. 2007;41:744-752.
72. Gill J, Vythilingam M, Page GG. Low cortisol, high DHEA, and high levels of stimulated TNF-alpha, and IL-6 in women with PTSD. *J Trauma Stress*. 2008;21:530-539.
73. von Känel R, Hepp U, Traber R, et al. Measures of endothelial dysfunction in plasma of patients with posttraumatic stress disorder. *Psychiatry Res*. 2008;158:363-373.
74. von Känel R, Begré S, Abbas CC, Saner H, Gander ML, Schmid JP. Inflammatory biomarkers in patients with posttraumatic stress disorder caused by myocardial infarction and the role of depressive symptoms. *Neuroimmunomodulation*. 2010;17:39-46.
75. von Känel R, Abbas CC, Begré S, Saner H, Gander ML, Schmid JP. Posttraumatic stress disorder and soluble cellular adhesion molecules at rest and in response to a trauma specific interview in patients after myocardial infarction. *Psychiatry Res*. 2010;179(3):312-317.
76. Heim C, Nemeroff CB. Neurobiology of posttraumatic stress disorder. *CNS Spectr*. 2009;14 (1 suppl 1):13-24.
77. Rohleder N, Karl A. Role of endocrine and inflammatory alterations in comorbid somatic diseases of post-traumatic stress disorder. *Minerva Endocrinol*. 2006;31:273-288.
78. Meewisse ML, Reitsma JB, de Vries GJ, Gersons BP, Olff M. Cortisol and post traumatic stress disorder in adults: systematic review and meta-analysis. *Br J Psychiatry*. 2007;191:387-392.
79. Strawn JR, Geracioti TD. Noradrenergic dysfunction and the psychopharmacology of post-traumatic stress disorder. *Depress Anxiety*. 2008;25:260-271.
80. von Känel R, Schmid JP, Abbas CC, Gander ML, Saner H, Begré S. Stress hormones in patients with posttraumatic stress disorder caused by myocardial infarction and role of comorbid depression. *J Affect Disord*. 2010;121:73-79.

81. von Känel R, Dimsdale JE. Effects of sympathetic activation by adrenergic infusions on hemostasis in vivo. *Eur J Haematol.* 2000;65:357-369.

82. von Känel R, Mills PJ, Fainman C, Dimsdale JE. Effects of psychological stress and psychiatric disorders on blood coagulation and fibrinolysis: a biobehavioral pathway to coronary artery disease? *Psychosom Med.* 2001;63:531-544.

83. Sack M, Hopper JW, Lamprecht F. Low respiratory sinus arrhythmia and prolonged psychophysiological arousal in posttraumatic stress disorder: heart rate dynamics and individual differences in arousal regulation. *Biol Psychiatry.* 2004;55:284-290.

84. Tracey KJ. Physiology and immunology of the cholinergic antiinflammatory pathway. *J Clin Invest.* 2007;117:289-296.

85. Rosas-Ballina M, Tracey KJ. Cholinergic control of inflammation. *J Intern Med.* 2009;265: 663-679.

86. von Känel R. Psychological distress and cardiovascular risk: what are the links [editorial]? *J Am Coll Cardiol.* 2008;52:2163-2165.

87. Kubzansky LD, Koenen KC. Is posttraumatic stress disorder related to development of heart disease? An update. *Cleve Clin J Med.* 2009;76(suppl 2):S60-S65.

88. Prins A, Ouimette PC, Kimerling R, et al. The Primary Care PTSD Screen (PC-PTSD): development and operating characteristics. *Prim Care Psychiatry.* 2004;9:9-14.

89. Zohar J, Sonnino R, Juven-Wetzler A, Cohen H. Can posttraumatic stress disorder be prevented? *CNS Spectr.* 2009;14(1 suppl 1):44-51.

90. Rose S, Bisson J, Churchill R, Wessely S. Psychological debriefing for preventing post traumatic stress disorder (PTSD). *Cochrane Database Syst Rev.* 2002;2:CD000560.

91. Bisson J, Andrew M. Psychological treatment of post-traumatic stress disorder (PTSD). *Cochrane Database Syst Rev.* 2007;3:CD003388.

92. Friedman MJ. Posttraumatic stress disorder among military returnees from Afghanistan and Iraq. *Am J Psychiatry.* 2006;163:586-593.

93. Stein DJ, Ipser J, McAnda N. Pharmacotherapy of posttraumatic stress disorder: a review of meta-analyses and treatment guidelines. *CNS Spectr.* 2009;14(1 suppl 1):25-31.

94. Shemesh E, Koren-Michowitz M, Yehuda R, et al. Symptoms of posttraumatic stress disorder in patients who have had a myocardial infarction. *Psychosomatics.* 2006;47:231-239.

95. Glassman AH, O'Connor CM, Califf RM, et al. Sertraline treatment of major depression in patients with acute MI or unstable angina. *JAMA.* 2002;288:701-709.

96. Lespérance F, Frasure-Smith N, Koszycki D, et al. Effects of citalopram and interpersonal psychotherapy on depression in patients with coronary artery disease: the Canadian Cardiac Randomized Evaluation of Antidepressant and Psychotherapy Efficacy (CREATE) trial. *JAMA.* 2007;297:367-379.

97. von Känel R, Begré S. Depression after myocardial infarction: unraveling the mystery of poor cardiovascular prognosis and role of beta-blocker therapy [editorial]. *J Am Coll Cardiol.* 2006;48:2215-2217.

Chapter 14
Sleep, Stress, and Heart Disease

Torbjörn Åkerstedt and Aleksander Perski

Keywords Brain metabolism • Glucose changes • Heart disease • Rapid eye movement sleep (REM) • Risk factors • Sleep • Sleep disorders • Stress

It is estimated that sleep problems affect around 20% of the adult population in the Western countries.[1,2] It has been shown that the short-term consequences of sleep problems lead to adverse physiological changes,[3] as well as to long-term health consequences. In experimental and epidemiological studies, both short and long sleep hours have been related to hypertension,[4] type-2 diabetes,[5,6] increased body mass index (BMI),[7] alterations in blood lipids,[8] and inflammatory markers[9] – all factors known to increase the risk of cardiovascular disease.[10]

Sleep disturbances (short, long sleep duration, stress-related insomnia, sleep apnea) have also been associated with manifestations and mortality due to coronary heart disease (CHD).[11] Stress research often refers to the observation that repeated stress with insufficient restitution in-between will lead to a gradual increase of physiological activation and eventually an allostatic upregulation of wear and tear.[12] While the duration or type of rest in-between may be important factors it is obvious that sleep is one of the major physiological means of restitution.[12] Thus one of the major mechanisms by which prolonged stress affects health is through limitation or disturbance of sleep.

The present chapter will try to summarize some of the knowledge about sleep physiology, the relationship between stress and disturbed sleep and implications of disturbed sleep for CHD. The possible ways of intervention against disturbed sleep will also be discussed.

T. Åkerstedt (✉) • A. Perski
Stress Research Institute, Stockholm University, 106 91 Stockholm, Sweden
e-mail: torbjorn.akerstedt@ki.se; aleksander.perski@ki.se

P. Hjemdahl et al. (eds.), *Stress and Cardiovascular Disease*,
DOI 10.1007/978-1-84882-419-5_14, © Springer-Verlag London Limited 2012

14.1   Sleep

There does not seem to exist a formal consensus definition of sleep but it has been argued that, behaviorally, sleep refers to a reversible condition of altered and decreased awareness.[13] The objective description of sleep is a combination of electroencephalography (EEG), electrooculography (EOG), and electromyography (EMG). Together they constitute polysomnography. The resulting polysomnogram identifies the stages of sleep across Stages 1, 2, 3, 4, and REM sleep.[14]

Stage 1 shows 6–8 Hz EEG frequency and low amplitude, relatively high muscle tonus, and often the presence of slow rolling eye movements. The recuperative value seems negligible. *Stage 2* is identified by the presence of so-called sleep spindles in the EEG (14–16 Hz short bursts) and occasional K-complexes against a background of 4–8 Hz activity. Muscle tonus has fallen further. This stage provides basic recovery and occupies 50% of the sleep period.

Stages 3 and 4, often grouped together under the label Slow Wave Sleep (SWS), show large amounts of 0.5–4 Hz high amplitude waves (present 20% of the time for stage 3 and 50% of the time for stage 4). Muscle tonus has decreased further. SWS is considered to represent the daily process of restitution, responds in a quantitative way to the time spent awake, and shows a large increase of growth hormone secretion, together with a suppression of cortisol secretion. Metabolism falls with the sleep stages and SWS is characterized by slow breathing, low heart rate, and low cerebral blood flow, etc.

Rapid eye movement sleep (REM) is a completely different sleep stage characterized by an EEG similar to that of stage 1, but with rapid eye movements, a virtual absence of muscle tonus in antigravity muscles, and a largely awake brain, particularly the hippocampus, amygdala, and occipital projection areas. Interestingly, the prefrontal areas are not involved in this awakened brain. It is evident that we normally dream in REM sleep (although dream reports may be elicited from other stages), and to prevent the acting-out of dreams the efferent signals to the muscles are blocked.

14.1.1   Development of Sleep Across the Night

The normal development across time involves a rapid descent from waking to stage 4 sleep in 15–25, 30–50 min of SWS, followed by a short (5–10 min) period of REM sleep. This cycle is repeated another 3–4 times during the night but with decreasing amounts of SWS and increasing amounts of REM sleep. The last two sleep cycles usually lack stages 3 and 4. This characteristic pattern is usually interpreted as a high level of recovery during the first hours of sleep, and a gradual reduction in speed of recovery during the later part of sleep, due to less need for sleep with time. This is evident in mathematical models that describe sleep regulation[15] and its effect on the parallel process of increased subjective and behavioral recovery.[16]

14.1.2   Brain Metabolism During Sleep

The physiological mechanism that turns sleep on and off involves a breakdown of adenosine triphosphate (ATP) in the central nervous system (CNS) as ATP is being used to provide energy to the waking brain. The CNS levels of extracellular adenosine will then increase.[17] The adenosine message is picked up by receptors in the hypothalamus. These receptors, in turn, suppress activity in the reticular activating system (the alertness inducer in the CSN). This reduced activity will trigger the thalamus to start inducing sleep.[18] Sleep will restore adenosine levels to baseline.[17]

14.2   The Regulation of Sleep

14.2.1   Homeostatic Regulation

The main determinants of sleep are the duration of time since prior sleep and the amount of prior sleep. Reduced prior sleep normally causes a homeostatic response during the next sleep opportunity, characterized by increased amounts of stage 3 and 4 (SWS – slow wave sleep).[19] This increase occurs at the expense of REM sleep, Stage 2 sleep, Stage 1 sleep, and Stage wake. Also, spectral power density in the 0.5–4 Hz band, called "delta power," which essentially corresponds to SWS, increases as SWS does. Recovery sleep becomes deeper and less fragmented. Essentially, there is a linear relation between the amount of prior time awake and SWS. This observation early led to the perception of SWS being the major restitutive component of sleep,[20] although this may be an oversimplification.

14.2.2   Circadian Influences

The other factor is circadian influences. The cells of the suprachiasmatic nuclei (SCN) in the hypothalamus produce a pronounced oscillation in most physiological parameters.[21] These nuclei drive the physiology in a daily cycle of high metabolic rate during daytime and a low rate during nighttime. The classical physiological indicator of this rhythmicity has been rectal temperature with a peak in the afternoon. Other typical indicators include the stress hormone cortisol, with a 6 a.m. peak and the hormone melatonin, with a peak around 4 a.m. The latter reduces metabolism and causes a certain amount of sleepiness.

The effect of circadian regulation on sleep is quite strong. The more sleep is postponed from the evening toward noon next day, the more truncated it becomes, and when noon is reached sleep duration is only around 5 h (despite the sleep loss), the trend then reverts and increase sleep is seen again.[22,23] Thus, sleep during the morning hours is strongly interfered with, despite the sizeable sleep loss that, logically, should enhance the ability to maintain sleep.[24]

Homeostatic influences also control sleep taken at the wrong time of day. For example, the expected 4–5 h of daytime sleep, after a night spent awake, will be reduced to 2 h if a normal night's sleep precedes it and to 3.5 h if a 2 h nap is allowed during the night.[25] Thus, the time of sleep termination depends on the balance between the circadian and homeostatic influences. The circadian homeostatic regulation of sleep has also been demonstrated in great detail in studies of forced or spontaneous desynchronization under conditions of temporal isolation and ad lib sleep hours.[24]

14.3   Stress and Sleep

One major obstacle to sleep is stress. Here we will focus on the role of stress in preventing recuperation through sleep. The core problem of stress with regard to sleep is that stress produces significant physiological activation, which is in conflict with the inherent requirement of physiological deactivation during sleep.

Long-term effects of stress are described by the term "*allostasis*" referring to the ability of the body to increase or decrease the activation level of vital functions to *new steady states* dependent on the characteristics of the challenge and the person's emotions and appraisal of the event.[26] The resulting "*allostatic load*" represents the cumulative cost to the body when the systems start to malfunction after a stressful event.[27] It is suggested that serious pathophysiology can occur if overload is not relieved in some way.[26] Clearly, one of the outcomes may be insomnia, as discussed below.

Considering the physiological activation involved in the stress response, it seems logical to expect a connection with sleep. The evidence is, however, surprisingly modest, at least in terms of studies of causal connections. There nevertheless exist a number of cross-sectional epidemiological studies which point to a strong link between stress and sleep.[28-32] In fact, stress is considered the primary cause of persistent psychophysiological insomnia.[33] In one study of life events, Cernovsky et al.[34] demonstrated a clear increase in negative life events before an outbreak of insomnia.

Stress as a predictor of later sleep disturbances has been the topic of rather few studies. One such is that of Jansson and Linton,[35] which showed effects of present stress on later complaints of disturbed sleep. Akerstedt et al.[32] showed that night time ratings of stress/worries at bedtime was related to reduced sleep efficiency, increased waking after sleep onset (WASO), and increased latency to SWS. In other polysomnographic (PSG) studies, sleep during the night before a big exam, before a day of skydiving, when on call, or sleep before an early awakening[36] have been studied. The results indicate a slight reduction of sleep efficiency and the amount of deep sleep. In addition, a number of laboratory studies of stress and sleep have been carried out, but the stressors have been rather artificial (e.g., an unpleasant movie) and the results unclear.[37] It is probably the case that the stressor needs to be of some significance to the individual in order to have any effect.

Sleep disturbances from stress seem to constitute a consistent response pattern. Drake et al.[38] for example, have shown that those who report higher habitual sleep vulnerability to stress also show longer sleep latency and lower sleep efficiency on the first night in the sleep laboratory.

The particular cause of stress-disturbed sleep has been addressed in several studies. Thus, Partinen et al.[39] investigated several occupational groups and found disturbed sleep to be most common among manual workers and much less so among physicians or managing directors. In a retrospective study of older individuals (above the age of 75), Geroldi et al.[40] found that former white collar workers reported better sleep than blue collar workers. Kupperman et al.[41] reported fewer sleep problems in persons who were satisfied with their work.

In one of the more detailed epidemiological studies so far, Ribet et al.[30] studied more than 21,000 persons in France, using a sleep disturbance index and logistic regression analysis. It was found that shift work, a long working week, exposure to vibrations, and "having to hurry" appeared to be the main risk factors, controlling for age and gender. Disturbed sleep was more frequent in women and in older age groups.[42]

The work stressor most closely linked to disturbed sleep may be "work under high demands."[28-32] In the study by Akerstedt et al.[43] it was found that the strongest item of the demand index was "having to exert a lot of effort at work" – not simply "having too much to do," for example. It was also found that when "not being able to stop thinking about work in the evening" was added to the regression this variable took over part of the role of work demands as a predictor. This suggests that it may not be work demands per se that are important, but rather their non-remitting character. It appears that rumination at bedtime may be one of the key factors behind difficulties sleeping.[44] Hall et al.[45] have demonstrated in a cross-sectional study that intrusive thoughts at bedtime are related to increased alpha and beta power in the sleep EEG. Similarly, increased cognitive arousal at bedtime is related to increased sleep latency[46,47] but the former study did not report on other sleep parameters and the latter only included actigraphy, which is only a very approximate indicator of physiological sleep.

Closely related to rumination is worrying and tension before sleep.[48,49] After times of worry and tension, sleep appears to contain less SWS, which supports the notion that it is the anticipation of difficulties that is important in the stress reaction. This was also found in the previously mentioned study on stress/worries at bedtime.[50] In that study, sleep recordings preceded by increased (moderately so) subjective "stress/worries" at bedtime were compared with sleep recordings preceded by low such levels.[50] The results showed an increased sleep latency, more stage wake and a longer latency to SWS, all of which were interpreted as indicating slight perturbation of sleep on nights when stress and worries and, by inference, rumination had been present at bedtime. Mean ratings of stress (every 2 h) during the same day and the day after were also significantly increased.

It has also been shown that sleep is disturbed under threats to national security, for example, after the nuclear accident at the facility at Three-Mile Island and during the scud missile attacks on Israel during the Gulf War.[51,52] The effect of losing a life partner has in one study been shown to have surprisingly modest effects, and then mainly an increase in REM intensity.[53]

Lack of social support at work is also a risk indicator for disturbed sleep.[32,54] Poor (general) social support has been associated for instance with sleep complaints in Viet Nam war veterans,[55] even if the amount of work available is rather limited.

Post-traumatic stress disorder (PTSD) is another well-established cause of disturbed sleep, even if many of the more common indicators of sleep quality (sleep latency, efficiency of sleep, total length of sleep, and amount of stage 3 and 4) are relatively moderately affected.[56-59] Instead, it appears that its major effect is to disturb REM sleep, in particular by either increasing or reducing its duration, and by increasing its intensity. It also increases the number of awakenings. The unpleasant dreams associated with traumatic memories also tend to produce conditioned avoidance responses in affected individuals, resulting in postponements on a daily basis of retiring or of even entering the sleeping area.

14.4 Sleep Disorders

Another major cause of disturbed sleep is the sleep disorders. Among the major categories are insomnia, hypersomnia, and parasomnias.[60] Insomnia is usually defined as difficulties in sleeping or complaints of non-restorative sleep at least half the days of the week and with the problem present for at least 3 months.[61] The difficulty in sleeping must be linked to daytime consequences such as sleepiness, fatigue, or performance impairment. The level of complaint must be of "clinical significance." The criteria are not quantitative with respect to specific sleep stages or other aspects of sleep, mainly because of the large overlap between poor and good sleepers. However, authoritative sources suggest a criterion for reported sleep latency of longer duration than 30 min or amount of time awake after sleep onset longer than 30 min.[62] Common criteria also include more than four awakenings per night as an indicator of insomnia. Polysomnographic criteria are presently not part of the official criteria, but many researchers use a sleep efficiency (sleep in percent of time in bed) of 85% as a cut-off between good and poor sleep. The international classification of sleep disorders provides more detailed diagnostic criteria.[60] A new addition to the diagnostic criteria is also that a complaint of non-restorative sleep can be used. The definition of this concept is not clear but obviously involves feelings of not having slept well enough to be in good shape in the morning.

In Europe, around 38% of the population suffer from insomnia DSM-IV symptoms and 6% meet the criteria for a diagnosis of insomnia.[63] Other estimates vary between 5% and 12%.[29,64,65] Excessive daytime sleepiness varies between 3.2% and 5.5%, whereas sleep apnea varies between 1.1% and 1.9%. Generally, sleep problems increase with increasing age, female gender, stressful work, and physical workload.[28,66,67]

In patients with primary insomnia, there is an increased incidence of stress markers, including elevated cortisol levels, increased heart rate, and above average body temperature, increased beta EEG intensity, etc.[68-72] have demonstrated increased overall oxygen use in insomnia patients and simulated insomnia by administering

400 mg of caffeine per day for 1 week. The results show increased uptake of oxygen VO_2, disturbed sleep, increased fatigue and anxiety, but decreased sleepiness, as measured by the multiple sleep latency tests. The results suggest that insomnia may be more of a metabolic disturbance than a disturbance of the sleep mechanism per se.

Also obstructive sleep apnea has profound effects on the recuperative value of sleep. Since the disease involves a sleep-related relaxation of the muscles of the upper respiratory system, the respiratory pathways become blocked. This requires the sleeper to wake up in order to breathe. When this happens repeatedly, as is usually the case, sleep becomes interrupted and recuperation may be totally absent depending on the frequency of awakenings. The immediate effects involve fatigue[73] and an increase of accident risk during the day.[74] However, the breathing effort also functions as a powerful stressor and results in increased levels of stress hormones, lipids, proinflammatory cytokines, etc.[75] Thus, Sleep apnea is a contributor to the metabolic syndrome[8,76] and directly related to workability.[77] Since sleep apnea and its contribution to CHD has been a subject of many reviews, we will not describe it in the present chapter.

Other types of insomnia include the "Restless legs syndrome," "Periodic limb movements," and those related to psychiatric disease and other medical disorders.

Another type of sleep disorder is that involving the circadian rhythm.[78] It includes advanced sleep phase disorder (early bedtime/awakening), delayed sleep phase disorder, non-24 h-sleep disorder, irregular sleep disorder, jet lag, and shift work disorder.

14.5   Sleep and Risk Factors for CHD

14.5.1   Cardiovascular System: Hypertension

Non-REM sleep is characterized by a progressive decrease in heart rate, blood pressure, cardiac output, peripheral vascular resistance mainly due to decrease in neural sympathetic activity, while in the REM periods dominated by vagal tone, sudden bursts of sympathetic activity lead to increases in the cardiovascular function as in the awake condition.[79] The parasymphatetic dominance leads to sinus arrhythmia and conduction disturbances in healthy people. There are also marked changes in the endothelial function, with attenuation more pronounced toward the morning hours.[80]

Circardian patterns affect coagulation, with increased coagulability in the early morning.[81] Since it has been observed that cardiovascular events such as myocardial ischemia, myocardial infarction, and stroke peak between 6 and 11 a.m.[82] the above sleep-related changes in autonomic nervous system activity and its influence on cardiac function as well as endothelial function and coagulation can explain this phenomenon. It has also has been observed that ventricular arrhythmia and sudden death are more frequent in the morning hours. Early morning ischemia and sympathetic nervous system surges during REM sleep may lay behind those phenomeneon.[83]

Since normal sleep influences cardiovascular function in a profound way, it is not surprising that sleep restriction, experimental or natural, as well as sleep disturbance due to stress, shift work, or sleep disorders will also affect cardiovascular function. The major research focus has been on the experimental sleep deprivation, which clearly demonstrated increased blood pressure due to increased sympathetic cardiac and blood pressure modulation as well as decreased baroreflex sensitivity.[84] Other studies with more naturally occurring sleep shortening has clearly demonstrated linkage with hypertension.[85,86]

14.5.2   Endocrine Effects: Increased Stress

Profound changes occur in the endocrine system during sleep.[87,88] During sleep, an interaction occurs between the electrophysiology and endocrinology. In adults, the first part of sleep is characterized by increased growth hormone (GH) release (together with increased SWS and low levels of REM sleep) and suppressed secretion of the hormones of the hypothalamic-pituitary-adrenocortical (HPA) system. This means that the corticotropin releasing hormone (CRH), the messenger to the adrenal cortex, corticotropin (ACTH), and the cortisol hormone itself are suppressed. These changes directly oppose the effects of stress. GH promotes protein synthesis, which means that it is essential for growing and for repairing tissue. It also prevents glucose from entering brain cells (for storage), which leads to high circulating levels of glucose during the first half of sleep. The reason is to ensure that the brain has a constant supply of energy during sleep, which is a period of fasting. During the second half of the night the HPA axis dominates and GH secretion is essentially absent. Thus, the first half of sleep is strongly anabolic.

When sleep is prevented, cortisol secretion will increase[3] and the rate of sleep fragmentation (microarousals) is related to increased levels of cortisol.[89] Thus, sleep reduction has effects similar to those of stress. In contrast, GH secretion is strongly reduced if no sleep occurs, but may to some extent reappear when it normally does not.[90]

Sleep does not only regulate hormone secretion, it is also affected by it. Thus GH-releasing hormone (GHRH) causes increased SWS and GH secretion, as well as reduced cortisol levels in males (not females).[87] CRH will exert the opposite effects. It appears that the quality of sleep partly depends on an interaction of GHRH and CRH. Changes in the balance between the two may be part of the sleep problems in depression and aging. Possibly, the differential response to GHRH in males and females can be related to the elevated risk of affective disorders in women. Also elevated glucocorticoid levels may contribute to the sleep EEG changes in depression and CRH antagonism normalizes sleep disturbances.

14.5.3   Glucose Changes: Diabetes and Obesity

Insulin and glucose levels are sensitive to manipulations of sleep.[3,91] In general, glucose levels during sleep are maintained at relatively normal levels and glucose infusion results in dramatically increased levels since insulin effects are impaired during sleep. Furthermore, sleep reduction down to 4 h for 6 days yields decreased glucose tolerance, increased evening cortisol, elevated sympathovagal balance, abnormal profiles of nocturnal growth hormone secretion and markedly decreased leptin levels, as well as a blunted response to influenza vaccination. Short sleepers (<6 h) show results consistent with the experimental results – decreased insulin sensitivity, largely due to the increased GH-secretion during sleep. Another observation in relation to experimental sleep reduction is that leptin levels are reduced and hunger markedly increased. The effects suggest links with the metabolic syndrome and may be related to (abdominal) obesity and poor lifestyle, often found in patients of lower socioeconomic background.[92,93]

One new and interesting aspect of sleep loss is the impact on glucose metabolism and diabetes.[94] Previous epidemiological studies have shown that patients with type 2 diabetes report more sleep problems than nondiabetic subjects.[95] This finding could be confounded by obesity or by obstructive sleep apnea. However, in a prospective follow-up study of healthy middle-aged men from Malmö, Sweden, it was recently shown that the 12 year risk of developing type 2 diabetes was independently predicted by self-reported difficulties in falling asleep and by elevated resting heart rate, after full adjustment for obesity, lifestyle factors, and other risk factors.[96] One possible explanation is sleep apnea, which was not measured in the Malmö study, but another possibility would be chronic low-grade inflammation, both linked to insomnia and risk of type 2 diabetes. Also, the weakening of insulin efficiency due to loss of sleep might contribute.[91]

14.5.4   The Immune System: Inflammation

The immune system shows strong effects of sleep.[97] During normal sleep, circulating cell counts for most major white blood cells decrease (monocytes, natural killer cells, T and B cells). The latter seem to accumulate in lymphoid tissue during sleep, facilitating local immune responses. However, the sleep process does not seem to affect the production of proinflammatory cytokines like IL-1, IL-6, or TNF-alpha; but IL-2 is markedly increased (compared to wakefulness) as is also IFNμ (also derived from T-cells).

However, reduced sleep causes increased levels of proinflammatory cytokines like IL-1ß, IL-6 and TNF-alpha. These are potent local sleep inducers and, at least the latter two, are elevated in patients with disorders of excessive daytime sleepiness (EDS).[98] There seems to be a correlation with BMI, and both cytokines are released by fat tissue. The same cytokines and leptin are increased in sleep apnea, independent of obesity, as is insulin resistance.[8] Sleep apnea (frequent awakenings due to respiratory pathways being blocked) is linked to both obesity and diabetes and it appears that insulin resistance, related to visceral obesity, may be partly responsible for sleep apnea. Possibly, sleep apnea, in turn, may accelerate such metabolic changes through elevation of stress hormones and cytokines (cortisol, IL-6, TNFα).

14.5.5 Sleep and CHD Morbidity and Mortality

Since reduced or disturbed sleep has been linked to the major risk factors for CHD like hypertension, obesity, diabetes, and inflammation, it is not surprising that poor sleep has been associated with an increased prospective risk of myocardial infarction, particularly when combined with increased resting heart rate – a marker of sympathetic over-activity.[99] In women under rehabilitation from a myocardial infarction, the risk of recurrent myocardial events is increased in self-reported poor sleepers.[100] In addition, frequent events of waking-up exhausted in the morning are a predictor of subsequent myocardial infarction.[101] The exhausted state is also associated with reduced amounts of sleep stages 3 and 4.[102] Also in the condition of work-related burnout, which is accompanied by sleep disturbances, there was an increased risk of future myocardial infarction.[103]

In the long-term follow-up of individuals with different amounts of habitual sleep,[104] it has been shown that large (3–4 h) deviations from the median (8 h), in apparently healthy individuals, yielded an increased mortality. This study was recently repeated with approximately the same results, even if the median with lowest risk turned out to be 7 h.[105] Similar results have been reported by others.[5,106,107] However, the association between sleep duration and CHD remains debatable.[79] In some studies, a positive, U shaped association between short and long sleep duration and manifestation of CHD or CHD mortality has been shown.[106,108-111]

In some studies, only short sleep duration[112,113] while in others, only long[105,114] sleep duration were found to affect CHD. Furthermore, some studies report associations only among men[108,114] while others only among women.[109,111] It is possible that these contradictory results may have occurred because sleep duration is not a sufficient measure of the disturbances in the recovery and physiological reinstitution of the body during sleep. Ekstedt et al.[115] reported an association between increased number of microarousals per hour in exhausted patients, and an increase in blood lipids, cortisol, and blood pressure; although the total sleep time was not affected. Microarousals during sleep are associated with increased levels of lipids, cortisol, and blood pressure.[89] Thus, one way of clarifying the debates on the sleep-CHD relationship may be to combine measures of short sleep and low sleep quality. A combination of sleep disturbance and short sleep duration together might be a much better measure of physiological disturbances during sleep than either one on its own. Such a combination may be a stronger predictor of coronary heart disease and cardiovascular mortality than its components. Complaints about disturbed sleep were linked to increased CHD risk in one study[113] but they were not combined with sleep duration.

Secondly, the variable results concerning association of sleep in men and women may be due to the nature of the CHD measures used in various studies, especially in working, younger populations. While fatal CHD and myocardial infarction is a more common expression of CHD in men,[116] nonfatal angina pectoris is more common in women.[117] Thus, studies that only examine myocardial infarction may be missing an important dimension of CHD among women. Analyses that include both myocardial infarction and angina may be important in understanding if there is a gender difference in the effect of sleep on CHD.

14.6   Implications for Physicians

1. Majority of people tend to sleep between 7 to 8 h. There is a health benefit in increasing sleep time from 5 to 7 or 8 h, but no benefit has been shown to increase sleep time from 7, 8 to 9 h or 10 h.
2. Disturbed sleep or extreme sleep time (too short or too long) should always be explored in patients with extreme tiredness.
3. Sleep apnea is considered as a major sleep disturbance affecting risk of CHD, but also the morbidity and mortality in CHD. It should be detected and treated promptly.
4. Insomnia due to stress is also a common sleep disturbance and by contributing to hypertension, obesity, and diabetes may affect the risk of CHD. However, it has not yet been shown that it constitutes an independent risk factor for CHD.
5. Insomnia is usually treated pharmacologically, with varied results depending on the choice of agents, treatment compliance, as well as the duration of treatment. The disadvantage being that the effect of treatment terminates often with the end of treatment.
6. As a rule, new, sleep-inducing agents should be preferred – due to less side effects and lower risk of tolerance development.
7. Cognitive therapy has been shown to be an effective treatment method for insomnia – with less side effects and a documented long-term effect. It may be combined with pharmacological treatment.
8. Cognitive therapy of sleep disturbances often addresses life style and stress issues – which may benefit the cardiac patients.

References

1. NSF. *Sleep in America Poll*. Washington DC: National Sleep Foundation; 2002.
2. Ohayon MM, Carskadon MA, Guilleminault C, Vitiello MV. Meta-analysis of quantitative sleep parameters from childhood to old age in healthy individuals: developing normative sleep values across the human lifespan. *Sleep.* 2004;27(7):1255-1273.
3. Spiegel K, Leproult R, Van Cauter E. Impact of sleep debt on metabolic and endocrine function. *Lancet.* 1999;354:1435-1439.

4. Gangwisch JE, Heymsfield SB, Boden-Albala B, et al. Short sleep duration as a risk factor for hypertension: analyses of the first National Health and Nutrition Examination Survey. *Hypertension.* 2006;47(5):833-839.

5. Gangwisch JE, Heymsfield SB, Boden-Albala B, et al. Sleep duration as a risk factor for diabetes incidence in a large U.S. sample. *Sleep.* 2007;30(12):1667-1673.

6. Yaggi HK, Araujo AB, McKinlay JB. Sleep duration as a risk factor for the development of type 2 diabetes. *Diabetes Care.* 2006;29(3):657-661.

7. Stranges S, Cappuccio FP, Kandala NB, et al. Cross-sectional versus prospective associations of sleep duration with changes in relative weight and body fat distribution: the Whitehall II Study. *Am J Epidemiol.* 2008;167(3):321-329.

8. Vgontzas AN, Bixler EO, Chrousos GP. Sleep apnea is a manifestation of the metabolic syndrome. *Sleep Med Rev.* 2005;9:211-224.

9. Vgontzas AN, Zoumakis E, Bixler EO, et al. Adverse effects of modest sleep restriction on sleepiness, performance, and inflammatory cytokines. *J Clin Endocrinol Metab.* 2004;89(5): 2119-2126.

10. Greenland P, Knoll MD, Stamler J, et al. Major risk factors as antecedents of fatal and nonfatal coronary heart disease events. *JAMA.* 2003;290(7):891-897.

11. Gallicchio L, Kalesan B. Sleep duration and mortality: a systematic review and meta-analysis. *J Sleep Res.* 2009;18:148-158.

12. McEwen BS. Sleep deprivation as a neurobiologic and physiologic stressor: allostasis and allostatic load [Suppl 2]. *Metabolism.* 2006;55:S20-S23.

13. Carskadon MA, Dement WC. Normal human sleep: an overview. In: Kryger MH, Roth T, Dement WC, eds. *Principles and practice of sleep medicine.* 3rd ed. Philadelphia: W.B. Saunders Company; 2000:15-25.

14. Rechtschaffe A, Kales A. *A manual of standardized terminology, techniques and scoring system for sleep stages of human subjects.* Bethesda: US Department of Health, Education and Welfare, Public Health Service; 1968.

15. Borbély AA. A two-process model of sleep regulation. *Hum Neurobiol.* 1982;1:195-204.

16. Åkerstedt T, Folkard S, Portin C. Predictions from the three-process model of alertness. *Aviat Space Environ Med.* 2004;75:A75-A83.

17. Porkka-Heiskanen T. Adenosine in sleep and wakefulness. *Ann Med.* 1999;31(2):125-129.

18. Saper CB, Chou TC, Scammell TE. The sleep switch: hypothalamic control of sleep and wakefulness. *Trends Neurosci.* 2001;24(12):726-731.

19. Webb WB, Agnew HW Jr. Stage 4 sleep: influence of time course variables. *Science.* 1971;174:1354-1356.

20. Horne JA. Functional aspects of human slow wave sleep. In: Wauquier A, Dugovic C, Radulovacki M, eds. *Slow Wave Sleep. Physiological, Pathophysiological, and Functional Aspects.* New York: Raven Press; 1989:109-119.

21. Saper CB, Lu J, Chou TC, Gooley J. The hypothalamic integrator for circadian rhythms. *Trends Neurosci.* 2005;28(3):152-157.

22. Foret J, Lantin G. The sleep of train drivers: an example of the effects of irregular work schedules on sleep. In: Colquhoun WP, ed. *Aspects of Human Efficiency. Diurnal Rhythm and Loss of Sleep.* London: The English Universities Press Ltd; 1972:273-281.

23. Åkerstedt T, Gillberg M. The circadian variation of experimentally displaced sleep. *Sleep.* 1981;4:159-169.

24. Czeisler CA, Weitzman ED, Moore-Ede MC, Zimmerman JC, Knauer RS. Human sleep: its duration and organization depend on its circadian phase. *Science.* 1980;210:1264-1267.

25. Åkerstedt T, Gillberg M. A dose-response study of sleep loss and spontaneous sleep termination. *Psychophysiology.* 1986;23:293-297.

26. McEwen BS, Wingfield JC. The concept of allostasis in biology and biomedicine. *Horm Behav.* 2003;43(1):2-15.

27. McEwen BS. Protection and damage from acute and chronic stress: allostasis and allostatic overload and relevance to the pathophysiology of psychiatric disorders. *Ann N Y Acad Sci.* 2004;1032:1-7.

28. Ancoli-Israel S, Roth T. Characteristics of insomnia in the United States: results of the 1991 National Sleep Foundation survey. I. *Sleep.* 1999;22 Suppl.2:S347-S353.
29. Morphy H, Dunn M, Lewis M, Boardman HF, Croft PR. Epidemiology of insomnia: a longitudinal study in a UK population. *Sleep.* 2007;30(3):274-280.
30. Ribet C, Derriennic F. Age, working conditions, and sleep disorders: a longitudinal analysis in the French Cohort E.S.T.E.V. *Sleep.* 1999;22:491-504.
31. Urponen H, Vuori I, Hasan J, Partinen M. Self-evaluations of factors promoting and disturbing sleep: an epidemiological survey in Finland. *Soc Sci Med.* 1988;26:443-450.
32. Åkerstedt T, Fredlund P, Gillberg M, Jansson B. Work load and work hours in relation to disturbed sleep and fatigue in a large representative sample. *J Psychosom Res.* 2002;53: 585-588.
33. Morin CM, Rodrigue S, Ivers H. Role of stress, arousal, and coping skills in primary insomnia. *Psychosom Med.* 2003;65:259-267.
34. Cernovsky ZZ. Life stress measures and reported frequency of sleep disorders. *Percept Mot Skills.* 1984;58:39-49.
35. Jansson M, Linton SJ. Psychosocial work stressors in the development and maintenance of insomnia: a prospective study. *J Occup Health Psychol.* 2006;11(3):241-248.
36. Holdstock TL, Verschoor GJ. Student sleep patterns before, during and after an examination period. *J Psychol.* 1974;4:16-24.
37. Åkerstedt T. Sleep and stress. In: Peter JH, Podszus T, von Wichert P, eds. *Sleep Related Disorders and Internal Diseases.* Heidelberg: Springer; 1987:183-191.
38. Drake C, Richardson G, Roehrs T, Scofield H, Roth T. Vulnerability to stress-related sleep disturbance and hyperarousal. *Sleep.* 2004;27:285-291.
39. Partinen M, Eskelinen L, Tuomi K. Complaints of insomnia in different occupations. *Scand J Work Environ Health.* 1984;10:467-469.
40. Geroldi C, Frisoni GB, Rozzini R, De Leo D, Trabucchi M. Principal lifetime occupation and sleep quality in the elderly. *Gerontology.* 1996;42:163-169.
41. Kuppermann M, Lubeck DP, Mazonson PD, et al. Sleep problems and their correlates in a working population. *J Gen Intern Med.* 1995;10:25-32.
42. Bixler EO, Kales A, Soldatos CR. Sleep disorders encountered in medical practice: a national survey of physicians. *Behav Med.* 1979;3:1-6.
43. Åkerstedt T, Knutsson A, Westerholm P, Theorell T, Alfredsson L, Kecklund G. Sleep disturbances, work stress and work hours. A cross-sectional study. *J Psychosom Res.* 2002; 53:741-748.
44. Harvey AG, Tang NK, Browning L. Cognitive approaches to insomnia. *Clin Psychol Rev.* 2005;25(5):593-611.
45. Hall M, Buysse DJ, Nowell PD, et al. Symptoms of stress and depression as correlates of sleep in primary Insomnia. *Psychosom Med.* 2000;62:227-230.
46. Haynes SN, Adams A, Franzen M. The effects of presleep stress on sleep-onset insomnia. *J Abnorm Psychol.* 1981;90:601-606.
47. Tang NKY, Harvey AG. Effects of cognitive arousal and physiological arousal on sleep perception. *Sleep.* 2004;27:69-78.
48. Kecklund G, Åkerstedt T. Objective components of individual differences in subjective sleep quality. *J Sleep Res.* 1997;6:217-220.
49. Kecklund G, Åkerstedt T, Lowden A. Morning work: effects of early rising on sleep and alertness. *Sleep.* 1997;20(3):215-223.
50. Akerstedt T, Kecklund G, Axelsson J. Impaired sleep after bedtime stress and worries. *Biol Psychol.* 2007;76(3):170-173.
51. Askenasy JJM, Lewin I. The impact of missile warfare on self-reported sleep quality. Part 1. *Sleep.* 1996;19:47-51.
52. Davidson L, Fleming R, Baum A. Chronic stress, catecholamines, and sleep disturbance at three Mile Island. *J Human Stress.* 1987;13:75-83.
53. Reynolds CF III, Hoch CC, Buysse DJ, et al. Sleep after spousal bereavement: a study of recovery from stress. *Biol Psychiatry.* 1993;34:791-797.

54. Nordin M, Knutsson A, Sundbom E. Is disturbed sleep a mediator in the association between social support and myocardial infarction? *J Health Psychol.* 2008;13(1):55-64.
55. Fabsitz RR, Sholinsky P, Goldberg J. Correlates of sleep problems among men: the Vietnam era twin registry. *J Sleep Res.* 1997;6:50-60.
56. Dow BM, Kelsoe JR, Gillin JC. Sleep and dreams in Vietnam PTSD and depression. *Biol Psychiatry.* 1996;39:42-50.
57. Mellman TA, Nolan B, Hebding J, Kulick-Bell R, Dominguez R. A polysomnographic comparison of veterans with combat-related PTSD, depressed men, and non-ill controls. *Sleep.* 1997;20:46-51.
58. Pillar G, Malhotra A, Lavie P. Post-traumatic stress disorder and sleep – what a nightmare! *Sleep Med Rev.* 2000;4:183-200.
59. Ross RJ, Ball WA, Dinges DF, et al. Motor dysfunction during sleep in posttraumatic stress disorder. *Sleep.* 1994;17:723-732.
60. AASM. *ICSD – International Classification of Sleep Disorders, Revised: Diagnostic and Coding Manual.* Chicago: American Academy of Sleep Medicine; 2005.
61. APA. *Diagnostic and Statistical Manual of Mental Disorders.* 4th ed. (DSM-IV). Washington DC: American Psychiatric Association; 1994.
62. Lichstein KL, Durrence HH, Taylor DJ, Bush AJ, Riedel BW. Quantitative criteria for insomnia. *Behav Res Ther.* 2003;41(4):427-445.
63. Ohayon M, Caulet M, Priest R, Guilleminault C. DSM-IV and ICSD-90 insomnia symptoms and sleep dissatisfaction. *Br J Psychiatry.* 1997;171:382-388.
64. Jansson-Frojmark M, Linton SJ. The course of insomnia over one year: a longitudinal study in the general population in Sweden. *Sleep.* 2008;31(6):881-886.
65. Roth T, Drake C. Evolution of insomnia: current status and future direction. *Sleep Med.* 2004;5(suppl 1):S23-S30.
66. Ohayon MM, Guilleminault C, Paiva T, et al. An international study on sleep disorders in the general population: methosological aspects of the use of the sleep-EVAL system. *Sleep.* 1997;20:1086-1092.
67. Sateia M, Doghramji K, Hauri PJ, Morin CM. Evaluation of chronic insomnia. *Sleep.* 2000;23:243-263.
68. Adam K, Tomeny M, Oswald I. Physiological and psychological differences between good and poor sleepers. *J Psychiatr Res.* 1986;20(4):301-316.
69. Bonnet MH, Arand DL. Heart rate variability in insomniacs and matched normal sleepers. *Psychosom Med.* 1998;60:610-615.
70. Monroe L. Psychological and physiological differences between good and poor sleepers. *J Abnorm Psychol.* 1967;72:255-264.
71. Perlis ML, Merica H, Smith MT, Giles DE. Beta EEG activity and insomnia. *Sleep Med Rev.* 2001;5(5):365-376.
72. Bonnet MH, Arand DL. Insomnia, metabolic rate and sleep restoration. *J Intern Med.* 2003; 254(1):23-31.
73. Wong KK, Marshall NS, Grunstein RR, Dodd MJ, Rogers NL. Comparing the neurocognitive effects of 40 h sustained wakefulness in patients with untreated OSA and healthy controls. *J Sleep Res.* 2008;17:322-330.
74. Terán-Santos J, Jimnénez-Gómez A, Cordero-Guevara J. The association between sleep apnea and the risk of traffic accidents. *N Engl J Med.* 1999;24:847-851.
75. Lopez-Jimenez F, Somers VK. Stress measures linking sleep apnea, hypertension and diabetes–AHI vs arousals vs hypoxemia. *Sleep.* 2006;29(6):743-744.
76. Lavie L. Sleep apnea syndrome, endothelial dysfunction, and cardiovascular morbidity. *Sleep.* 2004;27:1053-1055.
77. Mulgrew AT, Ryan CF, Fleetham JA, et al. The impact of obstructive sleep apnea and daytime sleepiness on work limitation. *Sleep Med.* 2007;9(1):42-53.
78. Zee PC, Manthena P. The brain's master circadian clock: implications and opportunities for therapy of sleep disorders. *Sleep Med Rev.* 2007;11(1):59-70.
79. Wolk R, Gami AS, Garcia-Touchard A, Somers VK. Sleep and cardiovascular disease. *Curr Probl Cardiol.* 2005;30(12):625-662.

80. Otto ME, Svatikova A, Barretto RB, et al. Early morning attenuation of endothelial function in healthy humans. *Circulation*. 2004;109(21):2507-2510.

81. Tofler GH, Brezinski D, Schafer AI, et al. Concurrent morning increase in platelet aggregability and the risk of myocardial infarction and sudden cardiac death. *N Engl J Med*. 1987; 316(24):1514-1518.

82. Muller JE, Stone PH, Zoltan GT, et al. Circadian variation in the frequency of onset of acute myocardial infarction. *N Engl J Med*. 1985;313:1315-1322.

83. Charkoudian N, Rabbitts JA. Sympathetic neural mechanisms in human cardiovascular health and disease. *Mayo Clin Proc*. 2009;84(9):822-830.

84. Mullington JM, Haack M, Toth M, Serrador JM, Meier-Ewert HK. Cardiovascular, inflammatory, and metabolic consequences of sleep deprivation. *Prog Cardiovasc Dis*. 2009;51(4): 294-302.

85. Gottlieb DJ, Redline S, Nieto FJ, et al. Association of usual sleep duration with hypertension: the Sleep Heart Health Study. *Sleep*. 2006;29(8):1009-1014.

86. Vgontzas AN, Liao D, Bixler EO, Chrousos GP, Vela-Bueno A. Insomnia with objective short sleep duration is associated with a high risk for hypertension. *Sleep*. 2009;32(4): 491-497.

87. Steiger A. Sleep and the hypothalamo-pituitary-adrenocortical system. *Sleep Med Rev*. 2002;6(2):125-138.

88. Steiger A, Antonijevic IA, Bohlhalter S, Frieboes RM, Friess E, Murck H. Effects of hormones on sleep. *Horm Res*. 1998;49:125-130.

89. Ekstedt M, Åkerstedt T, Söderström M. Microarousals during sleep are associated with increased levels of lipids, cortisol, and blood pressure. *Psychosom Med*. 2004;66: 925-931.

90. Van Cauter E, Latta F, Nedeltcheva A, et al. Reciprocal interactions between the GH axis and sleep. *Growth Horm IGF Res*. 2004;14:S10-S17.

91. Knutson KL, Spiegel K, Penev P, Van Cauter E. The metabolic consequences of sleep deprivation. *Sleep Med Rev*. 2007;11(3):163-178.

92. Hall MH, Muldoon MF, Jennings JR, Buysse DJ, Flory JD, Manuck SB. Self-reported sleep duration is associated with the metabolic syndrome in midlife adults. *Sleep*. 2008; 31(5):635-643.

93. Patel SR, Hu FB. Short sleep duration and weight gain: a systematic review. *Obesity (Silver Spring)*. 2008;16(3):643-653.

94. Tasali E, Leproult R, Spiegel K. Reduced sleep duration or quality: relationships with insulin resistance and type 2 diabetes. *Prog Cardiovasc Dis*. 2009;51(5):381-391.

95. Nilsson P, Rööst M, Engström G, Hedblad B, Janzon L, Berglund G. Incidence of diabetes in middle-aged men is related to resting heart rate and difficulties to fall asleep. (Abstract). Paper presented at: the 7th International Congress of Behavioural Medicine; 2002; Helsinki.

96. Nilsson PM, Rööst M, Engström G, Hedblad B, Berglund G. Incidence of diabetes in middle-aged men is related to sleep disturbances. *Diabetes Care*. 2004;27:2464-2469.

97. Bryant PA, Trinder J, Curtis N. Sick and tired: does sleep have a vital role in the immune system. *Nat Rev Immunol*. 2004;4:457-467.

98. Vgontzas AN, Papanicolaou DA, Bixler EO, Kales A, Tyson K, Chrousos GP. Elevation of plasma cytokines in disorders of excessive daytime sleepiness: role of sleep disturbance and obesity. *J Clin Endocrinol Metab*. 1997;82(5):1313-1316.

99. Nilsson P, Nilsson J-Å, Hedblad B, Berglund G. Sleep disturbances in association with elevated pulse rate for the prediction of mortality – consequences of mental strain? *J Intern Med*. 2001;250:521-529.

100. Leineweber C, Kecklund G, Janszky I, Åkerstedt T, Orth-Gomér K. Poor sleep increases the prospective risk for recurrent events in middle-aged women with coronary disease. The Stockholm Female Coronary Risk Study. *J Psychosom Res*. 2003;54:121-127.

101. Appels A, Schouten E. Waking up exhausted as risk indicator of myocardial infarction. *Am J Cardiol*. 1991;68:395-398.

102. van Diest R, Appels AWPM. Sleep physiological characteristics of exhausted men. *Psychosom Med*. 1994;56:28-35.

103. Melamed S, Shirom A, Toker S, Berliner S, Shapira I. Burnout and risk of cardiovascular disease: evidence, possible causal paths, and promising research directions. *Psychol Bull.* 2006;132(3):327-353.
104. Kripke DF, Simons RN, Garfinkel L, Hammond EC. Short and long sleep and sleeping pills. *Arch Gen Psychiatry.* 1979;36:103-116.
105. Kripke DF, Garfinkel L, Wingard DL, Klauber MR, Marler MR. Mortality associated with sleep duration and insomnia. *Arch Gen Psychiatry.* 2002;59:131-136.
106. Ferrie JE, Shipley MJ, Cappuccio FP, et al. A prospective study of change in sleep duration: associations with mortality in the Whitehall II cohort. *Sleep.* 2007;30(12):1659-1666.
107. Hublin C, Partinen M, Koskenvuo M, Kaprio J. Sleep and mortality: a population-based 22-year follow-up study. *Sleep.* 2007;30(10):1245-1253.
108. Amagai Y, Ishikawa S, Gotoh T, et al. Sleep duration and mortality in Japan: the Jichi Medical School Cohort Study. *J Epidemiol.* 2004;14(4):124-128.
109. Ayas NT, White DP, Manson JE, et al. A prospective study of sleep duration and coronary heart disease in women. *Arch Intern Med.* 2003;163(2):205-209.
110. Empana JP, Dauvilliers Y, Dartigues JF, et al. Excessive daytime sleepiness is an independent risk indicator for cardiovascular mortality in community-dwelling elderly: the three city study. *Stroke.* 2009;40(4):1219-1224.
111. Patel SR, Ayas NT, Malhotra MR, et al. A prospective study of sleep duration and mortality risk. *Sleep.* 2004;27:440-444.
112. Heslop P, Smith GD, Metcalfe C, Macleod J, Hart C. Sleep duration and mortality: the effect of short or long sleep duration on cardiovascular and all-cause mortality in working men and women. *Sleep Med.* 2002;3(4):305-314.
113. Meisinger C, Heier M, Lowel H, Schneider A, Doring A. Sleep duration and sleep complaints and risk of myocardial infarction in middle-aged men and women from the general population: the MONICA/KORA Augsburg cohort study. *Sleep.* 2007;30(9):1121-1127.
114. Mallon L, Broman JE, Hetta J. Sleep complaints predict coronary artery disease mortality in males: a 12-year follow-up study of a middle-aged Swedish population. *J Intern Med.* 2002;251(3):207-216.
115. Ekstedt M, Söderström M, Åkerstedt T, Nilsson J, Sondergaard H-P, Perski A. Disturbed sleep and fatigue in occupational burnout. *Scand J Work Environ Health.* 2006;32(2): 121-131.
116. Gopalakrishnan P, Ragland MM, Tak T. Gender differences in coronary artery disease: review of diagnostic challenges and current treatment. *Postgrad Med.* 2009;121(2):60-68.
117. Wenger NK. Preventing cardiovascular disease in women: an update. *Clin Cardiol.* 2008; 31(3):109-113.

Chapter 15
The Causal Role of Chronic Mental Stress in the Pathogenesis of Essential Hypertension

Murray Esler

Keywords Aversive stressors for hypertension • Chronic mental stress • Experimental models of stress-induced hypertension • Neurogenic hypertension • Pathogenesis of essential hypertension • Psychodynamic formulation • Public policy implementation • Sympathetic nervous system

The idea that essential hypertension may arise through psychosomatic mechanisms is an old one. Even before the standard methods of indirect blood pressure measurement were available, Geisbock (in 1905) wrote, concerning his male patients with polycythemia and hypertension (systolic pressure having been measured with a finger plethysmograph): "one finds an unusual frequency of those who as directors of big enterprises had a great deal of responsibility and demanding jobs, and who, after a long period of mental overwork, became nervous."[1] The lay public needs no convincing that chronic mental stress can cause hypertension, sometimes even using the word "hypertensive" as a psychological descriptor, for describing excitable or agitated behavior. Many personally relate to the "tense" in hypertension, and perhaps may be sometimes too ready to attribute their elevated blood pressure to stress in their job, or in their domestic life. Although providing proof that essential hypertension is a psychosomatic disorder has been difficult, the supporting evidence, elegantly reviewed by Folkow,[2] is now very persuasive.

M. Esler
Hypertension Thrombosis and Vascular Biology Division,
Baker IDI Heart and Diabetes Institute,
Melbourne, VIC, Australia
e-mail: murray.esler@bakeridi.edu.au

15.1   Experimental Models of Stress-Induced Hypertension

Because of logistic and ethical difficulties which exist in exploring the relation of chronic mental stress to the development of human hypertension, animal models have been developed. An acceptable animal model of presumed psychogenic human hypertension should meet the following criteria:

(i)   The blood pressure elevation should be permanent, persisting for at least months after removal of the stimulus
(ii) Cardiovascular complications of hypertension, such as strokes, atherosclerosis, left ventricular hypertrophy, and myocardial infarction should develop
(iii) The model should be plausible, and have points in common with human circumstances and behavior

The models of psychosocial hypertension developed in mice[3] and rats[4] by Henry and coworkers fulfilled these prerequisites. In Henry's mice experiments, colonies of animals were established from "asocial males," raised in isolation, and normally socialized females. Crowding was avoided. The male mice fought intensely over territories, failing to establish a stable social hierarchy. Blood pressure rose promptly and progressively in the males, associated with features of sympathetic nervous system overactivity and increased secretion of renin.[3] At first, the elevation in blood pressure was reversible when the mice were returned from the colony to isolation. But, after interacting in the colony for 6 months or more, the pressure rise was irreversible, and accompanied by cardiovascular complications.

15.2   Epidemiological and Clinical Evidence

While the studies with experimental stress in animals are interesting and important, in demonstrating that psychological stressors can cause permanent hypertension, and in identifying the crucial role of neural mechanisms in the development of the hypertension, it is another matter to demonstrate that essential hypertension is due to chronic mental stress.

The research by Brod and colleagues[5] in young men with normal or somewhat elevated blood pressure is important in this context. Hemodynamic measurements, of cardiac output, blood pressure and regional blood flow and vascular resistance suggested to Brod and his group that the "defence reaction," previously described in experimental animals,[6] could be invoked by laboratory mental stress in healthy men, and was actually chronically engaged at rest in mild hypertension.[5] Others, including Julius and colleagues also identified an elevated cardiac output as a common characteristic of early human hypertension.[7] In historic longitudinal studies, Lund-Johansen demonstrated that there was a reversal of this hemodynamic pattern over decades to the normal cardiac output, high peripheral vascular resistance form which is typical of more severe and longstanding essential hypertension.[8] The research of Folkow[2] and Korner[9] identified blood pressure-dependent arteriolar hypertrophy as central to this slow but progressive vascular remodeling.

15.2.1 Epidemiological Studies

Clinical and epidemiological studies provide increasingly strong support for the notion that behavioral and psychological factors are of importance in the pathogenesis of human hypertension.[10-13] Importantly, Henry and Grim[14] and Harburg et al.[12] have linked the increased prevalence of hypertension in Afro-Americans to high levels of psychosocial stress, the former authors providing evidence that what is in play here is an underlying genetic propensity to sodium retention by the kidneys (perhaps attributable to the survival benefit this might have provided at times of severe dietary sodium shortage on slave ship voyages) interacting with mental stress exposure. Sharma and colleagues[15] have identified greater cardiovascular responses to laboratory mental stress in "salt sensitive" humans.

Also influential have been long-term follow-up studies of human populations, such as the celebrated study of cloistered nuns in Umbria[16] who lived in a secluded and unchanging environment, and in whom blood pressure did not show the expected rise with age. Also important are studies linking coronary heart disease, hypertension, and metabolic syndrome development to chronic mental stress in the workplace.[17-19] Additional key observations have been made on human populations who demonstrate blood pressure elevation soon after migration,[20] this rise in pressure being attributed primarily to mental stress, although changes in physical activity and diet are also operative. Also pertinent is the observation that panic disorder and essential hypertension are commonly comorbid conditions. Patients with panic disorder have recurring and often severe stress responses with sympathetic nervous system activation, surges of adrenaline secretion, and acute blood pressure elevation.[21] The inference is that the recurring stress responses in panic disorder can initiate the development of persistently elevated pressure.

15.2.2 A Hypertensive Personality?

Research on the possible psychosomatic origins of essential hypertension, in addition to focusing on the external stress as the stimulus, has assessed the personality characteristics of hypertensive patients, which determine responsiveness to the external environment. As a group, hypertensive patients commonly exhibit a behavioral pattern, suppression of hostility, that is particularly associated with activation of the sympathetic nervous system and hypertension development.[10,12,13] Alexander[22] first drew attention to this: "Our society requires that the individual should have complete control over all his hostile impulses. While everyone is subjected to this restriction some people are more inhibited in their faculty to express aggressive and self-assertive tendencies.... consequently they live in a chronically inhibited hostile state." Links have been made between measured levels of suppressed aggression in hypertensive patients and the pathophysiology of their hypertension. Young hypertensive patients with suppression of hostility tend to have sympathetic nervous system activation, neural stimulation of renin release from the kidneys, and high renin hypertension.[10,13,23]

15.2.3   Public Policy Implementation?

A recent research approach breaks radically with the epidemiological methodology of the past, in searching for the presence of stress biomarkers in patients with essential hypertension.[24] Stress biomarkers have been identified in patients with essential hypertension (see below). This biological evidence of chronic mental stress exposure in essential hypertension patients, coupled with the epidemiological evidence, provided the lynchpin for a judgment by an Australian Government Committee that mental stress is a proven cause of high blood pressure, published in the March 27, 2002 Government of Australia Gazette (Members of Specialist Medical Review Council, 2002) following a request for adjudication on this matter by the Health Minister. This was an unpopular ruling in the corridors of political power, and was subsequently reversed by a second adjudicating committee appointed by the Minister!

In short, although the concept that in some patients essential hypertension may be psychogenic in origin is not definitively proven, there is a wealth of supporting experimental and clinical evidence. As discussed below, long-term neural effects of stress on renal function could possibly be the principal blood pressure elevating mechanism.[11,25,26]

15.3   A Psychodynamic Formulation of Stress-Induced Hypertension

What might be the mechanism by which chronic mental stress leads to essential hypertension? Figure 15.1 presents a general scheme for the path to stress-induced illnesses, including high blood pressure. An ongoing aversive stimulus, which can be modified, extinguished, or perpetuated in particular circumstances, can lead to illness. As indicated in this generic formulation, the existence of strong social support in a person's life, or their possession of good coping strategies can dampen the stressor impact, minimizing its transfiguration into pathophysiology or psychopathology. Also impacting on this is the presence or absence of genetic predisposition. In the unfavorable circumstances of poor coping strategies, absent social supports and genetic predisposition, the effects of the aversive stimulus can be perpetuated with the development of stress-induced illness. For essential hypertension, information is available on both the aversive stimuli, and the mediating pathophysiology, but not the genetically predisposing factors.

15.3.1   Aversive Stressors for Hypertension

Two well-documented patterns of adverse work environment are demonstrated to be causal for high blood pressure (and also coronary heart disease).[17-19,27-30] First, the

Psychodynamics of Mental Stress-Induced Illness

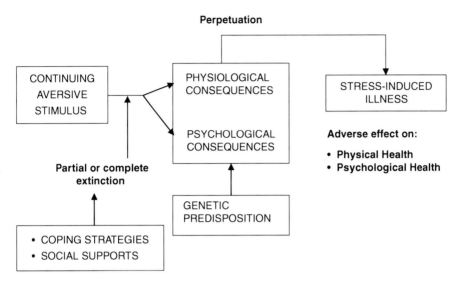

Fig. 15.1 Psychodynamics of mental stress-induced illness. What might be the mechanism by which chronic mental stress leads to essential hypertension? The figure presents a general scheme for the path to stress-induced illnesses, including high blood pressure. An ongoing aversive stimulus, which can be modified, extinguished, or perpetuated in particular circumstances can lead to illness. As indicated in this generic formulation, the existence of strong social supports in a person's life, or their possession of good coping strategies can dampen the stressor impact, minimizing its transfiguration into pathophysiology or psychopathology. For hypertension, there are two well-documented aversive patterns of work environment demonstrated to be causal for high blood pressure.[17-19,27-30] The first is the "*High Job Strain*" workplace, characterized by lack of control over the pace of work and its targets and deadlines. The second is the "*Effort-Reward Imbalanced*" workplace, typified by demanding work, which causes little personal gratification. Additionally, inescapable time pressure constitute a unique stressor of the present day,[31] this being intensified by the immediacy demands of the electronic age. The mediating pathophysiology most probably involves ongoing activation of the sympathetic nervous system

"*High Job Strain*" workplace, characterized by lack of control over the pace of work and its targets and deadlines. And second, the "*Effort-Reward Imbalanced*" workplace, typified by demanding work, which causes little personal gratification because of lack of appreciation and unjustified criticism by workplace superiors. The scientific case for causality here is very strong indeed.

The clichéd response of skeptics often takes the form: "surely life was more stressful for hunter-gatherer societies in paleolithic times than in the present." Not necessarily so. Klein[31] emphasizes that inescapable time pressure constitute the unique stress of the present day, this being intensified by the immediacy demands of the electronic age. Time pressures, coupled with difficulties in adjusting to the societal changes, which are relentless in contemporary living, is claimed to be pivotal. The probable mediating mechanisms are discussed below, but do seem to involve ongoing activation of the sympathetic nervous system.

15.4 Stress Biological Markers in Essential Hypertension

Testing for the presence of stress biomarkers in patients with essential hypertension[24] supplements the evidence drawn from epidemiology sources in affirming the importance of chronic mental stress in pathogenesis.

In searching for biological evidence that essential hypertension is caused by chronic mental stress, parallels have been noted with panic disorder, which provides an explicit clinical model of recurring stress responses[24]:

(i) There is clinical comorbidity; panic disorder prevalence is increased threefold in essential hypertension.[21]

(ii) Plasma cortisol is elevated in both.

(iii) In panic disorder and essential hypertension, but not in health, single sympathetic nerve fibers commonly fire repeatedly within an individual cardiac cycle.[32] Salvoes of single fiber sympathetic nerve firing of this type is seen as a "signature" of mental stress exposure.[24]

(iv) For both, adrenaline cotransmission is present in sympathetic nerves.[24] This also occurs with chronic mental stress exposure in experimental animals.[33]

(v) Tissue nerve growth factor in biopsied subcutaneous veins is increased in both conditions (nerve growth factor is a stress reactant).[24]

(vi) There is induction of the adrenaline synthesizing enzyme, PNMT, in sympathetic nerves in essential hypertension and panic disorder, an explicit indicator of mental stress exposure.[24]

Observations (iv) to (vi) were based on a study where biopsied forearm veins served as a source of sympathetic nerves; sympathetic nerve proteins were extracted and subjected to Western blot analysis.

15.5 Pathophysiological Mechanisms of the Hypertension

The weight of evidence supports the importance of neural mechanisms involving the sympathetic nervous system in the pathogenesis of essential hypertension,[34-36] and doubly so in hypertension attributable to chronic mental stress.[24] Surprisingly, cortisol is not the prime mover here, unlike in some other medical settings.

15.5.1 The Renin-Angiotensin System

Given that antihypertensive drugs antagonizing the renin-angiotensin system are the dominant therapy, how can a case for preeminence of sympathetic neural origins of human hypertension be sustained? Drug prescribing practices in hypertension are, however, not based on tailoring to the individual patient's pathogenesis. In any era, the drug class used most widely for an illness commonly dictates which research stream is followed for the illness (especially if the drug patents have not expired!), and aspects of pathophysiology relevant to that drug class. Despite the current dominance of therapy with drugs antagonizing the renin-angiotensin system, plasma renin levels in essential hypertension are often low.[37] When plasma renin activity is high this typically has a neural mechanism, with high sympathetic outflow to the kidneys stimulating renin release[23,38]; the importance of a cellular, extrarenal renin-angiotensin system, often invoked since plasma renin values are unremarkable in hypertension, is disputed.[39] There is no doubting the physiological importance of an intrarenal RAS system in humans, but studying the intrarenal RAS in essential hypertension, of course, is difficult. When this has been attempted, high rates of renin release within the kidneys, and overflow into the renal veins have been detected in some patients, but this is neural, resulting from stimulation of renin release by activation of the renal sympathetic outflow.[23,38] In the touted reciprocal sympathetic nervous system/RAS stimulation in patients with essential hypertension, demonstrating sympathetic stimulation of renin release is easy,[3] demonstrating the converse, angiotensin augmentation of sympathetic activity, is much more difficult.[40]

15.5.2   The Sympathetic Nervous System

Application of sympathetic nerve recording and norepinephrine spillover methodology has demonstrated activation of sympathetic nervous outflows to the kidneys, heart, and skeletal muscle vasculature, typically a doubling or trebling overall, in patients with essential hypertension.[32,34,36,41-43] The syndrome of neurogenic essential hypertension appears to account for no less than 50% of all cases of high blood pressure. This estimate is based on both the proportion of patients with essential hypertension who have demonstrable sympathetic excitation, and the number in whom substantial blood pressure lowering is achieved with antiadrenergic drugs or devices.[44,45] Multiple studies from different research groups[32,34,36,41-43] identify activated sympathetic outflow to the skeletal muscle vasculature, heart, and kidneys in 40–65% of patients. Single fiber sympathetic recording demonstrates increased firing frequencies[32,43] and multiple firings within a cardiac cycle (firing salvos), not seen in health.[32]

15.5.2.1   Does This Sympathetic Activation Cause the Blood Pressure Elevation?

There is strong evidence, both historical and contemporary, that the answer to this question is "yes." In earlier times, prior to the availability of antihypertensive drugs, extensive surgical sympathectomy was effectively used as a treatment for severe hypertension.[46] Of the antihypertensive drugs subsequently developed from the mid-twentieth century, many were antiadrenergic.

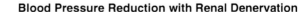

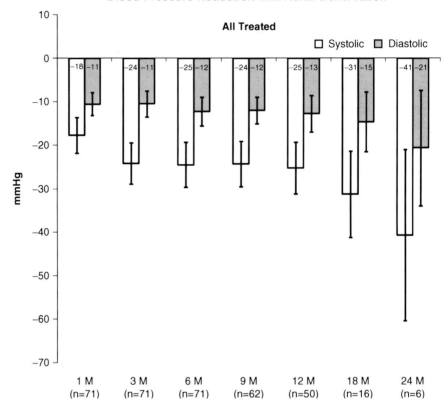

Fig. 15.2 Blood pressure reduction with renal denervation. Fall in blood pressure following an endovascular bilateral renal sympathetic denervation procedure in patients with hypertension resistant to treatment with multiple antihypertensive drugs, including a diuretic. Notably, all patients were under treatment with an ACE inhibitor or angiotensin receptor blocker (or both). The patients shown represent the initial treatment cohort from the proof-of-principle study,[44] with ongoing surveillance of these patients, and additional recruitment. The histogram depicts the changes in clinic systolic and diastolic pressures during follow-up (M = months post-procedure), the number of patients at each time point being indicated in brackets

Once it was thought that the sympathetic nervous system exerts minute by minute circulatory control only, and was not of importance in the pathogenesis of hypertension. The regulatory effects of the renal sympathetic nerves on renin release, glomerular filtration rate, and renal tubular reabsorption of sodium are, however, now seen to provide a range of potential hypertension-producing mechanisms. Experimental studies establish the important concept that sub-vasoconstrictor levels of renal sympathetic activity can increase renin secretion and renal sodium retention, without changing renal hemodynamics.[35] In human hypertension, an adverse interaction of high renal sympathetic activity and high dietary sodium consumption is probably often key.

15.6   Neurogenic Hypertension: A Final Common Pathway for "Lifestyle Hypertension"?

Hypertension commonly arises from societal ills, from the obesity epidemic, from sedentary lifestyle, and apparently from chronic mental stress in community life,[12] in the workplace[17] (although such an association of workplace mental stress with hypertension is not uniformly found[47]), and in the life of nations,[20] There is evidence that each elevates blood pressure primarily through neural mechanisms, and in particular, through activation of the renal sympathetic outflow.[34-36] The renal sympathetic outflow is chronically activated in obesity-related hypertension.[48] Exercise training in sedentary individuals lowers renal sympathetic activity and blood pressure.[49]

No doubt it would be best to catch this pathophysiological fault of chronic renal sympathetic activation at its roots, applying non-pharmacological treatment measures. The application of relaxation and stress reduction therapies (Chap. 18) has a helpful antihypertensive effect, but perhaps surprisingly this effect is outstripped by weight loss from calorie restriction, and by aerobic exercise training. For minimal elevations of blood pressure, these preventive and treatment modalities may be powerful enough. In more severe hypertension, although chronic mental stress may be an important causal factor, rather than changing the world, my colleagues and I have used a new device-based antihypertensive treatment, inhibiting what might be the common final pathway, the renal sympathetic nerves, by ablating them using an intravascular radiofrequency catheter. In patients with resistant hypertension, now very much the mainstream as target blood pressures get lower by the day, this technique has produced very favorable results[44,45] (Fig. 15.2).

References

1. Geisbock F. The nervous system. In: Julius S, Esler M, eds. *Arterial Hypertension*. Springfield: Charles C Thomas; 1976:xii.
2. Folkow B. Considering the "mind" as a primary cause. In: Robertson JIS, Zanchetti A, eds. *Handbook of Hypertension*, Hypertension in the Twentieth Century: Concepts and Achievements, vol. 22. Amsterdam: Elsevier; 2004:59-79.
3. Henry JP, Stephens PM, Santisteban GA. A model of psychosocial hypertension showing reversibility and progression of cardiovascular complications. *Circ Res*. 1975;36:156-164.
4. Henry JP, Wissam EN, Qian C, et al. Psychosocial stress can induce chronic hypertension in normotensive strains of rats. *Hypertension*. 1993;21:714-723.
5. Folkow B. Physiological aspects of primary hypertension. *Physiol Rev*. 1982;62:348-504.
6. Folkow B. Physiological organization of neurohormonal responses to psychological stimuli: implications for health and disease. *Ann Behav Med*. 1993;15:234-236.
7. Julius S, Conway J. Hemodynamic studies in patients with borderline blood pressure elevation. *Circulation*. 1968;38:282-288.
8. Lund-Johansen P. Haemodynamics of essential hypertension. In: Swales JD, ed. *Textbook of Hypertension*. Oxford: Blackwell Science Publication; 1994:61-76.
9. Korner PI. *Essential Hypertension and Its Causes. Neural and Non-Neural Mechanisms*. Oxford: Oxford University Press; 2007.

10. Esler M, Julius S, Zweifler A, et al. Mild high-renin essential hypertension: a neurogenic human hypertension? *N Engl J Med.* 1977;296:405-411.

11. Light KC, Obrist PA. Cardiovascular reactivity to behavioral stress in young males with and without marginally elevated casual systolic pressures: comparison of clinic, home, and laboratory measures. *Hypertension.* 1980;2:802-808.

12. Harburg E, Erfurt JC, Hauenstein LS, et al. Socio-ecological stress, suppressed hostility, skin colour, and black-white male blood pressure: Detroit. *Psychosom Med.* 1973;35:276-296.

13. Perini C, Muller FB, Rauchfleisch U, et al. Hyperadrenergic borderline hypertension is characterized by suppressed aggression. *J Cardiovasc Pharmacol.* 1986;8(Suppl 5):53-56.

14. Henry JP, Grim CE. Psychosocial mechanisms of primary hypertension. *J Hypertens.* 1990; 8:783-793.

15. Deter HC, Bucholz K, Schorr U, Schachinger H, Turan S, Sharma AM. Psychophysiological reactivity of salt-sensitive normotensive subjects. *J Hypertens.* 1997;15:839-844.

16. Timio M, Verdechioa P, Rononi M, et al. Age and blood pressure changes: a 20 year follow-up study of nuns of a secluded order. *Hypertension.* 1988;12:457-461.

17. Steptoe A, Willemsen G. The influence of job control on ambulatory blood pressure and perceived stress over the working day in men and women from the Whitehall II cohort. *J Hypertens.* 2004;22:915-920.

18. Rosengren A, Hawken S, Ounpuu S, INTERHEART investigators, et al. Association of psychological risk factors with risk of acute myocardial infarction in 11,119 cases and 13,648 controls from 52 countries (the INTERHEART study): a case-control study. *Lancet.* 2004; 364:953-962.

19. Chandola T, Brunner E, Marmot M. Chronic stress at work and the metabolic syndrome. *Br Med J.* 2006;332:521-524.

20. Poulter NR, Khaw KT, Hopwood BEC, et al. The Kenyan Luo migration study: observations on the initiation of the rise in blood pressure. *BMJ.* 1990;300:967-972.

21. Davies SJ, Ghahramani P, Jackson PR, et al. Association of panic disorder and panic attacks with hypertension. *Am J Med.* 1999;107:310-316.

22. Alexander F. Emotional factors in essential hypertension. *Psychosom Med.* 1939;1:173-179.

23. Esler M. Hyperadrenergic and "labile" hypertension. In: Swales J, ed. *Textbook of Hypertension.* London: Blackwell; 1994:741-749.

24. Esler M, Eikelis N, Schlaich M, et al. Chronic mental stress is a cause of essential hypertension: presence of biological markers of stress. *Clin Exp Pharmacol Physiol.* 2008;35: 498-502.

25. Koepke JP, Jones S, DiBona GF. Stress increases renal nerve activity and decreases sodium excretion in Dahl rats. *Hypertension.* 1988;11:334-338.

26. DiBona GF, Kopp UC. Neural control of renal function: role in human hypertension. In: Laragh JH, Brenner BM, eds. *Hypertension. Pathophysiology, Diagnosis and Management.* New York: Raven; 1995:1349-1358.

27. Karasek R, Baker D, Marxer F, et al. Job decision latitude, job demands, and cardiovascular disease: a prospective study of Swedish men. *Am J Public Health.* 1981;71:694-705.

28. Karasek R, Theorell T, Schwartz JE, et al. Job characteristics in relation to prevalence of myocardial infarction in the US Health Examination (HES) and the Health and Nutrition Survey (HANES). *Am J Public Health.* 1988;78:910-918.

29. Pieper C, LaCroix AZ, Karasek RA. The relation of psychological dimensions of work with coronary heart disease risk factors: a meta-analysis of five United States data bases. *Am J Epidemiol.* 1989;129:483-499.

30. Siegrist J. Adverse health effects of high-effort/low-reward conditions. *J Occup Health Psychol.* 1996;71:694-705.

31. Klein S. *The Secret Pulse of Time.* Berlin: S. Fischer Verlag; 2006; (Translation, Avalon Publishing Group, USA, 2007).

32. Lambert E, Straznicky N, Schlaich MP, et al. Differing patterns of sympathoexcitation in normal weight and obesity-related hypertension. *Hypertension.* 2007;50:862-868.

33. Micutkova L, Krepsova K, Sabban E, et al. Modulation of catecholamine-synthesizing enzymes in the rat heart by repeated immobilization stress. *Ann N Y Acad Sci*. 2004;1018:424-429.
34. Esler M. The 2009 Carl Ludwig Lecture. Pathophysiology of the human sympathetic nervous system in cardiovascular diseases: the transition from mechanism to medical management. *J Appl Physiol*. 2010;108:227-237.
35. DiBona GF, Esler M. Translational medicine: the antihypertensive effect of renal denervation. *Am J Physiol Regul Integr Comp Physiol*. 2010;298:R245-R253.
36. Esler M, Lambert E, Schlaich M. Point Counterpoint: chronic activation of the sympathetic nervous system is the dominant contributor to systemic hypertension. *J Appl Physiol*. 2010; 109:1996-1998.
37. Buhler FR, Laragh JH, Baer L, Vaughan ED, Brunner HR. Propranolol inhibition of renin secretion. *N Engl J Med*. 1972;287:1209-1214.
38. Esler M, Lambert G, Jennings G. Regional norepinephrine turnover in human hypertension. *Clin Exp Hypertens*. 1989;11(suppl 1):75-89.
39. Reudelhuber TL. Truncated prorenin comes up … short. *Hypertension*. 2009;54:1216-1217.
40. Krum H, Lambert E, Windebank E, Campbell DJ, Esler M. Effect of angiotensin II receptor blockade on autonomic nervous system function in patients with essential hypertension. *Am J Physiol*. 2006;290:H1706-H1712.
41. Grassi G, Colombo M, Seravalle G, Spaziani D, Mancia G. Dissociation between muscle and skin sympathetic nerve activity in essential hypertension, obesity, and congestive heart failure. *Hypertension*. 1998;31:64-67.
42. Grassi G, Dell'Oro R, Quarti-Trevano F, et al. Neuroadrenergic and reflex abnormalities in patients with the metabolic syndrome. *Diabetologia*. 2005;48:1359-1365.
43. Greenwood JP, Stoker JB, Mary DASG. Single-unit sympathetic discharge. Quantitative assessment in human hypertensive disease. *Circulation*. 1999;100:1305-1310.
44. Krum H, Schlaich MP, Whitbourn R, et al. Catheter-based renal sympathetic denervation for resistant hypertension: a multicentre safety and proof-of-principle cohort study. *Lancet*. 2009;373:1275-1281.
45. Symplicity HTN-2 Investigators. Renal sympathetic denervationin patients with treatment-resistant hypertension (The Symplicity HTN-2 Trial): a randomized controlled trial. *Lancet*. 2010;376:1903-1909.
46. Smithwick RH, Bush RD, Kinsey D, Whitelaw GP. Hypertension and associated cardiovascular disease; comparison of male and female mortality rates and their influence on selection of therapy. *J Am Med Assoc*. 1956;160:1023-1026.
47. Kivimaki M, Head J, Ferrie JE, et al. Hypertension is not the link between job strain and coronary heart disease in the Whitehall II Study. *Am J Hypertens*. 2007;20:1146-1153.
48. Rumantir MS, Vaz M, Jennings GL, et al. Neural mechanisms in human obesity-related hypertension. *J Hypertens*. 1999;17:1125-1133.
49. Meredith IT, Friberg P, Jennings GL, et al. Regular exercise lowers renal but not cardiac sympathetic activity in man. *Hypertension*. 1991;18:575-582.

Chapter 16
Metabolic Syndrome and Diabetes

Annika Rosengren

Keywords Cardiovascular disease • Diabetes • Metabolic syndrome • Premature death • Psychosocial factors

16.1 Introduction

The last century has witnessed profound changes in living conditions and health for the global population. Rapid urbanization and industrialization have led to changes in nutrition, transportation, and psychosocial environment. Whereas, throughout the history of mankind, the availability of enough food to subsist has been a major concern, the present era is characterized by abundant availability of food, particularly energy-dense food, for large proportions of the world's population. At the same time, the changing of job types, increased mechanization at work and at home, increased sedentariness in leisure time, and less energy expenditure in transportation are increasingly shifting the situation for many people toward reduced energy expenditure. In the wake of the obesity epidemic the number of people with diabetes has increased sevenfold in just over 20 years, and is estimated to reach 380 million within another 20 years (http://www.idf.org). Even though caloric imbalance is likely the main driving force behind the current obesity epidemic, increasing evidence indicates that psychosocial factors, through various mechanisms, may influence the development of obesity, adipose tissue distribution, and complications of obesity. Psychosocial stress and sleep deprivation, features of modern society, have been proposed to contribute to the increased prevalence of obesity through chronic activation of the neuroendocrine systems.[1] The purpose of this chapter is to review

A. Rosengren
Institute of Medicine, Sahlgrenska Academy, Sahlgrenska University Hospital, Ostra,
Gothenburg, Sweden
e-mail: annika.rosengren@hjlgu.se

P. Hjemdahl et al. (eds.), *Stress and Cardiovascular Disease*,
DOI 10.1007/978-1-84882-419-5_16, © Springer-Verlag London Limited 2012

existing evidence with respect to psychosocial factors and the development of obesity, the metabolic syndrome, and diabetes.

16.2   The Metabolic Syndrome

The metabolic syndrome refers to a cluster of aberrations in glucometabolic and lipid balance, which is strongly associated with cardiovascular diseases and the development of diabetes. Characteristics of the metabolic syndrome include abdominal obesity, dyslipidemia (elevated triglyceride levels, small dense low density lipoprotein particles, and low levels of high density lipoprotein cholesterol), hypertension, insulin resistance/impaired glucose tolerance, and diabetes. Several definitions of the syndrome have been provided, resulting in widely varying prevalence rates.[2]

Although early researchers had observed a clustering of hyperglycemia, hypertension, and gout, it was Vague who first drew attention to the association between abdominal, or android, obesity, and the metabolic abnormalities associated with type 2 diabetes and cardiovascular disease.[3] This line of thought was further developed by Reaven[4] who was the first to indicate the role of insulin resistance in the cluster. However, it was not until 1998 that there was an initiative to develop an internationally recognized definition. With the objective to achieve some agreement on definition, and to provide a tool for clinicians and researchers, a WHO consultation proposed a set of criteria.[5] Subsequently, there have been several updated definitions.[6] The most important ones are summarized in Table 16.1. All the definitions agree on the essential components – glucose intolerance, obesity, hypertension, and dyslipidemia – but they differ in detail and criteria, with later definitions being wider, and having lower thresholds for glucose and accordingly defining larger subsets in the population with the syndrome.

The syndrome is multifactorial in origin, but obesity and sedentary lifestyle coupled with dietary, epigenetic and genetic factors[7,8] are key players. With the dramatic increase in overweight and obesity worldwide, there has been a striking increase in the prevalence of the metabolic syndrome, which now affects up to a third of men and women in the USA and Europe.[6,9] However, there is considerable variation across different cultural and geographical settings.[10] The worldwide obesity epidemic has been the most important driving force in the recognition of the syndrome.

The metabolic syndrome is linked to increased risk of premature death, cardiovascular disease, and diabetes.[11] In individuals with the metabolic syndrome, the relative risk of suffering atherosclerotic vascular disease ranges from 1.5 to 3, depending on the stage of progression.[12,13] In people free of diabetes, the risk for progression to type 2 diabetes is about fivefold compared with those without the syndrome.[14,15] Estimates suggest that the population-attributable fraction for the metabolic syndrome is 6–7% for all-cause mortality, 12–17% for cardiovascular disease, and 30–52% for diabetes.[16]

Table 16.1 Different definitions of the metabolic syndrome

WHO 1999	ATP III 2001	IDF
Abnormal glucose metabolism (type 2 diabetes, glucose intolerance, or insulin resistance)	3 or more of	Central obesity defined by ethnic-specific waist circumference criteria ($\geq$94 cm in Europid men and $\geq$80 cm in Europid women)
Plus 2 or more of the following		Plus any 2 or more of the following 4 components:
Obesity: BMI $\geq$ 30, or waist-to-hip ratio >0.9 in men and >0.85 in women	Increased waist circumference (>102 cm in men and >88 cm in women)	
Dyslipidemia: triglycerides $\geq$1.7 mmol/L or HDL cholesterol <0.9 (male) or <1.0 (female)/mmol/L	Elevated triglycerides ($\geq$1.7 mmol/L/$\geq$150 mg/dL)	Elevated triglycerides ($\geq$1.7 mmol/L/$\geq$150 mg/dL), or specific treatment for this lipid abnormality
	HDL cholesterol Men < 1 mmol/L/40 mg/dL Women < 1.3 mmol/L/50 mg/dL	HDL cholesterol Men <1 mmol/L/40 mg/dL Women < 1.3 mmol/L/50 mg/dL
Hypertension: blood pressure >140/90 mmHg	Elevated blood pressure ($\geq$ 130 systolic and/or $\geq$85 mmHg diastolic or on treatment for hypertension)	Elevated blood pressure ($\geq$ 130 systolic and/or $\geq$ 85 mmHg diastolic or on treatment for hypertension)
Microalbuminuria: albumin excretion >20 μg/min	Fasting glucose ($\geq$6.1 mmol/L/$\geq$110 mg/dL), or known diabetes	Fasting glucose ($\geq$5.6 mmol/L/$\geq$100 mg/dL), or previously recognized diabetes

It is important, however, to understand that the metabolic syndrome is more of a way to understand the clustering of risk factors (i.e., pathophysiology) than a diagnostic entity in itself. When the syndrome is used as endpoint in drug treatment studies (e.g., rimonabant, but also other drugs) one may be led astray by changes in the prevalence of the metabolic syndrome – someone who lowered one of the defining components from just above to below threshold can be "cured," without appreciably altering the absolute cardiovascular risk.

Ultimately, obesity, diabetes, and the metabolic syndrome are caused by caloric imbalance. Intake of calories in excess of expenditure results in accumulation of fat tissue. While obesity is usually the result of complex interactions between genetic predisposition and individual life style, with decreased physical activity and/or overeating, these behaviors are to a great extent a result of environmental factors which affect entire populations. The structure of the community affects individual choices at work and at home. Accordingly, obesity with resulting comorbidities is not just a matter of individual choices, but one where societal and environmental factors produce populations where predisposed individuals may develop risk factors and, ultimately, disease.

16.3 Psychosocial Factors in the Development of Obesity and Its Complications

Whether psychosocial factors contribute to the development of obesity, and by which mechanisms have been fairly extensively investigated. An increasing body of literature links both the development of obesity itself, as well as diabetes and the metabolic syndrome, with stress and other psychosocial variables. It has been put forward that environmental stress, together with elements of modern society such as westernization of the diet and sedentary lifestyle, may induce obesity through dys-regulation of the hypothalamic-pituitary-adrenal (HPA) axis.[17] Still, psychosocial factors are not yet among the established risk factors for either obesity or diabetes. The physiological mechanisms for the HPA axis and cardiovascular disease are described in greater detail in Chap. 5 (Chrousos).

There are some methodological problems in the study of psychosocial factors and health outcomes. Compared to other biological and life style risk factors, psychosocial factors represent a more problematic construct in that there is little uniformity with respect to either definition, or measurement of these factors. Additionally, most of the dimensions involved are subjective, and hence potentially open to biases and confounding. Psychosocial variables are also more difficult to define objectively, because several different dimensions are involved. Despite this, separate constructs within the broad conceptual framework of psychosocial factors are increasingly considered as being causally related to various outcomes. Stress at work and in family life, life events, low perceived control, lack of social support, socioeconomic status, and depression are some of the dimensions that have been studied.

Psychosocial factors influence health both directly and indirectly. Direct effects include influences on lipids, blood pressure, insulin sensitivity, or coagulation/fibrinolysis, but also, potentially, the central regulation of appetite. Indirect effects are mediated by changes in lifestyle, such as poor diet, less physical activity, less time for sleep, use of alcohol and nicotine, habits which, either one by one or jointly, increase the risk of adverse health outcomes.

Stressful experiences include a multitude of external influences, such as life events, or demands from the workplace or the family. The individual experience of stress is not only determined by external stimuli but also by the perception of stress and coping mechanisms. The response to a stress challenge involves both turning on a response initiating a complex adaptive pathway as well as shutting off this response when the threat is past.[18] The ability to achieve stability through change is some-times referred to as allostasis. Through allostasis we are able to cope with noxious stimuli. Allostatic systems respond to stress by initiating the adaptive response, sustaining it until the stress ceases, and then shutting it off (recovery). Allostatic responses are initiated by increases in sympathetic nerve activity and circulating catecholamines from the autonomic nervous system and glucocorticoids from the adrenal cortex, setting into motion adaptive processes. These processes are initiated through intracellular receptors for steroid hormones, and plasma-membrane recep-tors and second-messenger systems for catecholamines.[18] Maladaptive changes to allostatic load include lack of adaptation to repeated exposure to stressors of the same type, resulting in prolonged exposure to stress hormones, inability to shut off allostatic responses when no longer needed, and inadequate responses by some allostatic systems triggering compensatory increases in others. One speculation is that allostatic load over a lifetime may cause these systems to wear out or become exhausted.

One of the first to propose a link between psychosocial factors and the development of the metabolic syndrome was Björntorp.[19] Based on experimental studies, an initial defense reaction characterized by high levels of noradrenaline, gonadotrophins, and sex hormones was, if prolonged or repeated, suggested to be followed by a defeat reaction, with an activation of the HPA axis and increased levels of ACTH and cortisol secretion. As a consequence, sex steroid and growth hormone secretions are inhibited, with accumulation of intra-abdominal fat and insulin resistance, similar to a mild Cushing's syndrome. Thus, with frequent or repetitive stress stimuli, the response to stress becomes maladaptive.

Support for Björntorp's theory was first derived from animal studies. Female cynomolgus monkeys that were socially subordinate were more likely than dominants to exhibit a central fat deposition pattern.[20] In a recent, elegant study[21] it was found that female monkeys with visceral obesity assessed by computed tomography were relatively subordinate, socially isolated, and were desensitized to circulating glucocorticoids. They also had more coronary artery atherosclerosis, consistent with the hypothesis that stress may cause coronary disease partly by increasing the ratio of visceral to subcutaneous abdominal fat.

Recent experimental studies have also indicated a mechanism through which stress and obesity could be related to the hypothalamic control of food intake and metabolism.[22,23] Stress was found to exaggerate diet-induced obesity through a peripheral mechanism in the abdominal white adipose tissue mediated by neuropeptide Y (NPY). Stressors such as exposure to cold or aggression lead to increased release of NPY relative to that of noradrenaline from sympathetic nerves, and upregulates its Y2 receptors (NPY2R) in a glucocorticoid-dependent manner in the abdominal fat. This positive feedback response by NPY led to abdominal obesity and a metabolic syndrome-like condition in animals.

Several lines of evidence support the relevance of these findings to humans. First, human white adipose tissue expresses NPY2R, which mediate angiogenic and adipogenic responses. Second, a common silent NPY2R gene variant recently found in the Swedish population seems to protect against obesity, whereas the gain-of-function Leu7Pro7 NPY gene polymorphism is associated with human obesity.

16.4   Cross-Sectional Studies

In humans, several cross-sectional studies have demonstrated that features associated with the metabolic syndrome, such as obesity or diabetes, cluster in socially disadvantaged groups,[24-28] which is of interest because this may contribute to explain the social gradient in cardiovascular diseases. For example, in the Whitehall II study[24], the odds ratios among British civil servants for having the metabolic syndrome, or for occupying the highest versus the lowest quintile for waist-hip ratio, post-load glucose, triglycerides and fibrinogen ranged from 1.4 to 2.2. Health-related behaviors explained only a small fraction of the differences in metabolic syndrome prevalence.

Even so, it must be pointed out that this pattern is not universal, but depends on the type of the country. In a comprehensive review published in 1989, a strong direct relationship between socioeconomic status and obesity was found in developing societies,[29] as opposed to the inverse gradient found in developed societies, particularly for women, but less consistently so for men and children. In a recent update[30] this pattern still prevails, but with signs that the burden of obesity even in low- and middle income countries is being shifted onto the poor.

Other than low socioeconomic status, several other psychosocial factors have been associated with obesity and other metabolic risk factors. Short sleep duration, a feature of modern life, was investigated in a meta-analysis involving over 600,000 subjects from 17 studies.[31] The pooled odds ratio for short sleep duration in relation to obesity was 1.55 (1.43–1.68), with no evidence of publication bias. Lower job control, higher job strain, and higher effort-reward imbalance were associated with higher body mass index in a large cohort of Finnish employees,[32] although an association between weight and job strain has not been universally found. A review of ten cross-sectional studies, all published no later than the year 2000, did not find support for an association between workload and obesity.[33] Poor characterization of exposure and cross-sectional designs were thought to underlie these null findings, with prospective designs being needed.[34]

Work stress and low sense of coherence has been cross-sectionally associated with a higher risk of developing diabetes in women[35] Another study found that obesity and other features of the metabolic syndrome tended to cluster together more often in shift workers than in day workers.[36]

To investigate these cross-sectional associations further, Brunner and coworkers[37] performed a nested case-control study among working men in the Whitehall II cohort on potential associations between markers of neurohormonal and inflammatory activity and presence of the metabolic syndrome. The authors applied two definitions of the metabolic syndrome to their material, and obtained similar results with the two sets of criteria. They found that cases with the metabolic syndrome, compared to controls, had raised urinary excretion of cortisol metabolites and normetanepinephrine (a marker for sympathetic activity), and also a strong association with cardiac autonomic activity (reduced heart rate variability, suggesting reduced vagal activity). Additionally, elevated levels of interleukin-6 (IL-6) and C-reactive protein were found in cases, compared to controls, but not of other markers of inflammatory activity (serum amyloid A and plasma fibrinogen). Psychosocial factors explained a substantial part of the increase in sympathetic activity. Adverse cardiac autonomic function related to the syndrome was attributable both to psychosocial factors and to the degree of obesity. This study represents one of the first steps toward establishing empirical evidence that an adverse psychosocial environment contributes to the development of the metabolic syndrome.

16.5 Prospective Studies

Interpretation of cross-sectional studies is problematic because temporal sequences cannot be determined, nor can causality. Longitudinal studies are needed in order to establish causality. Over the last few years, several prospective studies have investigated psychosocial factors with respect to weight gain, metabolic disturbances, and overt or latent diabetes.

In a study of Danish nurses, those who reported often being busy at work gained more weight over 6 years than those who were less often busy, as did those reporting a low influence over their job.[38] In a Finnish study of employed people the overall weight gain over time was considerable, with a third of participants gaining at least 15 kg from youth to middle age, but working conditions exerted only a weak effect.[39] Working overtime was associated with weight gain among men, whereas high work pace was associated with weight gain among women. Multiple domains of psychosocial stress were investigated in a nationally representative sample of US citizens.[40] Among men with a high baseline body mass index, weight gain was associated with increasing levels of psychosocial stress related to job-related demands, lack of skill discretion, lack of decision authority, and difficulty in paying bills. Among women with a high baseline body mass index, weight gain was associated with job-related demands, perceived constraints in life, strain in relations with family, and difficulty in paying bills. Kivimaki et al.[41] used the Whitehall study to analyze a potential association between job stress and weight change over a period of 5 years. Among men who were lean at baseline, high job strain and low job control were associated with weight loss at follow-up, whereas among men who were overweight or obese these stress indicators were associated with subsequent weight gain. No corresponding interaction was seen among women. Brunner et al.[34] reported, with a more extended follow-up of the above-mentioned cohort after 19 years, a dose-response relation between work stress and risk of both general and central obesity that was largely independent of covariates. The imputed odds ratios of body mass index obesity for one, two, and three or more reports of work stress adjusted for age, sex, and social position were 1.17, 1.24, and 1.73 (trend $p < 0.01$), respectively. For waist obesity, the corresponding findings were 1.17, 1.41, and 1.61 (trend $p < 0.01$). The work stress effect was modestly attenuated after exclusion of obese individuals at baseline and further adjustments for smoking, dietary factors, and physical activity.

Other than work stress, one study examined whether anger and hostility predicted visceral obesity over a period of 13 years in a population-based sample of 157 postmenopausal healthy women. Trait anger and hostility predicted increases in visceral adipose tissue during the follow-up, independently of weight gain.[42]

There is also emerging evidence that adverse psychosocial factors are related to the development of the metabolic syndrome. In still another investigation from the Whitehall cohort,[43] work stress measured on four occasions showed a dose-response relation between work stressors and the risk of developing the metabolic syndrome, independently of other relevant risk factors. Employees with chronic work stress (three or more exposures) were more than twice as likely to have the metabolic syndrome compared to those without work stress. These findings were confirmed in a recent study in Belgian workers,[44] where rotating shift work increased the risk of developing the metabolic syndrome. Depressive symptoms and stressful life events were associated with increased risk among middle-aged healthy women.[45] Likewise, reports of marital dissatisfaction, divorce, and widowhood were associated with increased risk in women.[46]

Even though psychosocial factors are not among the established risk factors for the development of type 2 diabetes, there is an emerging field of research suggesting such associations; however with conflicting results. Studies on work hours and diabetes have yielded inconsistent results. A Japanese study of male industrial workers found a higher risk of developing type 2 diabetes among those working more than 50 h versus those working less than 25 h per week or more than 11 h versus less than 8 h per day.[47] A second study,[48] however, found a strong negative association between hours of paid work and type 2 diabetes in male office workers.

Work characteristics and the risk of developing diabetes were investigated in the Nurse's Health Study.[49] This was a prospective study of 62,574 young and middle-aged women, where 365 new cases of type 2 diabetes were identified over 6 years of follow-up. Women working less than 20 h per week had a 20% lower risk of developing diabetes whereas those working in excess of 40 h per week had a 23% increase in risk compared with women working 21–40 h per week in paid employment. Job strain, however, was unrelated to this risk. In contrast, a Swedish study found that work stress and low emotional support increased the risk of developing type 2 diabetes in women, but not in men.[50] Similarly, another investigation from the Whitehall II cohort study, found an effect of work stress among women, but again not in men.[51] However, in a Swedish study of middle-aged men and women with normal glucose tolerance at baseline[52], a score measuring psychological distress predicted the development of prediabetes or diabetes 8–10 years later among men, but not in women. High scores for insomnia, apathy, anxiety, and fatigue also predicted diabetes among men but not women. These interaction effects (gender-stress) may obviously be due to chance, particularly because they are so incongruous. Further exploration seems warranted.

16.6   Conclusion

Even though psychosocial factors are not currently among the established risk factors for developing obesity, the metabolic complications of obesity, or diabetes, increasing evidence from prospective studies indicates that they are important. Chronic activation of the neuroendocrine systems has been implicated as a plausible mechanism, but there is still insufficient evidence to back this up. Future research needs to investigate the role of appetite regulation and physical activity in relation to the accumulation and distribution of excess adipose tissue in the presence of adverse psychosocial factors. From a societal perspective, however, there is clearly a need to increase the perception of stress and other psychosocial factors as a problem with respect to the achievement of a lifestyle conducive to optimal cardiovascular health.

References

1. Siervo M, Wells JC, Cizza G. The contribution of psychosocial stress to the obesity epidemic: an evolutionary approach. *Horm Metab Res.* 2009;41(4):261-270.
2. Eckel RH, Grundy SM, Zimmet PZ. The metabolic syndrome. *Lancet.* 2005;365(9468): 1415-1428.
3. Vague J. La différenciation sexuelle, facteur déterminant des formes de l'obésité. *Presse Med.* 1947;55(30):339-340.
4. Reaven GM. Banting lecture 1988. Role of insulin resistance in human disease. *Diabetes.* 1988;37(12):1595-1607.
5. Alberti KG, Zimmet PZ. Definition, diagnosis and classification of diabetes mellitus and its complications. Part 1: diagnosis and classification of diabetes mellitus provisional report of a WHO consultation. *Diabet Med.* 1998;15(7):539-553.
6. Ford ES, Giles WH, Dietz WH. Prevalence of the metabolic syndrome among US adults: findings from the third National Health and Nutrition Examination Survey. *JAMA.* 2002;287(3):356-359.
7. Nestel P. Nutritional aspects in the causation and management of the metabolic syndrome. *Endocrinol Metab Clin North Am.* 2004;33(3):483-492. v.
8. Symonds ME et al. Nutritional programming of the metabolic syndrome. *Nat Rev Endocrinol.* 2009;5(11):604-610.
9. Balkau B et al. Frequency of the WHO metabolic syndrome in European cohorts, and an alternative definition of an insulin resistance syndrome. *Diabetes Metab.* 2002;28(5):364-376.
10. Cameron AJ, Shaw JE, Zimmet PZ. The metabolic syndrome: prevalence in worldwide populations. *Endocrinol Metab Clin North Am.* 2004;33(2):351-375.
11. Grundy SM. Metabolic syndrome: connecting and reconciling cardiovascular and diabetes worlds. *J Am Coll Cardiol.* 2006;47(6):1093-1100.
12. Isomaa B et al. Cardiovascular morbidity and mortality associated with the metabolic syndrome. *Diabetes Care.* 2001;24(4):683-689.
13. Lakka HM et al. The metabolic syndrome and total and cardiovascular disease mortality in middle-aged men. *JAMA.* 2002;288(21):2709-2716.
14. Klein BE, Klein R, Lee KE. Components of the metabolic syndrome and risk of cardiovascular disease and diabetes in Beaver Dam. *Diabetes Care.* 2002;25(10):1790-1794.
15. Lorenzo C et al. The metabolic syndrome as predictor of type 2 diabetes: the San Antonio heart study. *Diabetes Care.* 2003;26(11):3153-3159.
16. Ford ES. Risks for all-cause mortality, cardiovascular disease, and diabetes associated with the metabolic syndrome: a summary of the evidence. *Diabetes Care.* 2005;28(7):1769-1778.
17. Bose M, Olivan B, Laferrere B. Stress and obesity: the role of the hypothalamic-pituitary-adrenal axis in metabolic disease. *Curr Opin Endocrinol Diabetes Obes.* 2009;16(5):340-346.
18. McEwen BS. Protective and damaging effects of stress mediators. *N Engl J Med.* 1998;338(3): 171-179.
19. Bjorntorp P. Stress and cardiovascular disease. *Acta Physiol Scand Suppl.* 1997;640:144-148.
20. Shively CA, Clarkson TB. Regional obesity and coronary artery atherosclerosis in females: a non-human primate model. *Acta Med Scand Suppl.* 1988;723:71-78.
21. Shively CA, Register TC, Clarkson TB. Social stress, visceral obesity, and coronary artery atherosclerosis in female primates. *Obesity (Silver Spring).* 2009;17(8):1513-1520.
22. Kuo LE et al. Chronic stress, combined with a high-fat/high-sugar diet, shifts sympathetic signaling toward neuropeptide Y and leads to obesity and the metabolic syndrome. *Ann N Y Acad Sci.* 2008;1148:232-237.
23. Kuo LE et al. Neuropeptide Y acts directly in the periphery on fat tissue and mediates stress-induced obesity and metabolic syndrome. *Nat Med.* 2007;13(7):803-811.
24. Brunner EJ et al. Social inequality in coronary risk: central obesity and the metabolic syndrome. Evidence from the Whitehall II study. *Diabetologia.* 1997;40(11):1341-1349.
25. Lawlor DA, Ebrahim S, Davey SG. Socioeconomic position in childhood and adulthood and insulin resistance: cross sectional survey using data from British women's heart and health study. *BMJ.* 2002;325(7368):805.

26. Lidfeldt J et al. Socio-demographic and psychosocial factors are associated with features of the metabolic syndrome. The Women's Health in the Lund Area (WHILA) study. *Diabetes Obes Metab.* 2003;5(2):106-112.

27. Parker L et al. A lifecourse study of risk for hyperinsulinaemia, dyslipidaemia and obesity (the central metabolic syndrome) at age 49–51 years. *Diabet Med.* 2003;20(5):406-415.

28. Wamala SP et al. Education and the metabolic syndrome in women. *Diabetes Care.* 1999; 22(12):1999-2003.

29. Sobal J, Stunkard AJ. Socioeconomic status and obesity: a review of the literature. *Psychol Bull.* 1989;105(2):260-275.

30. McLaren L. Socioeconomic status and obesity. *Epidemiol Rev.* 2007;29:29-48.

31. Cappuccio FP et al. Meta-analysis of short sleep duration and obesity in children and adults. *Sleep.* 2008;31(5):619-626.

32. Kouvonen A et al. Relationship between work stress and body mass index among 45,810 female and male employees. *Psychosom Med.* 2005;67(4):577-583.

33. Overgaard D, Gyntelberg F, Heitmann BL. Psychological workload and body weight: is there an association? A review of the literature. *Occup Med (Lond).* 2004;54(1):35-41.

34. Brunner EJ, Chandola T, Marmot MG. Prospective effect of job strain on general and central obesity in the Whitehall II Study. *Am J Epidemiol.* 2007;165(7):828-837.

35. Agardh EE et al. Work stress and low sense of coherence is associated with type 2 diabetes in middle-aged Swedish women. *Diabetes Care.* 2003;26(3):719-724.

36. Karlsson B, Knutsson A, Lindahl B. Is there an association between shift work and having a metabolic syndrome? Results from a population based study of 27,485 people. *Occup Environ Med.* 2001;58(11):747-752.

37. Brunner EJ et al. Adrenocortical, autonomic, and inflammatory causes of the metabolic syndrome: nested case-control study. *Circulation.* 2002;106(21):2659-2665.

38. Overgaard D et al. Psychological workload is associated with weight gain between 1993 and 1999: analyses based on the Danish Nurse Cohort Study. *Int J Obes Relat Metab Disord.* 2004;28(8):1072-1081.

39. Lallukka T et al. Working conditions and weight gain: a 28-year follow-up study of industrial employees. *Eur J Epidemiol.* 2008;23(4):303-310.

40. Block JP et al. Psychosocial stress and change in weight among US adults. *Am J Epidemiol.* 2009;170(2):181-192.

41. Kivimaki M et al. Work stress, weight gain and weight loss: evidence for bidirectional effects of job strain on body mass index in the Whitehall II study. *Int J Obes (Lond).* 2006;30(6): 982-987.

42. Raikkonen K et al. Anger, hostility, and visceral adipose tissue in healthy postmenopausal women. *Metabolism.* 1999;48(9):1146-1151.

43. Chandola T, Brunner E, Marmot M. Chronic stress at work and the metabolic syndrome: prospective study. *BMJ.* 2006;332(7540):521-525.

44. De Bacquer D et al. Rotating shift work and the metabolic syndrome: a prospective study. *Int J Epidemiol.* 2009;38(3):848-854.

45. Raikkonen K, Matthews KA, Kuller LH. Depressive symptoms and stressful life events predict metabolic syndrome among middle-aged women: a comparison of World Health Organization, Adult Treatment Panel III, and International Diabetes Foundation definitions. *Diabetes Care.* 2007;30(4):872-877.

46. Troxel WM et al. Marital quality and occurrence of the metabolic syndrome in women. *Arch Intern Med.* 2005;165(9):1022-1027.

47. Kawakami N et al. Overtime, psychosocial working conditions, and occurrence of non-insulin dependent diabetes mellitus in Japanese men. *J Epidemiol Community Health.* 1999;53(6): 359-363.

48. Nakanishi N et al. Hours of work and the risk of developing impaired fasting glucose or type 2 diabetes mellitus in Japanese male office workers. *Occup Environ Med.* 2001;58(9):569-574.

49. Kroenke CH et al. Work characteristics and incidence of type 2 diabetes in women. *Am J Epidemiol.* 2007;165(2):175-183.

50. Norberg M et al. Work stress and low emotional support is associated with increased risk of future type 2 diabetes in women. *Diabetes Res Clin Pract.* 2007;76(3):368-377.
51. Heraclides A et al. Psychosocial stress at work doubles the risk of type 2 diabetes in middle-aged women: evidence from the Whitehall II study. *Diabetes Care.* 2009;32(12):2230-2235.
52. Eriksson AK et al. Psychological distress and risk of pre-diabetes and type 2 diabetes in a prospective study of Swedish middle-aged men and women. *Diabet Med.* 2008;25(7): 834-842.

Part IV
Treatment

Chapter 17
Stress Management and Behavior: From Cardiac Patient to Worksite Intervention

Daniela Lucini and Massimo Pagani

Keywords Active role • Adaptation • Arousal • Autonomic nervous system • Baroreflex sensitivity • Behavior • Breathing • Cardiovascular risk • Cognitive restructuring • Control system • Coping • Coronary artery disease • Downsizing • Functional syndromes • Life style • Multidimensional approach • Occupational health • Parasympathetic activity • Relaxation training • Respiratory techniques • Spectral analysis • Autoregressive • Stress • Sympathetic activity • Symptom • Unexplained symptoms • Vagal activity • Worksite

17.1   Introduction: A Clinical Model of Stress

In this period of my life I feel very tired, I cannot sleep well, I have difficulties in concentrating and getting by my job with enough attention... and what is worrying me most is that I feel that there is something wrong with my heart.... Sometimes, especially at night as soon as I go to bed, it starts beating faster and faster... sometimes I perceive an alteration in the rhythm of the heart beat....two beats very close and then a short pause.... Sometimes I feel pain, here... just in the middle of my chest... Six months ago I talked about these problems with my family doctor. He ordered me an ECG: it was normal. He then suggested that I reduce my body weight and consult a cardiologist like you, because my blood pressure was a little bit elevated, in his opinion...140/95 mmHg. I had too much work to do, too many problems at work.... So I had no time but managed to get here now... I'm 45 years old, my father suffered a heart attack when he was 65, I tried to keep a diet... but it is not possible for me in this period of my life, I am too stressed, I need to eat to calm myself and to have enough energy... I'm very worried also because in this period I need to be healthy....I have a lot of problems to solve at work! Doctor....can you help me?.

Stress is one of the most used, or abused, words in the world, at least in the western part. There are many meanings attached to the concept of stress, reflecting its psychological, physiological, behavioral, or social aspects. When defining stress it is

D. Lucini (✉) • M. Pagani
Department of Clinical Science, L. Sacco, University of Milan, Milan, Italy
e-mail: daniela.lucini@unimi.it; massimo.pagani@ctnv.unimi.it

P. Hjemdahl et al. (eds.), *Stress and Cardiovascular Disease,*
DOI 10.1007/978-1-84882-419-5_17, © Springer-Verlag London Limited 2012

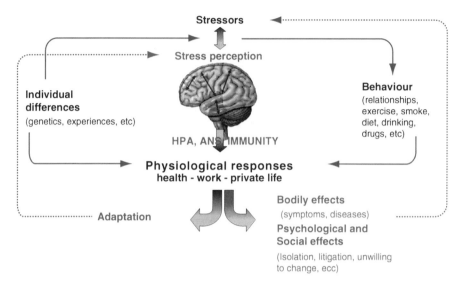

Fig. 17.1 Model of stress (adapted from McEwen,[2] Fig. 1). The effects of stressors on health, work, and private life depend on hypothalamic-pituitary-adrenal (HPA) axis, autonomic nervous system (ANS), and immunity responses mediated by individual stress perception, individual differences, and behavior. The final result may be adaptation (eustress) or maladaptation (distress), represented by negative organic (somatic symptoms or increased risk of diseases) or psychosocial consequences. These latter ones may per se become new stressors initiating a vicious cycle

important to consider all these facets.[1-3] The definition to which we will refer in this chapter, in full awareness that it might be improved, is: "Stress may be considered as the psychological, behavioral and physiological (or pathophysiological) consequence of the interaction between a subject and a 'stressor' which may be anything (acute or chronic) in the environment or in the subject's mind that could be perceived as important, dangerous, or potentially capable of modifying, either negatively or positively, the subject's life (Fig. 17.1)."

Stress[4] induces a physiological, often useful, response[2] to reestablish homeostasis through a complex process. This includes regulatory systems (HPA axis, autonomic nervous system, and immunity), which are modulated by subjective perceptions of stress, individual (genetic, biological, psychological) differences, and behavior. The negative nature of stress appears when the final result is not adaptation, homeostasis, and when instead bodily (somatic symptoms or diseases such as coronary heart disease (CHD), and functional syndromes[3,5-7]) or psychosocial effects (change of mood, unwillingness to change, isolation, etc.[8]) appear. As depicted in Fig. 17.1 (modified from McEwen[2]) these negative consequences may depend more on individual characteristics, the personal way of perceiving the stressor and behavior, than on the initial stressor. Moreover, in some situations these consequences may worsen the clinical picture becoming themselves new stressors. This is the case with patients who are extremely worried because of chronic unexplained somatic symptoms (such as altered heart beat, gastrointestinal disturbances, chronic pain, etc.)[5,6] or subjects who unconsciously change their behavior to an unhealthy lifestyle (smoking, incorrect nutrition, abuse of alcohol or drugs, etc.).[9] These subjects may, again unconsciously, change their social behavior by isolating themselves, increasing conflict in the family or on the job, etc., reducing their work and social performance, and thus deteriorating their quality of life.

Following this stress model, it is clear that therapeutic approaches must have the goal to drive the subject toward adaptation by avoiding the chronic negative consequences of the stress response, by modulating the perception of the stressor (i.e., psychotherapy, counseling), by reducing when possible the enhanced physiological response (i.e., drug therapy, mental relaxation), and by promoting useful coping strategies to help the subject to change his/her behavior (i.e., unhealthy lifestyle reduction, acquisition of new internal or external resources, etc.). The therapeutic approach, therefore, should help the subjects to initiate a process of personal change, enhancing internal and external resources, reducing real or imaginary barriers, considering at any level of intervention both physiological and psychosocial sides of stress. Only when the subject has gained enough resources to manage the stressful situation will he/she no longer suffer the chronic negative consequences of stress.[10]

17.2 Stress: From Symptoms to Diseases

Stress is gaining more and more clinical and social attention, because it is significantly linked to impaired health and to reductions of quality of life, social well-being, and productivity.[11,12] But at what point in time does stress become a real clinical problem? When must a physician take care of it?

There are many reports showing that stress is an independent risk factor for CHD,[3,7,9,13-17] and data on associations between stress and other diseases such as hypertension; arrhythmias; depression; cancer; and immunological, infective, or gastrointestinal disorders are continuously growing.[16,18,19]

An interesting area is the link between stress and physical symptoms.[5,6,20] Some patients report one or a few symptoms related to a specific bodily system, while other patients report several nonspecific symptoms. In the first case it is easy to define specific conditions, defined as "functional" syndromes, which are characterized by the presence of somatic symptoms without clinical evidence for their explanation, like irritable bowel syndrome or fibromyalgia, chronic fatigue syndrome, etc. (almost every medical specialty has at least one!).[21] To date, no clear etiology for functional conditions is available. They are often attributed to single causes,[6] either biological (such as a viral infection in the case of chronic fatigue syndrome), or psychological (such as stress). A multidimensional approach to these conditions may be more useful from the clinician's point of view.[5,6,19,21] Thus, a somatic symptom may not have an organic cause, but arise as a consequence of an increased awareness of physiological changes associated with a stressor or variations of normal physiology (like in the case of mitral valve prolapse syndrome), all mediated by regulatory systems like the autonomic nervous system, or of an increased awareness of the physiological process (like digestion). Individual experience or biological and psychological predispositions may facilitate the occurrence of specific symptoms. Importantly, medically unexplained symptoms are not necessarily due to a psychiatric disorder[5,6,22] (even though several psychiatric diseases present with unexplained somatic symptoms), but may reflect a condition of stress.

17.2.1   Autoregressive Spectral Analysis of Cardiovascular Variabilities

Emerging techniques for the study of autonomic regulation, not only in the clinic but also in real life, employing autoregressive spectral analysis of cardiovascular variability (Fig. 17.2),[20,25-28] offer a new window for the study of functional syndromes, and of patients who report medically unexplained symptoms. This noninvasive technique, based on indices derived from beat-to-beat RR variability, furnishes markers of sympathetic and vagal modulation of the sinoatrial (SA) node, represented by the low frequency (LF$_{RR}$ expressed in normalized units, nu) and high frequency (HF$_{RR}$ expressed in normalized units) components, respectively, of RR interval variability.[23] Moreover, if a continuous arterial pressure signal is also simultaneously available, a marker of the sympathetic modulation of the vasculature may be obtained by the low frequency component of systolic arterial pressure variability (LF$_{SAP}$), and an overall marker of baroreflex sensitivity is furnished by the frequency domain alpha index (or by the baroreflex slope[29,30]).

Employing this technique, we studied otherwise healthy patients who asked our clinical advice because of unexplained somatic symptoms, and compared them to asymptomatic controls.[20] The patients showed a significantly higher perception of stress compared with the controls, and the autonomic assessment suggested cardiovascular dysregulation, with higher arterial pressures and altered markers of autonomic control. In particular, the LF component of RR variability (LF$_{RR}$ nu) was significantly higher (see Fig. 17.3), whereas (HF$_{RR}$, nu) was significantly smaller in patients than in controls. Patients were also characterized by a greater LF component of SAP variability and by a reduced alpha index, indicating impaired baroreflex sensitivity. Systolic and diastolic arterial pressure, although still in the normal range, were significantly higher in patients compared with controls. Interestingly, both the overall stress perception score and symptoms perception scores showed significant correlations with arterial pressure and several autonomic indices. Similar results were observed in a group of caregivers of cancer patients[28] and among patients affected by chronic fatigue syndromes.[26,31]

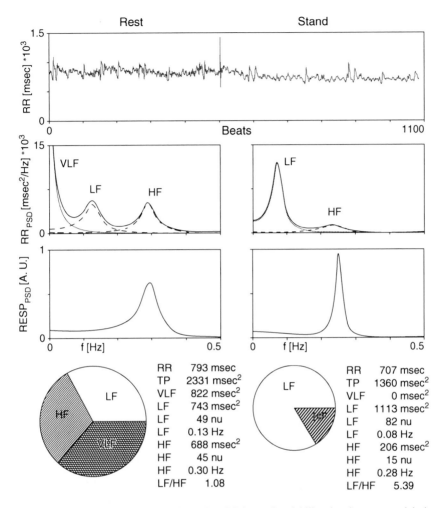

Fig. 17.2 Example of the analysis performed on RR interval variability signals, at rest and during standing up (i.e., during sympathetic activation). This illustration highlights the usual presence of three major components (very low frequency *VLF*, low frequency *LF*, high frequency *HF*), as seen in the *middle left panel*, during a resting condition. Conversely, no VLF is present in the *right middle panel* when the individual is standing. The *bottom panels*, representing the spectrum of the respiratory signals, show that the RR HF component is synchronous with respiration. At the bottom of the figure all major computed indices pertaining to LF and HF components are indicated, together with a pie chart showing the relative powers of VLF, LF, and HF. Note that when VLF is absent (such as during standing in this example) the normalized units, computed as Pf[nu] = Pf [ms]^2/(total power − VLF) [ms]^2*100, coincide with the % value. A key advantage of the autoregressive approach[23] derives from its capacity to detect for each component not only the associated power but also its center frequency. Practical software solutions[24] can also handle conditions where more than three components are detected. To this end, bands of interest may be set. We employ a setting of 0.03–0.14 Hz for LF and of 0.15–0.35 Hz for HF. The software allocates individual components of RR variability spectrum to either LF or HF, and provides a sum of all major components pertaining to either frequency band, while disregarding minor components as noise. Accordingly, the sum of LF and HF powers in nu is usually close to 100

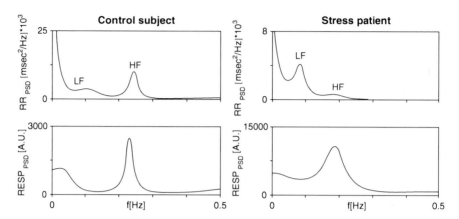

Fig. 17.3 Examples of spectral profiles obtained in a control subject (*left panels*) and a stressed patient (*right panels*) for RR interval (*top panels*) and respiration (*bottom panels*) variabilities at rest. Note the greater amplitude of the low frequency (*LF*) component (reflecting sympathetic modulation of heart rate) and conversely the low amplitude of the high frequency (*HF*) component (reflecting vagal modulation of heart rate) in the stressed patient's spectral profile

17.3   Stress and Behavior

Behavior represents one of the main factors in the genesis of stress responses and also in the management of stress. In fact, as Lazarus[8] pointed out, as soon as an individual has to deal with a stressful situation, either acutely or chronically, he or she reverts, consciously or unconsciously, to coping strategies that are the complex result of past experience, personality, genetics, biological characteristics, cognitive and emotional involvements, and autonomic nervous system and HPA axis activation. The subject's capability to overcome the stressful situation will depend more upon coping strategies and behavior than the stressor itself.[32,33] The stress response per se[1,2,4] is a physiological response, involving both psychological and biological mechanisms. Its main goal is to reestablish homeostasis. The behavioral response may be a positive reaction (e.g., the gazelle that escapes as soon it realizes the presence of a lion). However, in the clinical setting, especially with chronic stressful conditions, complexity is much greater and the resulting behavior may be deleterious, even if the subject considers it as positive response or an almost unique chance in that specific moment (e.g., to ask a moneylender for help).[10] One of the main goals of stress management is to help the individual to develop skills, and to discover or find enough internal or external resources to choose a positive behavior, in order to overcome the stressful situation (see also the Chap. 19).

Negative behavioral responses due to chronic psychosocial factors may be related both to choices of unhealthy life styles (such as smoking, poor nutrition, sedentary life, abuse of alcohol or drugs), and to psychosocial/relational changes like reduced compliance with medical prescriptions, isolation, litigation, poor social relationships, reduced self-esteem, etc., that in the long term may lead to a worsening of somatic symptoms, and to reductions of quality of life and productivity.[7,9,34-36]

17.3.1   Unhealthy Life Styles

Unhealthy lifestyle behaviors should be of interest to the cardiologist because they increase cardiovascular risk due to the association between psychosocial factors and CHD[3,7,9,17,37,38] and affect major bodily regulatory systems, such as the HPA axis and the autonomic nervous system.[39]

Stress frequently promotes food-seeking behavior (but may also cause loss of appetite, especially when acute), inducing individuals to chose progressively more palatable food, generally containing more sugar, fats, and salt[36,40-42], hence increasing body weight, and worsening lipid and glucose profiles. Stress also promotes sedentary life,[35] generally increasing tiredness, the feeling of "lack of time" to exercise and the desire to rest. Stress promotes smoking,[35,43] and increases the number of cigarettes smoked per day in smokers, induces ex smokers to restart, and sometimes induces nonsmokers (in particular young susceptible subjects) to start the habit. Reasons are probably that nicotine may reduce stress symptoms and anxiety, modulate arousal and mood control, and increase feelings of concentration and attention.[43] Stress may also, in susceptible individuals, induce a craving for alcohol and/ or drugs.[44] Recent preclinical and clinical studies[36,40-44] are disentangling a critical mechanism responsible for these behavioral choices: the seeking of pleasure or "gratification." Thus, under stress, patients tend to chose behaviors that interfere with the brain reward systems.

17.3.2   Psychosocial Coping

Stress may also determine changes in psychosocial coping. These strategies are defined as thoughts and behaviors used to manage the internal and external demands of situations appraised as stressful.[45] They help the individual to overcome the stressful situation when he/she has all the necessary resources to do so. The simple example is beneficial competition at work or during a sports match, pushing subjects to find more efficacious strategies allowing victory. When the stressful situation lasts longer, or is perceived as too important or dangerous, or when the subject has poor control over it and/or inadequate resources, the resulting behavior (even to do nothing!) may be counterproductive. A typical example is a subject who perceives him/herself as being a victim of bullying at work, while he or she (and perhaps his/her colleagues or managers too) is just having a very stressful period, and misinterprets unusual, perhaps unkind, reactions from colleagues as voluntarily directed against him/herself. In this example, the negative consequences of stress are twofold: the change in colleagues' behavior (unkind reactions) and the misinterpretation of this behavior and attendant thoughts or actions of the subject (the belief of being a victim of bullying and deciding to stop the usual and fruitful collaboration with colleagues). The psychological mechanisms underlying this kind of behavior are very complex and are not within the objectives of this chapter.

Here, we will only summarize a few principles and basic therapeutic approaches that may be employed to manage or prevent stress in subjects complaining of stress and related symptoms either in a clinical setting, for example, in cardiac patients, or outside of the hospital, for instance at the worksite.

There are several theories describing psychological processes experienced by a subject when he/she must cope with a stressful situation that represents a "change" in his/her life.[34,46] Simplifying, when a subject has to deal with a challenge, before assuming a given behavior, he/she experiences emotions that represent a first psychological phase. These emotions depend on individual perception, meaning (logically) attributed to the stressor and its possible consequences, previous experiences, etc., and (implicit) autonomic nervous system activation. Then the subject may experience a second psychological phase where problem-focused cognitive processes may become much more important. Among these are: reality check, determination of own desires, limits and goals, individualization of resources, etc. The subject's psychological coping is the result of these two phases. In this model, the final result depends not only on the stressor but also on the subject's psychological process and the ensuing behaviors.

17.4 Stress Management: The Example of Worksite Intervention

17.4.1 Stress and Work

Over recent decades, emphasis has been placed on the changing nature of work and attendant new forms of risk that could negatively affect employees' health and safety[47] (see also Chap. 11). These have been termed psychosocial risks and have been defined in terms of the interaction between job content, work organization and management, and other environmental and organizational conditions on one hand, and the employees' capabilities and needs on the other. Issues like work-related stress, bullying, and harassment are receiving attention on a global basis and efforts have been made to address them. Moreover, the rapid changes in organizational structures caused by globalization have introduced new types of stress, generally related to new forms of employment contracts, job insecurity, the ageing workforce, work intensification, high emotional demands at work, and poor work-life balance[11] that impose growing challenges to the site management and employees confronted with diminishing resources. The consequence is that, according to the WHO,[48] mental health problems and stress-related disorders are becoming the major overall cause of early death in Europe, and are among the major health concerns with great economic cost for society, being in Europe responsible for at least 20 billion Euros per year in lost time and health bills.

European Community surveys have identified stress-related disorders among the most commonly reported sources of work-related illnesses, second only to back pain (a problem that per se may also be related to stress).[49] They are primarily related to the presence of somatic symptoms like sleep problems, tiredness, anxiety,[50,51] muscular tension and pain, palpitations, gastrointestinal dysfunction, and, in general, various functional syndromes.[50] In addition, they tend to increase the risk of cardiovascular disease[3,13,17,52-55] and mental illnesses,[56] in particular when associated with unhealthy lifestyle behaviors.[36] Of particular importance are the economic and social consequences of stress at work, related to a loss of quality of life and productivity mainly due to absenteeism,[11,57] presenteeism (decreased on the job performance due to presence despite health problems),[58] and worsening of human relationships both at the worksite and in private life, with attendant isolation, increased litigation, etc.

17.4.2   Principles of Stress Assessment and Management at Work

Several psychological tools may be employed to obtain indicators related to stress. They are generally based on questionnaires that provide measures of several factors involved in the genesis, response, and consequences of stress.[13,59-62] In particular, worksite stress assessment is usually directed toward both the organizational and the individual level and its utility derives from the help in planning possible and realistic therapeutic approaches to the management and/or prevention of stress.

The two leading models in occupational health psychology are the demand-control model[59] and the effort-reward imbalance model.[60] In the first one, high demand but low decision latitude characterizes job strain. In the effort-reward imbalance model, increased job effort may result from either extrinsic demands or personal overcommitment, and "reward" may occur in the form of money, recognition, prestige, security, or career opportunities. High effort with low reward characterizes job imbalance. These two conceptual models of work stress were used to create psychological tools widely employed, alone or with other tools that point out other key psychological dimensions as change,[62] individual stress perception,[17] stress-related somatic symptom perception,[12,13,57,63] or behaviors[32,35,64]; moreover, the literature abounds with tools that assess multiple psychological dimensions all together.

Due to the multidimensional and complex nature of stress, psychological tools to assess stress are useful particularly in nonpsychiatric populations, or when used at the group level, for example, at worksites, or for research purposes. However, they may present many limits when applied in a clinical setting on (single) individuals. The use of tools to measure indicators of physiological responses to stress, like hormonal changes or autonomic nervous system involvement (see other chapters in this book), may be useful. Of particular interest is the observed correlation between subjective somatic stress-related symptom scores and subjective stress perception scores (very simple psychological indicators) and indices of autonomic regulation in healthy subjects,[27] in chronic stressed patients complaining of somatic symptoms,[20] in close caregivers of cancer patients,[28] and in healthy employees experiencing a chronic stressful situation due to work downsizing.[13]

If stress assessment is complex, its clinical management may be even more complex and challenging.[33,65-69] In this section we will consider some basic therapeutic principles that are applicable in the management/prevention of stress in subjects/patients who do not present with psychiatric disorders like depression, hypochondria, or panic disorder (who require ad hoc treatment), even though these conditions may also present overlapping behavior and symptoms to the ones observed in patients suffering from chronic stress. Obviously, stress can exacerbate depression, and there is an overlap between the symptoms of stress and depression (see Chap. 12).

Although there are several models of stress, the division between external stressors and the stress response of the individual is common to all.[70] Stress management techniques thus can be divided into two kinds: environmental management, which attempts to modify work or private life environments to reduce the sources of stress, and approaches that aim to support subjects to deal effectively with stressful situations.[69] This concept is applicable to every kind of stress, on the job or outside the worksite.

Some clinical studies[13,68,71] suggest that assessments and interventions aimed at providing personal support and resources, are more effective than environmental management to reduce stressors. This may be due to the novel nature of work stressors[11]: fear of losing one's job, excessive speed in procedural changes, types of contracts, etc., as compared to "traditional" work stressors like reduced safety, organizational and communicational problems, etc. These kinds of stress may also be reduced by organizational initiatives such as improvements in decision making and time management.[67] This principle is also valid for stressors outside work life, such as caregiving for chronic untreatable diseases, when it is impossible to remove the stressor.

Among the various approaches to stress management, cognitive-behavioral models seem to be more effective than other interventions, both at the worksite[69] and among patients complaining of somatic symptoms.[5,6] Stress prevention and management programs also utilize interventions such as cognitive restructuring, relaxation, and behavioral modification to improve individual skills and lifestyle choices.[66] These issues are further discussed by Talbot-Ellis and Linden in the chapter on psychological treatment. Drug treatment may obviously be considered in some individuals to reduce symptoms (e.g., beta-blockers for palpitations or anxiolytics to reduce anxiety) and antidepressants may (but not always) help in reducing unexplained symptoms, even when there are no clear symptoms of depression.[6]

17.4.3 An Example of a Worksite Intervention Program

In recent years, following the model of stress patterned by integrating behavioral observations with autonomic measures,[25] we developed a clinical approach for the management of chronic stress[13,20,28] in ambulant patients, combining[72] conventional with complementary techniques. It is based on a multidimensional approach[13]: body–mind interventions such as mental restructuring (focusing on the patient's point of view) and relaxation techniques[72] (focusing on autonomic arousal) are combined with eating re-education and exercise training, and integrated with more orthodox drug regimens[13,34,65,73] when indicated. This method has been applied in a working population[13] and was capable of improving stress symptom perception, slightly reducing arterial pressure and improving autonomic cardiac regulation (see Fig. 17.4). Ninety-one white-collar workers at the Italian site of an American

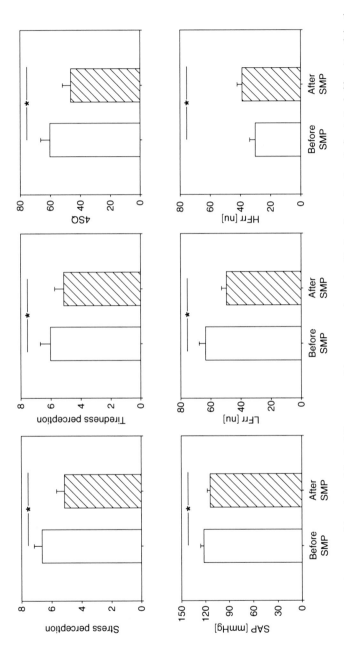

Fig. 17.4 Psychological (*top panels*) and physiological (*bottom panels*) parameters determined before (*open bars*) and after (*stippled bars*) participation in the 1 year stress management program (*SMP*) described in Table 17.1.[13] Note the reductions of all psychological scores, and of systolic arterial pressure (SAP), and the LF component of RR interval variability (LFrr, reflecting sympathetic modulation of heart rate) after the SMP intervention. Conversely, note the increase of the high frequency component of RR interval variability (HFrr, marker of prevalent vagal modulation to the SA node)

multinational Company were compared with 79 healthy control subjects enrolled outside the company. All subjects were assessed by a clinical psychologist through semistructured interviews to establish the possible presence of chronic psychosocial stress and stress-related symptoms, and to exclude patients with psychiatric illness (with particular attention to depression, hypochondria, and somatoform disorders). Moreover, they filled in questionnaires[20] to assess individual perceptions of stress and somatic symptoms. Spectral analysis of RR interval variability was used to assess autonomic nervous system regulation.

On the basis of self-selection, a subgroup of workers ($n = 26$) elected to participate in an active Stress Management Program (see Table 17.1a) lasting 1 year and the remainder participated in a sham program (involving annual information sessions and short articles published in the house magazine and in e-mail messages sent approximately once a month).

Workers presented with an elevated level of stress-related symptoms and an altered variability profile as compared with control subjects (the low-frequency component of RR variability was, respectively, 65.2 ± 2 vs 55.3 ± 2 normalized units; $P < 0.001$; opposite changes were observed for the high-frequency component). These alterations were largely reversed (low-frequency component of RR variability from 63.6 ± 3.9 to 49.3 ± 3 normalized units; $P < 0.001$) by the stress management program, which also slightly lowered systolic arterial pressure and significantly reduced score of stress and somatic symptom measures. No changes were observed in the sham program group.

The simple relaxation technique,[74,75] which is easy to learn and to apply also at the worksite, focuses mostly on the active modulation of respiration, and resulted in a reduced respiratory frequency at rest after 1 year of intervention. Other more complex techniques, like transcendental meditation, yoga, autogenic training, etc., combining the respiratory modulation with other tools, like imagination, muscular stretching and relaxation, music listening, etc., also seem to be useful in reducing stress appraisal. We cannot completely define the mechanisms responsible for this. However, the active training of respiration might play a role, as corroborated by recent studies with slow breathing training in hypertension[76] and heart failure,[77] also using respiratory-driven biofeedback devices. The relaxation technique we employed seems to be capable of reducing subjective components of stress, like somatic symptoms perception, as well as to promote a more balanced autonomic profile, with reduced sympathetic and increased vagal modulation of the SA,[13] an increased baroreflex gain,[75] and a reduction of arterial blood pressure.[13]

Neuropsychological research[44] seems to indicate that relaxation techniques can elicit pleasurable experiences or sensations activating natural brain reward systems and senses of pleasure that seem to possess a coordinating influence on a network of cortical and subcortical limbic and paralimbic structures which are intimately involved in the regulation of cognition, emotion and autonomic, endocrine or vegetative function.

Table 17.1 Main components of worksite intervention program

(a) *Stress management program*

Cognitive restructuring	Cognitive/behavioral model: – Emotions and behavior are largely determined by individual's cognitive perceptions[66] – Problem-focused psychological coping styles may be more helpful than emotion-focused ones in managing stress and in helping the subject to reach his own real goals. It comprises:
• Educational component	Participants are provided with information about the causes of stress, its consequences on bodily and psychological functioning (in particular the role of regulatory systems), and the importance of behavior in bettering or worsening psychological and physical well-being.
• Open discussions	Permit to the subjects to declare their emotion-focused psychological coping strategies in a controlled clinical environment where the trainer may promote discussions and reflections on them.
• Skills training	Instructions in specific skills to reduce the affective, behavioral, cognitive, and psychological components of stress and help the subjects to develop positive psychological coping strategies.
Relaxation training	Weekly encounters of 1 h duration with an expert technician, unsupervised daily exercises at home. Based on:
• Active respiratory techniques	[13,72,74,75] Focus attention on the breathing pattern and rate. Progressively, the patient is asked to deepen, regularize, and slow respiration to reach the most comfortable mix. On average, the nominal rate is about 8–10 breaths/min.
• Muscular relaxation	Patients are asked to relax their musculature progressively and to disregard any interfering thoughts.

(b) *Life style interventions program*

• Health assessment	It comprises:
• Medical evaluation:	Medical history, physical assessment (BMI, blood pressure determinations, etc.)
• Venous blood determination	Fasting glucose, total, HDL, LDL cholesterol, triglycerides, liver function, and blood cell counts.
• Lifestyle intervention	Based on:
• Group training	Focusing on healthy nutrition, physical activity, and quitting smoking
• Individual consultations	To manage specific risks factors

Our initial investigations, although suggestive, need further confirmation in clinical settings with large populations, and employing randomized, controlled study designs. A possible further clinical advantage of active treatments is that patients learn to actively relax[5,13,73] and focus on a personally chosen breathing pattern, which can be maintained without the need for specific instrumentation[75] or special setting, thus including the relaxation technique as a component of their usually daily routine. Relaxation becomes a chosen positive behavior, and a useful psychological coping strategy. Even passive relaxation treatment, like massage, seems to be useful in reducing stress appraisal, at least according to patients' self-report. Recent data[74] point out that these techniques allow improvement of psychological indices while showing no effect on physiological variables. This suggests a role for nonspecific factors[78] in relieving the perception of stress and arousal, altering the personal experience of stress. Among these factors, we may consider the belief that the chosen technique is effective,[79] personal expectations, relaxing clinical setting, the pleasant feeling of the massage, the positive value of dedicating time to own personal care. Studies with functional MRI[80,81] suggest that this psychological involvement mirrors the activity of placebo in altering expectations of pain in patients.

Regarding the lifestyle intervention (see Table 17.1b) 44 participated and modified their nutrition pattern, while 52 served as control group receiving only monthly educational messages by e-mail or in the local house magazine regarding healthy life styles. After 2 years, only the intervention group showed an improvement in metabolic profile; in particular, a reduction in triglyceride and total cholesterol levels (Lucini et al., work in progress). Not all employees who participated in the cognitive restructuring and relaxation protocol[13] took part to this lifestyle intervention program and vice versa, as consequence of individual needs, the presence of behavioral risk factors, and time restrictions. Despite its methodological limitations, the study shows that lifestyle interventions are possible at the worksite, even during a very stressful period caused by downsizing of the company.

In general a combination of medical and psychological skills may provide the best results in lifestyle intervention programs at worksites, thereby improving health,[71,82,83] saving money[84], and helping the employees to manage stress.[85,86]

Lifestyle modification may also be important in the patient's approach to managing stress. As noted above, it is not always possible to eliminate the stressor but a complex psychological and behavioral process may modify stress perception, lead to acquisition of psychological and practical skills to overcome it or at least to minimize its consequences. This entire process requires the patient's problem-focused active role, which is more difficult to assume if the stressor is perceived as hazardous, or if coping strategies are emotion focused. Experiencing that a change, previously considered impossible, is indeed possible (like to lose weight, reduce a somatic symptom, reduce or even quit smoking, or to be less tired doing physical activity, etc.) can be a motivational tool. The patient experiences that he/she can change, possibly enabling further psychological, cognitive changes associated with useful problem-focused coping strategies.

17.5   Conclusions

What is stress? Now, we may argue that it is "an issue that doctors, even cardiologists, have to deal with." It may cause cardiovascular disease and/or symptoms and these consequences may themselves become a source of stress. Stress management and prevention approaches are possible and effective, and should not be underestimated or considered to be outside the realm of regular clinical care. To integrate psychology with biology may be of great help both in understanding the complex links between stress and illnesses, and in delivering therapy. Work may represent an important source of stress that merits attention from cardiologists. In addition, the worksite may be a proper environment in which to promote and realize cardiovascular and metabolic prevention.

References

1. Engel BT. Stress is a noun! No, a verb! No, an adjective! In Field TM, McCabe PM, Schneiderman N, (eds), *Stress and Coping*. Hillsdale, NJ, Erlbaum, 1985, pp3-12.
2. McEwen BS. Protective and damaging effects of stress mediators. *N Engl J Med*. 1998;338: 171-179.
3. Rozanski A, Blumenthal JA, Saab PG, et al. The epidemiology, pathophysiology, management of psychosocial risk factors in cardiac practice: the emerging field of behavioural cardiology. *J Am Coll Cardiol*. 2005;45:637-651.
4. Selye H. *The Stress of Life*. New York: McGraw Hill; 1956.
5. Hatcher S, Arroll B. Assessment and management of medically unexplained symptoms. *BMJ*. 2008;336:1124-1128.
6. Mayou R, Farmer A. ABC of psychological medicine: functional somatic symptoms and syndromes. *BMJ*. 2002;325:265-268.
7. Brotman D, Golden SH, Wittstein IS. The cardiovascular toll of stress. *Lancet*. 2007;370: 1089-1099.
8. Lazarus RS, Folkman S. *Stress Appraisal and Coping*. New York: Springer; 1984.
9. Hamer M, Molloy GJ, Stamatakis E. Psychological distress as risk factor for cardiovascular events. *J Am Coll Cardiol*. 2008;52:2156-2162.
10. Lucini D. *Super Stress – Come superare la crisi senza che il tuo lavoro ti rovini la salute*. Milano: Rizzoli; 2009.
11. Brun E, Milczarek M, Gonzales ER. *Expert Forecast on Emerging Psychosocial Risks Related to Occupational Safety and Health*. Luxembourg: European Agency for Safety and Health at Work; 2007.
12. Iellamo F, Pigozzi F, Spataro A, Malcarne M, Pagani M, Lucini D. Autonomic and psychological adaptations in Olympic rowers. *J Sports Med Phys Fitness*. 2006;46:598-604.
13. Lucini D, Riva S, Pizzinelli P, Pagani M. Stress management at the worksite: reversal of symptoms profile and cardiovascular dysregulation. *Hypertension*. 2007;49:291-297.
14. Curtis BM, O'Keefe JHJ. Autonomic tone as a cardiovascular risk factor: the dangers of chronic fight or flight. *Mayo Clin Proc*. 2002;77:45-54.
15. Wilbert-Lampen U, Leistener D, Greven S, Pohl T, Sper S, Völker C. Cardiovascular events during world cup soccer. *N Engl J Med*. 2008;358:475-483.
16. Lampert R, Shusterman V, Burg M, et al. Anger-induced T-wave alkternans predicts future ventricular arrhythmias in patients with implantable cardioverter-defibrillators. *J Am Coll Cardiol*. 2009;73:774-778.

17. Rosengren A, Hawken S, Ôunpuu S, et al. Association of psychosocial risk factors with risk of acute myocardial infarction in 11119 case and 13648 controls from 52 countries (The INTERHEART study): case control study. *Lancet.* 2004;364:953-962.
18. Vissoci Reiche AM, Vargas Nunes SO, Kaminami MH. Stress depression, the immune system, and cancer. *Lancet.* 2004;5:617-695.
19. Horwitz BJ, Fisher RS. The irritable bowel syndrome. *N Engl J Med.* 2001;344:1846-1850.
20. Lucini D, DiFede G, Parati G, et al. Impact of chronic psychosocial stress on autonomic cardiovascular regulation in otherwise healthy subjects. *Hypertension.* 2005;46:1201-1206.
21. Kanaan RAA, Lepine JP, Wessely SC. The association or otherwise of the functional somatic syndromes. *Psychosom Med.* 2007;69:855-859.
22. Mayou R. Are treatments for common mental disorders also effective for functional symptoms and disorders? *Psychosom Med.* 2007;69:876-880.
23. Pagani M, Lombard F, Guzzetti S, et al. Power spectral analysis of heart rate and arterial pressure variabilities as a marker of sympatho-vagal interaction in man and conscious dogs. *Circ Res.* 1986;58:178-193.
24. Badilini F, Pagani M, Porta A. HeartScope: a software tool addressing autonomic nervous system regulation. *Comput Cardiol.* 2005;32:259-262.
25. Pagani M, Lucini D. Cardiovascular physiology, emotions, and clinical applications: are we ready for prime time? *Am J Physiol Heart Circ Physiol.* 2008;295:H1-H3.
26. Pagani M, Lucini D. Chronic fatigue syndrome. A perspective focusing on the autonomic nervous system. *Clin Sci.* 1999;96:117-125.
27. Lucini D, Norbiato G, Clerici M, et al. Hemodinamic and autonomic adjustments to real life stress conditions in humans. *Hypertension.* 2002;39:184-188.
28. Lucini D, Cannone V, Malacarne M, et al. Evidence of autonomic dysregulation in otherwise healthy cancer caregivers: a possible link with health hazard. *Eur J Cancer.* 2008;44:2437-2443.
29. Lucini D, Mela GS, Malliani A, et al. Impairment in cardiac autonomic regulation preceding arterial hypertension in humans: insight from spectral analysis of beat-by-beat cardiovascular variability. *Circulation.* 2002;19:2673-2679.
30. Pagani M, Somers VK, Furlan R, et al. Changes in autonomic regulation induced by physical training in mild hypertension. *Hypertension.* 1988;12:600-610.
31. Pagani M, Lucini D, Mela GS, et al. Sympathetic overactivity in subjects complaining of unexplained fatigue. *Clin Sci.* 1994;87:655-661.
32. O'Donnell K, Badrick E, Kumari M, Steptoe A. Psychological coping styles and cortisol over the day in healthy older adults. *Psychoneuroendocrinology.* 2009;33:601-611.
33. Rozanski A. Integrating psychologic approaches into the behavioural management of cardiac patients. *Psychosom Med.* 2005;67:567-573.
34. Lazarus RS. *Emotion and Adaptation.* New York: Oxford University Press; 1991.
35. Chen WQ, Wong TW, Tak-Sun YuI. Association of occupational stress and social support with health-ralated behaviors among Chinese offshore oil workers. *J Occup Health.* 2008;50:262-269.
36. Volkow ND, Wise RA. How can drug addiction help us understand obesity? *Nat Neurosci.* 2005;8:555-560.
37. Hjemdahl P. Stress and the metabolic syndrome. An interesting but enigmatic association. *Circulation.* 2002;106:2634-2636.
38. Lavie CJ, Milani RV. Adverse psychological and coronary risk profiles in young patients with coronary artery disease and benefits of formal cardiac rehabilitation. *Arch Intern Med.* 2006;166:1878-1883.
39. Lucini D, Bertocchi MA, Pagani M. Autonomic effects of nicotine patch administration in habitual cigarette smokers: a double-blind, placebo-controlled study using spectral analysis of RR interval and systolic arterial pressure variabilities. *J Cardiovasc Pharmacol.* 1998;31:714-720.
40. Kesseler D. *The End of Overeating: Taking Control of the Insatiable American Appetite.* New York: Rodale; 2009.

41. Spiegel A, Nabel E, Volkow N, et al. Obesity on the brain. *Nat Neurosci.* 2005;8:552-553.
42. Volkow N, Li TK. The neuroscience of addiction. *Nat Neurosci.* 2005;8:1429-1430.
43. Benowitz NL. Neurobiology of nicotine addiction: implications for smoking cessation treatment. *Am J Med.* 2008;121:S3-S10.
44. Esch T, Stefano GB. The neurobiology of pleasure, reward processes, addiction and their health implications. *Neuro Endocrinol Lett.* 2004;25:235-251.
45. Folkman S, Moskowitz JT. Coping: pitfalls and promise. *Annu Rev Psychol.* 2004;55:745-774.
46. Bridges W. *Managing Transitions: Making the Most of Change.* 2nd ed. Cambridge: Da Capo Press – Perseus Books Group; 2003.
47. Leka S, Kortum E. A European framework to address psychosocial hazards. *J Occup Health.* 2008;50:294-296.
48. WHO: Fact Sheet No 220. Mental health: Strengthening mental health promotion. Geneva: World Health Organization, 2001.
49. European Agency for Safety and Health at Work. *Research on Work-Related Stress* 2002.
50. Ungin P. Functional disorders – a cause of increasing work absence? *Occup Med.* 2007;57: 2-3.
51. Kawano Y. Association of job-related stress factors with psychological and somatic symptoms among Japanese hospital nurses: effect of departmental environment in acute care hospitals. *J Occup Health.* 2008;50:79-85.
52. Kivimäki M, Leino-Arja P, Luukkonen R, Riihimäki H, Vahtera J, Kirjonon J. Work stress and risk of cardiovascular mortality: prospective cohort study of industrial employees. *BMJ.* 2002;325:1-5.
53. Chandola T, Britton A, Brunner E, et al. Work stress and coronary heart disease: what are the mechanisms? *Eur Heart J.* 2008;29:640-648.
54. Yarnell J. Stress at work – an independent risk factor for coronary heart disease? *Eur Heart J.* 2008;29:579-580.
55. Elovainio A, Kivimäki M, Puttonen S, et al. Organisational injustice and impaired cardiovascular regulation among female employees. *Occup Environ Med.* 2006;63:141-144.
56. Langlieb AM, DePaulo JR. Etiology of depression and implications on work environment. JOEM. 2008;50(4):391-395.
57. Fourth European Working Conditions Survey. *European Foundation for the Improvement of Living and Working Conditions.* 2007.
58. Schultz AB, Edington DW. Employee health and presenteeism: a systematic review. *J Occup Rehabil.* 2007;17:547-579.
59. Karasek R, Baker D, Marxer F, Theorell T, et al. Job decision latitude, job demands, and cardiovascular disease: a prospective study of Swedish men. *Am J Public Health.* 1981;71: 694-705.
60. Siegrist J. Adverse health effects of high-effort/low-reward conditions. *J Occup Health Psychol.* 1996;71:694-705.
61. Fliege H, Rose M, Arck P, Walter OB, et al. The perceived stress questionnaire (PSQ) reconsidered: validation and reference values from different clinical and healthy adult samples. *Psychosom Med.* 2005;67:78-88.
62. Smith P, Beaton D. Measuring change in psychosocial working conditions: methodological issues to consider when data are collected at baseline and one follow-up time point. *Occup Environ Med.* 2008;65:288-296.
63. Jackson J, Fiddler M, Kapur Navneet K, et al. Number of bodily symptoms predicts outcome more accurately than health anxiety in patients attending neurology, cardiology, and gastroenterology clinics. *J Psychosom Res.* 2006;60:357-363.
64. Carver CS, Scheier MF, Weintraub JK. Assessing coping strategies: a theoretically based approach. *J Pers Soc Psychol.* 1989;56:267-283.
65. Milani RV, Lavie CJ. Stopping stress at its origins. *Hypertension.* 2007;49:268-269.
66. Blumenthal JA, Sherwood A, Babyak MA, et al. Effects of exercise and stress management training on markers of cardiovascular risk in patients with ischemic heart disease: a randomized controlled trial. *JAMA.* 2005;293:1626-1634.

67. Michie S, Williams S. Reducing work related psychological ill health and sickness absence: a systematic literature review. *Occup Environ Med*. 2003;60:3-9.
68. Mimura C, Griffiths P. The effectiveness of current approaches to workplace stress management in the nursing profession: an evidence based literature review. *Occup Environ Med*. 2003; 60:10-15.
69. Verbeek J. The evidence for workplace counselling is in medicine. *Occup Environ Med*. 2004;61:558-559.
70. Payne RL. Stress at work: a conceptual framework. In: Firth-Cozens J, Payne RL, eds. *Stress in Health Professionals: Psychological and Organisational Causes and Interventions*. Chichester: Wiley; 1999:3-16.
71. Goetzel RZ, Ozminkowski RJ. The health and cost benefits of work site health-promotion programs. *Annu Rev Public Health*. 2008;29:303-323.
72. Vogel JHK, Bolling SF, Costello RB, et al. Integrating complementary medicine into cardiovascular medicine. A report of the American College of Cardiology Foundation Task Force on Clinical Experts Consensus Document (Writing Committee to develop an Expert Consensus on Complementary and Integrative Medicine). *J Am Coll Cardiol*. 2005;45:184-221.
73. Henningsen P, Zipfel S, Herzog W. Management of functional somatic syndromes. *Lancet*. 2007;396:946-955.
74. Lucini D, Malcarne M, Solaro N, et al. Complementary medicine for the management of chronic stress: superiority of active versus passive techniques. *J Hypertens*. 2009;27(12): 2421-2428.
75. Lucini D, Covacci G, Milani RV, et al. A controlled study of the effects of mental relaxation on autonomic excitatory responses in healthy subjects. *Psychosom Med*. 1997;59:541-552.
76. Parati G, Carretta R. Device-guided slow breathing as a nonpharmacological approach to antihypertensive treatment efficacy, problems and perspectives. *J Hypertens*. 2007;25:57-61.
77. Parati G, Malfatto G, Boarin S, et al. Device-guided paced breathing in the home setting. *Circ Heart Fail*. 2008;1:178-183.
78. Kaptchuk T, Kelley JM, Conboy LA, et al. Components of placebo effect: randomised controlled trial in patients with irritable bowel syndrome. *BMJ*. 2008;336:999-1003.
79. Hrobjartsson A, Getzsche PC. Is the placebo powerless? An analysis of clinical trials comparing placebo with no treatment. *N Engl J Med*. 2009;344:1594-1602.
80. WagerTD RJK, Smith EE, et al. Placebo-induced changes in fMRI in the anticipation and experience plan. *Science*. 2004;204:1162-1167.
81. Diederich NU, Goetz CG. The placebo treatments in neurosciences: new insights from clinical and neuroimaging studies. *Neurology*. 2008;71:677-684.
82. Prabhakaran D, Jeemom P, Goenka S, et al. Impact at a worksite intervention program on cardiovascular risk factors: a demonstration project in an Indian Industrial population. *J Am Coll Cardiol*. 2009;53:1718-1728.
83. Okie S. The employer as health coach. *N Engl J Med*. 2007;357:1465.
84. American College of Occupational and Environment Medicine. Healthy workforce/healthy economy: the role of health, productivity, and disability management in addressing the nation's health care crisis. *J Occup Environ Med*. 2009;51:114-119.
85. Kuhn K. *Managing Stress by Promoting Health. Working on Stress*. European Agency for Safety and Health at Work. 2002.
86. Graveling RA, Crawford JO, Cowie H, et al. *A Review of Workplace Interventions that Promote Mental Wellbeing in the Workplace*. Edinburgh: IOM; 2008. www.iom-world.org

Chapter 18
Exercise to Reduce Distress and Improve Cardiac Function: Moving on and Finding the Pace

Hugo Saner and Gunilla Burell

Keywords Exercise • Reduce distress • Improve cardiac function • Physical activity • Primary prevention • Group interventions • Psychosocial risk factors • Stress management programs

18.1 Introduction

There is now clear scientific evidence linking regular aerobic physical activity to a significant cardiovascular risk reduction, and a sedentary lifestyle is currently considered one of the major risk factors for cardiovascular disease. Several behavioral profiles, including depression, hostility, anxiety, and overall psychosocial stress, are prevalent in patients with coronary artery disease and have been shown to independently confirm a high risk for subsequent myocardial infarction and death. It has been demonstrated that exercise training during cardiac rehabilitation can markedly reduce these high-risk behaviors. Exercise also reduces the psychophysiological response to psychological stress. Therefore, exercise has become an important component of stress management in conjunction with, and as a supplement to psychological counseling.

H. Saner (✉)
Cardiovascular Prevention and Rehabilitation,
University Hospital Inselspital,
CH-3010 Bern, Switzerland
e-mail: hugo.saner@insel.ch

G. Burell
Department of Public Health and Caring Sciences, University Hospital of Uppsala,
Uppsala, Sweden
e-mail: gunilla.burell@pubcare.uu.se

P. Hjemdahl et al. (eds.), *Stress and Cardiovascular Disease*,
DOI 10.1007/978-1-84882-419-5_18, © Springer-Verlag London Limited 2012

18.2 Physical Activity in Primary Prevention

In healthy subjects, aerobic physical activity and cardiorespiratory fitness are associated with a significant reduction in risk of all-cause mortality in a dose–response fashion.[1-7] Evidence suggests that the risk of dying during a given period declines with increasing levels of physical activity and cardiorespiratory fitness; this seems to be true both for men and women and across a broad range of ages from childhood to the very elderly. As these conclusions are based on the results of observational studies, selection bias may be linked to the existence of subclinical, undiagnosed diseases that may have made some individuals decrease their physical activity levels before the beginning of the study; alternatively, there is the tendency of associating more healthy habits (such as nonsmoking and eating a healthier diet) with physically active individuals. However, studies controlling these potential confounders also observe the inverse association between physical activity or cardiorespiratory fitness and all-cause mortality. Most of the mortality reduction seems to be due to a decrease of cardiovascular and coronary heart disease (CHD) mortality, and the level of decreased coronary risk attributable to regular aerobic physical activity is similar to that of other lifestyle factors, such as nonsmoking. Available data comprising 2,286,806 person-years for studies of physical activity and 317,908 person-years for studies of cardiorespiratory fitness[8] indicate that the risk of suffering cardiovascular disease (including CHD and stroke) or CHD alone is significantly reduced among more physically active or fit persons; the relative risk reduction is nearly twice as great for cardiorespiratory fitness compared with physical activity increases above the 25th percentile of the parameter used (Fig. 18.1). A possible explanation for the stronger dose–response gradient for fitness than for activity is that fitness is measured objectively, whereas physical activity is assessed by self-reports that may lead to misclassification and bias toward finding weaker physical activity/health benefit associations[9].

The reduction of cardiovascular and CHD mortality in physically active or fit individuals finds its biological plausibility in the effects of aerobic exercise on the cardiovascular system and cardiovascular risk factors. Regular aerobic physical activity results in improved exercise performance, which depends on an increased ability to use oxygen to derive energy for work. Improvements in both maximal cardiac output and peripheral oxygen extraction contribute to such increases of maximal oxygen uptake. These effects are attained for regular aerobic physical activity intensities, which range between 40% and 85% of maximal heart rate or oxygen uptake (VO2), with higher intensity levels being needed the higher the initial level of fitness, and vice versa.[11-13] Aerobic exercise also results in decreased myocardial oxygen demands for the same level of external work performed, as demonstrated by a decrease in the product of heart rate x systolic blood pressure, thus reducing the likelihood of myocardial ischemia.[3,12] Moreover, animal studies have demonstrated that the coronary circulation may also be modified by aerobic exercise, with an increase of the interior diameter of major coronary arteries and formation of new myocardial capillaries and arterioles.[14] Additional reported effects of aerobic exercise are beneficial effects on several hemostatic mechanisms (see Chap. 6 on hemostasis),

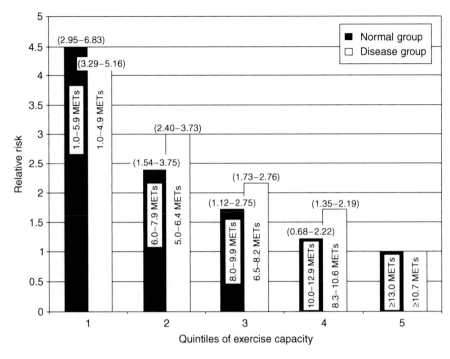

Fig. 18.1 Age-adjusted relative risks of mortality by quintiles of exercise capacity among normal subjects and patients with cardiovascular disease. The subgroup with the highest exercise capacity (group 5) is the reference category. For each quintile, the range of values for exercise capacity represented appears within each bar; 95% confidence intervals for the relative risks appear above each bar[10]

a reduction of arrhythmic risk by a favorable modulation of autonomic balance,[15] and an improvement of endothelial function.[16]

Physical activity also has a positive effect on many of the established risk factors for cardiovascular diseases, preventing or delaying the development of high blood pressure in normotensive subjects and reducing blood pressure in people with hypertension, increasing high-density lipoprotein cholesterol levels, helping to control body weight, and lowering the risk of developing non-insulin-dependent diabetes mellitus.[3,12] Overall, the above-mentioned effects tend to ameliorate the coronary risk profile and curtail the development of atherosclerosis, thus reducing the risk of cardiovascular and CHD mortality.

18.3   Physical Activity in Secondary Prevention

Aerobic physical activity in the secondary prevention setting is included in structured and comprehensive cardiac rehabilitation programs. The available data deal almost exclusively with cardiovascular fitness measurements and not with habitual physical activity evaluations. There is, however, a need for both a formal evaluation of the exercise associated risk and a lifestyle behavioral change in patients with established cardiac, and especially coronary, disease. Cardiac rehabilitation has thus been defined as the coordinated sum of interventions required to ensure the best possible physical, psychological, and social conditions so that patients with chronic or post-acute cardiovascular disease may, by their own efforts, preserve or resume optimal functioning in society and, through improved health behaviors, slow or reverse progression of disease.[17-20]

According to a Position Paper on Secondary Prevention through Cardiac Rehabilitation from the Cardiac Rehabilitation Section of the European Association of Cardiovascular Prevention and Rehabilitation (EACPR),[21] cardiac rehabilitative interventions should be integrated in a multifactorial and comprehensive long-term program including: clinical assistance and optimized medical or interventional treatment, appropriate cardiovascular risk evaluation, education and counseling, adequate follow-up, and exercise training. In this context, the effects of physical activity alone on cardiovascular risk may not be easily discernible. However, a recent meta-analysis,[22] which included 8,440 patients (mainly middle-aged men), most of whom had a history of previous acute myocardial infarction, previous coronary artery bypass, percutaneous transluminal coronary angioplasty, or were affected by stable angina pectoris, showed 31% and 26% reductions of total cardiac mortality for exercise only and comprehensive rehabilitation programs, respectively. These figures rose to 35% and 28%, respectively, when only deaths from CHD were considered. Neither exercise only nor comprehensive rehabilitation interventions showed any effect on the occurrence of nonfatal myocardial infarction, whereas insufficient data were available as to effects of physical activity alone and cardiac rehabilitation on revascularization rates. The reason for the apparent absence of difference between exercise alone and comprehensive rehabilitation programs on cardiac mortality rates reduction is not clear. The extreme heterogeneity between the available secondary prevention trials in terms of study design and quality, type, and duration of exercise and nonexercise interventions, and study populations must be considered. In addition, the mean follow-up period of the available trials was only 2.4 years; as physical activity is a human behavior highly affected by sociopsychological factors and compliance with exercise programs is usually poor and strictly dependent on appropriate counseling and educational interventions,[23] it seems likely that longer follow-up may better underscore the utility of the comprehensive rehabilitation approach.

It must also be considered that the more extensive use of thrombolysis, improved myocardial revascularization techniques, and aggressive pharmacological treatments over the past 15 years has progressively resulted in a relatively low-risk general population of cardiac patients, in which significant survival improvements are less obvious as a result of any added intervention. In this clinical setting, mortality and reinfarction should probably not be the only endpoints to be evaluated when measuring the effectiveness of physical activity interventions; other descriptors focusing on quality of life, functional independence and performance of daily activities, as well as coronary risk factors should be part of the standard outcome measures for all cardiac patients (Table 18.1). In any case, recent data confirm the existence of an inverse dose–response relationship between

Table 18.1 Changes in risk factors influenced by exercise training

Decrease in blood pressure
Increase in high-density lipoprotein cholesterol level
Reduction in plasma inflammatory risk markers (C-reactive protein, homocysteine)
Augmented weight reduction efforts
Psychological effects:
  Less depression
  Reduced anxiety
Improved glucose tolerance
Improved fitness level

cardiovascular fitness (evaluated by treadmill stress testing and expressed in METs) and all cause mortality in a population of 3,679 cardiovascular patients, defined as having a history of angiographically documented coronary artery disease, myocardial infarction, coronary bypass surgery, coronary angioplasty, congestive heart failure, peripheral vascular disease, or signs or symptoms suggestive of coronary artery disease during exercise testing; the results were the same irrespective of use of beta-blocking agents.[10]

The mechanisms thought to justify the positive effects of aerobic physical activity in the secondary prevention setting are the same as for primary prevention; that is decreased myocardial oxygen demands for the same level of external work, favorable modulation of autonomic and coronary endothelial function, improved cardiovascular risk factors profile, improved cardiovascular fitness, and increased patient surveillance.[24] This, together with technological advances leading to early detection of atherosclerosis in asymptomatic individuals tends to weaken the dividing line between primary and secondary prevention interventions. Indeed, recent clinical indications for in-patient and out-patient cardiac rehabilitation programs from the American College of Sports Medicine[25] comprehend both established cardiac disease and presence of coronary risk factors in otherwise healthy subjects.

18.4   Psychosocial Risk Factors for Cardiovascular Disease

Behavioral factors, including depression, hostility, anxiety, and overall psychosocial stress, have been demonstrated to be potent risk factors for the development of myocardial infarction and death, yet remain underappreciated as contemporary coronary risk factors[26-29] (see also Chaps. 12 and 19). The INTERHEART study evaluated cardiovascular risk factors in 29,972 people from 52 countries to investigate the risk of first myocardial infarction.[30] Nine independent risk factors including psychosocial factors accounted for 90% of the population-attributable risk in men and 94% in women. The psychosocial factors, which included depression and psychosocial stress, increased the odds of first myocardial infarction by approximately threefold and accounted for 33% of the population-attributable risk for the development of myocardial infarction, a magnitude similar to standard risk factors such as smoking, diabetes, and hypertension[31]. Physiological responses and cardiac effects of neutral stress are shown in Fig. 18.2.

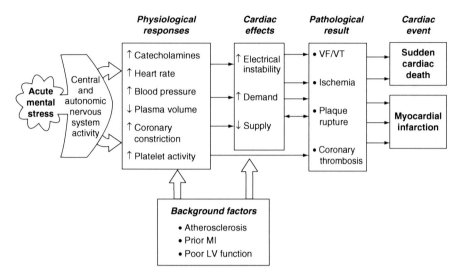

Fig. 18.2 Physiological responses and cardiac effects of neutral stress

In patients with known CHD, particularly after a major coronary event, the risk of subsequent myocardial infarction and death related to psychosocial factors appears much higher.[32-34] Frasure-Smith et al.[24] reported that depression was associated with a more than fourfold increase risk of mortality during the first 6 months after an acute myocardial infarction after adjustment for other risk factors. In that study, the magnitude of depression as a risk factor for mortality postmyocardial infarction was similar to that of left ventricular dysfunction and previous myocardial infarction. Several epidemiologic studies suggest that hostility and unexpressed anger are risk factors for coronary artery disease.[23,35-38] Allison et al.[39] demonstrated that among patients referred for cardiac rehabilitation, those with high psychologic stress had a 2.5-fold increased risk of rehospitalization, a fivefold increased risk of major cardiac events, and a fourfold increase in medical costs compared with patients with low levels of psychologic stress.[27] Frasure-Smith et al.[40] demonstrated that high-stress men with non-Q-wave myocardial infarction exhibited a 5-year mortality of more than 50%, threefold greater than in patients with low stress.[41] Shibeshi et al.[42] recently reported the effect of anxiety, measured using the Kellner Symptom Questionnaire used in this study, in 516 stable patients with coronary artery disease who were followed for an average of 3.4 years. They reported that anxiety scores were strong independent predictors of subsequent nonfatal myocardial infarction and total mortality.

18.5   Exercise and Psychophysiological Responses to Mental Stress

Exercise reduces the psychophysiological response to psychological stress.[43-45] Explanations include a reduction of arousal; hedonic properties; emotional effects; neurochemical changes; and effects on anxiety-like behavior, learning, and memory.[45-47] Exercise also seems to protect against stress-induced health complaints.[48] Age and gender may moderate this effect.[44]

The hypothalamic-pituitary-adrenal (HPA) axis plays a central role in the physiological response to acute physical stress by secreting glucocorticoids in addition to the sympathoadrenal activation which is important for the immediate cardiovascular response. The increased secretion of cortisol helps mobilize stored energy in response to perturbation, thus increasing the individual's chance for surviving or enduring the physical challenge. In today's society, however, stress is more likely to be psychological. Interestingly, the stress response to a psychological challenge is similar to the response to a physical challenge (i.e., increases in ACTH and cortisol secretion, heart rate, and blood pressure). However, psychological stress is different in that it is not tied to an increased metabolic demand, nor is there a clear beginning or end. Frequent stress-related activation of the HPA axis with concomitant increase in cortisol has been linked to visceral obesity, hypertension, hyperlipidemia, and insulin resistance,[49,50] and an increased risk for chronic conditions such as cardiovascular disease, diabetes, and atherosclerosis.[41]

Exercise training leads to adaptations in the HPA axis response to acute exercise including a higher threshold for activation, resulting in a blunted response to exercise at the same absolute intensity, but also a greater maximal capacity for cortisol secretion.[51-53] This occurs to a similar extent in older individuals.[54] What is not known is whether these HPA axis adaptations to physical stress also translate into similar adaptations to psychological stress since studies of whether fitness is associated with greater resistance to psychosocial stress have primarily focused on cardiovascular reactivity and catecholamine responses. More importantly, the few studies that did include measures of cortisol were not able to demonstrate an increase in cortisol in connection with the challenge.[55-57] Cardiovascular responses to laboratory stressors have been found to be decreased in fit individuals compared to unfit individuals in some studies[56-58] but not in others.[59,60]

Overall, exercise and psychological stress management has shown better results with regard to markers of cardiovascular risks than medical care alone.[61] The strongest positive effect can be achieved with a combination of exercise and psychological stress management.[62] Behavioral interventions are important to increase and maintain physical activity.[46] Therefore, "body tuning" has been proposed as important part of stress management.[63]

18.6 Exercise and Psychological Problems in Patients with Coronary Artery Disease

As noted above, exercise training improves endothelial function, favorably modulates autonomic balance, and has an antithrombotic effect through various mechanisms. Furthermore, exercise training reduces psychosocial stress and may even reduce mortality in patients with CHD.[64]

Effects of exercise on psychiatric disorders in patients with CHD have been well demonstrated. This includes reductions of depression, hostility, anxiety, somatization, and all aspects of psychological distress.[65] In particular, exercise improves both mental and physical stress symptoms in patients with depression.[66] The efficacy of exercise intervention in patients with depression is comparable to the effects of anti-depressant drugs better than the effects of placebo.[67] Because somatic and affective symptoms are associated with myocardial infarction severity and cardiovascular prognosis, exercise is an appropriate intervention under such circumstances.[68] Whether a reduction of high risk behaviors can lead to a subsequent reduction in mortality was recently explored by Milani et al.[69] They found that depressed patients with coronary disease completing exercise training demonstrated a 73% lower mortality than depressed controls. The same group demonstrated the salutary effects of exercise training on high-risk behaviors among which indices of hostility, depression, and overall psychosocial stress could be reduced by 50–70%.[70-76] In a recent prospective randomized study in the setting of cardiac rehabilitation, mortality was approximately fourfold greater in patients with high psychosocial stress than in those with low psychosocial stress (22% vs 5%; $P=0.003$).[36] Exercise training decreased the prevalence of psychosocial stress from 10% to 4% ($P<0.001$) and improved peak oxygen uptake similarly in patients with high and low psychosocial stress. Mortality in patients who improved exercise capacity by $\geq 10\%$ was 60% lower than in patients who had $\leq 10\%$ improvement in exercise capacity and this was also highly significant. Mortality was lower in patients with high psychosocial stress plus greater improvement of exercise capacity compared to patients with high psychosocial stress but little improvement of exercise capacity (0% vs 19%; $P=0.009$). In contrast, there was no significant reduction of mortality in patients with improvement of exercise capacity in patients with low psychosocial stress (4% vs 8%; $P=0.14$).

18.7   Stress Management Programs

Psychological treatment and in particular stress management is an important and mandatory component of cardiac rehabilitation according to the guidelines in Europe, the USA and Canada, and around the world.[77-80] Secondary prevention through exercise-based cardiac rehabilitation is, second to quitting smoking, the behavioral intervention with the best scientific evidence for a contribution to decreased morbidity and mortality in coronary artery disease, in particular after myocardial infarction but also in chronic stable heart failure. The term cardiac rehabilitation describes a broad class of interventions targeting risky behaviors, namely, smoking, lack of exercise, poor eating habits, and often also targets psychological stress. Cardiac rehabilitation programs that focus on psychological factors are largely similar in that they use cognitive-behavioral interventions to reduce distress[19,28] and teach psychophysiological self-regulation skills.[81-83] While previous meta-analytic reviews[84-89] document the effectiveness of multicomponent cardiac rehabilitation programs for reducing mortality and secondary event rates, there are two meta-analyses showing the benefit of adding psychological treatment.[86,90] These issues are further discussed in the Chap. 19 by Talbot-Ellis and Linden.

18.8   Beliefs and Behaviors: Clinical Perspectives on Motivation and Adherence

Stress management programs in cardiac rehabilitation and secondary prevention of CHD have shown mixed results. Based on failures and successes, some general conclusions can be drawn regarding treatment components that increase the likelihood of positive effects on disease outcomes.

Frasure-Smith et al.[91] evaluated the effects of a nurse-based psychosocial support intervention on depression and cardiac endpoints. The nurses had no special training in management of depression and anxiety, purposely in order to evaluate a model that could be implemented in usual care. Depression entails a considerably increased risk of recurrence and cardiac death, independently of other risk factors.[24,27] The hypothesis was that help to manage depression and anxiety would decrease the risk of recurrence. Male and female post-MI patients were offered telephone support and home visits in order to cope with increased anxiety and depression. At follow-up, there were no differences in depression, anxiety, and mortality between male patients in the intervention and usual care control condition. However, the female patients in the intervention had a significantly increased mortality.

The ENRICHD trial[92] evaluated the effects on depression, social support, and mortality of a combined individual and group intervention aimed at reducing depression and increasing social support. The treatment program was based on the Beck model of Cognitive therapy for depression. The overall results showed a significant but small difference in depression scores between intervention and control patients but no differences in mortality. There was a tendency toward increased mortality for the female patients in the intervention, and this unfavorable difference was more pronounced in minority women. The group component had a beneficial effect in white male patients, but the individual sessions had no overall impact. An elevated depression score was required for inclusion in the group treatment, and a majority of patients did not attain that and were thus never included in a group.

The RCPP trial[93] demonstrated a significant difference in CHD mortality between patients receiving stress management in groups and control patients in alternative group treatment. The SUPRIM project also demonstrated significant differences in recurrent MI and mortality between patients in stress management groups and usual care controls.[94] These two treatment programs are similar with respect to group format, longer treatment periods (1–3 years), and focus on stress behavior and reactivity. In order to have an effect on actual behavior, just talk is obviously not enough. In the SUPRIM program, there were separate groups for men and women but results were the same.

Conclusions from the above trials are:

- Group interventions are generally more effective than individual sessions.
- Men and women may need different focus and strategies in stress management.
- Staff conducting the treatment need specialist training.
- The duration of treatment should be at least several months to impact on behavior.
- Most importantly, there must be a focus on *behavioral skills training*.

In this last respect, stress management shares the basic conditions with physical exercise, change of diet, smoking cessation, and other lifestyle changes included in comprehensive cardiac rehabilitation. Actual *behavior change* is needed to obtain an impact on disease progression and medical endpoints. Thus, factors that facilitate behavioral change must be included and applied in the setup of lifestyle interventions. That includes motivation, self-efficacy, practice, modeling, social support, self-monitoring, feedback, a long-term perspective, and a supportive environment (see also Chap. 20 by Rozanski).

The Health Belief Model[95] states that when the individual perceives a threat to health, and believes that there are actions that are under his or her control that can reduce the threat, he or she will engage in that behavior. Most cardiac patients are indeed aware of the threat. However, studies show that it is not uncommon that they hold misconceptions and maladaptive beliefs about their disease.[96] Misconceptions have been shown to be associated with reductions in both functional and psychological status.[96] Patients with misconceptions following MI were less likely to return to work[97] and had more readmissions with chest pain.[98] In a study by Furze et al.,[96] change in angina beliefs over 1 year was the most significant predictor of physical functioning, independently of angina frequency. Reductions of misconceptions were associated with increases in physical functioning. Furze et al.[96] conclude that "health professionals could improve their patients' activity levels and psychological status by spending just a few minutes seeking out and, if necessary, discussing any of these maladaptive beliefs." Such maladaptive beliefs can be changed, and the best evidence has been demonstrated for cognitive-behavioral therapy (CBT) interventions,[99], which should be included in comprehensive cardiac rehabilitation to strengthen patients' beliefs in their own ability to influence disease progression.

The key issue is *self-efficacy*,[100] which means the patient believes that he or she can perform and succeed with the behaviors needed to influence the disease. The treatment program offered to the patient must therefore be organized and scheduled such that the patient perceives that it is realistic for him or her. Many studies have shown that self-efficacy is of great importance for the success and outcome of the behavior change efforts. Gradual practice, beginning with small steps, is realistic for most patients. The first goal is *behavioral*. Then, increasingly larger "doses" of practice will eventually lead to effects on biological and medical parameters.

According to the Transtheoretical Model of motivation and behavior change,[101] individuals often experience a period of ambivalence toward lifestyle change, and it may be important to help patients explore the pros and cons of the new lifestyle versus the old. The opportunity to explore the important needs and reasons for change can strengthen commitment to the program and support long-term motivation and adherence. It is also important to include strategies for reducing the risk of relapsing to old habits. Relapse prevention strategies help the patient to maintain the new lifestyle beyond the time of the active treatment period and to include it as a natural and automatic behavior pattern in everyday life. Important for long-term maintenance is also the mobilization of family support and ensuring a generally health-promoting environment in work and family life.

Among success factors is the specific feedback provided by professionals to the patients on their progress. Self-monitoring techniques such as simple diaries, pedometers, etc., are of great help. Groups have the advantage of offering different perspectives as well as modeling of problem solving. All staff in the cardiac rehabilitation team could serve this function, and follow-up visits also provide social support. The enthusiasm and enduring trust in the patient's ability and potential is a vital reinforcer for the patient's efforts and progress.

18.9 Clinical Implications and Recommendations

Physical activity and exercise training is a cornerstone in comprehensive prevention and rehabilitation. Exercise reduces the psychophysiological response to psychological stress. Stress management programs including physical activity should therefore be considered as an important part of preventive measures in cardiovascular disease management. However, motivation and patient's beliefs are important predictors of adherence to cardiac rehabilitation and secondary prevention programs, and should be taken into consideration when establishing such programs.

References

1. Physical Activity and Cardiovascular Health. NIH consensus development panel on physical activity and cardiovascular health. *JAMA*. 1996;276:241-246.
2. Pate RR, Pratt M, Blair SN, et al. Physical activity and public health. A recommendation from the Centers for Disease Control and Prevention and the American College of Sports Medicine. *JAMA*. 1995;273:402-407.
3. US Department of Health and Human Services. *Physical Activity and Health: A Report of the Surgeon General*. Atlanta: US Department of Health and Human Services, Centers for Disease Control and Prevention, National Center for Chronic Disease Prevention and Health Promotion; 1996.
4. Myers J. Exercise and cardiovascular health. *Circulation*. 2003;107:e2-e5.
5. Lee I-Min, Skerret PJ. Physical activity and all-cause mortality: what is the dose-response relation? *Med Sci Sports Exerc*. 2001;33:S459-S471.
6. Fagard RH. Physical exercise and coronary artery disease. *Acta Cardiol*. 2002;57:91-100.
7. Thompson PD, Buchner D, Piña IL, et al. Exercise and physical activity in the prevention and treatment of atherosclerotic cardiovascular disease. A Statement from the Council on Clinical Cardiology (Subcommittee on Exercise, Rehabilitation, and Prevention) and the Council on Nutrition, Physical Activity, and Metabolism (Subcommittee on Physical Activity). *Circulation*. 2003;107:3109-3116.
8. Williams PT. Physical fitness and activity as separate heart disease risk factors: a meta-analysis. *Med Sci Sports Exerc*. 2001;33:754-761.
9. Blair SN, Cheng Y, Holder JS. Is physical activity or physical fitness more important in defining health benefits? *Med Sci Sports Exerc*. 2001;33:S379-S399.
10. Myers J, Prakash M, Froelicher V, et al. Exercise capacity and mortality among men referred for exercise testing. *N Engl J Med*. 2002;346:793-801.

11. ACSM position stand on the recommended quantity and quality of exercise for developing and maintaining cardiorespiratory and muscular fitness, and flexibility in healthy adults. *Med Sci Sports Exerc.* 1998;30:975-991.

12. Fletcher GF, Balady GJ, Amsterdam EA, et al. Exercise standards for testing and training: a statement for healthcare professionals from the American Heart Association. *Circulation.* 2001;104:1694-1740.

13. Durstine JL, Painter P, Franklin BA, et al. Physical activity for the chronically ill and disabled. *Sports Med.* 2000;30:207-219.

14. Franklin BA, Kahn JK. Delayed progression or regression of coronary atherosclerosis with intensive risk factors modification. Effects of diet, drugs, and exercise. *Sports Med.* 1996;22: 306-320.

15. Billman GE. Aerobic exercise conditioning: a non-pharmacological antiarrhythmic intervention. *J Appl Physiol.* 2002;92:446-454.

16. Hambrecht R, Wolf A, Gielen S, et al. Effect of exercise on coronary endothelial function in patients with coronary artery disease. *N Engl J Med.* 2000;342:454-460.

17. Wenger NK, Froelicher ES, Smith LK, et al. *Cardiac Rehabilitation.* Clinical Practice Guideline No. 17. Rockville: US Department of Health and Human Services, Public Health Service, Agency for Health Care Policy and Research and the National Heart, Lung, and Blood Institute. AHCPR Publication No. 96-0672. October 1995.

18. American Association of Cardiovascular & Pulmonary Rehabilitation. *Guidelines for Cardiac Rehabilitation and Secondary Prevention Programs.* 3rd ed. Champaign: Human Kinetics; 1999.

19. Ades PA. Cardiac rehabilitation and secondary prevention of coronary heart disease. *N Engl J Med.* 2001;345:892-902.

20. Williams MA, Fleg JL, Ades PA, et al. Secondary prevention of coronary heart disease in the elderly (with emphasis on patients Z75 years of age). An American Heart Association scientific statement from the council on clinical cardiology subcommittee on exercise, cardiac rehabilitation, and prevention. *Circulation.* 2002;105:1735-1743.

21. Piepoli MF, Corrá U, Benzer W et al. Secondary prevention through cardiac rehabilitation: from knowledge to implementation. A position paper from the Cardiac Rehabilitation Section of the European Association of Cardiovascular Prevention and Rehabilitation. *Eur J Cardiovasc Prev Rehabil.* 2010;17:1-17.

22. Jolliffe JA, Rees K, Taylor RS, et al. Exercise-based rehabilitation for coronary heart disease (Cochrane review). In: *The Cochrane Library,* vol. 1. Oxford: Update Software; 2003.

23. Mittleman MA, Maclure M, Sherwood JB, et al. Triggering of acute myocardial infarction onset by episodes of anger. Determinants of myocardial infarction onset study investigators. *Circulation.* 1995;92:1720-1725.

24. Frasure-Smith N, Lesperance F, Talajic M. Depression following myocardial infarction. Impact on 6-month survival. *JAMA.* 1993;270:1819-1825.

25. American College of Sports Medicine. *Guidelines for Exercise Testing and Prescription.* 6th ed. Baltimore: Lippincott Williams & Wilkins; 2000.

26. Rozanski A, Blumenthal JA, Davidson KW, et al. The epidemiology, pathophysiology, and management of psychosocial risk factors in cardiac practice: the emerging field of behavioral cardiology. *J Am Coll Cardiol.* 2005;45:637-651.

27. Frasure-Smith N, Lesperance F, Talajic M. Depression and 18-month prognosis after myocardial infarction. *Circulation.* 1995;91:999-1005.

28. Rozanski A, Blumenthal JA, Kaplan J. Impact of psychological factors on the pathogenesis of cardiovascular disease and implications for therapy. *Circulation.* 1999;99: 2192-2217.

29. Rumsfeld JS, Ho PM. Depression and cardiovascular disease: a call for recognition. *Circulation.* 2005;111:250-253.

30. Yusuf S, Hawken S, Ounpuu S, et al. Effect of potentially modifiable risk factors associated with myocardial infarction in 52 countries (the INTERHEART study): case-control study. *Lancet.* 2004;364:937-952.

31. Rosengren A, Hawken S, Ounpuu S, et al. Association of psychosocial risk factors with risk of acute myocardial infarction in 11119 cases and 13648 controls from 52 countries (the INTERHEART study): case control study. *Lancet.* 2004;364:953-962.
32. Blumenthal JA, Lett HS, Babyak MA, et al. Depression as a risk factor for mortality after coronary artery bypass surgery. *Lancet.* 2003;362:604-609.
33. Carney RM, Blumenthal JA, Catellier D, et al. Depression as a risk factor for mortality after acute myocardial infarction. *Am J Cardiol.* 2003;92:1277-1281.
34. Milani RV, Littman AB, Lavie CJ. Psychological adaptation to cardiovascular disease. In: Messerli FH, ed. *Cardiovascular Disease in the Elderly.* 3rd ed. Boston: Kluwer; 1993:401-412.
35. Koskenvuo M, Kaprio J, Rose RJ, et al. Hostility as a risk factor for mortality and ischemic heart disease in men. *Psychosom Med.* 1988;50:330-340.
36. Dembroski TM, MacDougall JM, Costa PT Jr, Grandits GA. Components of hostility as predictors of sudden death and myocardial infarction in the multiple risk factor intervention trial. *Psychosom Med.* 1989;51:514-522.
37. Kawachi I, Sparrow D, Spiro A 3rd, et al. A prospective study of anger and coronary heart disease. The normative aging study. *Circulation.* 1996;94:2090-2095.
38. Kawachi I, Sparrow D, Kubzansky LD, et al. Prospective study of a self-report type a scale and risk of coronary heart disease: test of the MMPI-2 type a scale. *Circulation.* 1998;98:405-412.
39. Allison TG, Williams DE, Miller TD, et al. Medical and economic costs of psychologic distress in patients with coronary artery disease. *Mayo Clin Proc.* 1995;70:734-742.
40. Frasure-Smith N, Lesperance F, Juneau M. Differential long-term impact of in-hospital symptoms of psychological stress after non-Q wave and Q-wave acute myocardial infarction. *Am J Cardiol.* 1992;69:1128-1134.
41. Bjorntorp P. Stress and cardiovascular disease. *Acta Physiol Scand Suppl.* 1997;640:144-148.
42. Shibeshi WA, Young-Xu Y, Blatt CM. Anxiety worsens prognosis in patients with coronary artery disease. *J Am Coll Cardiol.* 2007;49:2021-2027.
43. Thorne LC, Bartholomew JB, Craig J, Farrar RP. Stress reactivity in fire fighters: an exercise intervention. *Int J Stress Manag.* 2000;7:235-246.
44. Bond DS, Lyle RM, Tappe MK, Seehafer RS, D'Zurilla J. Moderate aerobic exercise, t'ai chi, and social problem-solving ability in relation to psychological stress. *Int J Stress Manag.* 2002;9:329-343.
45. Salmon P. Effects of physical exercise on anxiety, depression, and sensitivity to stress: a unifying theory. *Clin Psychol Rev.* 2001;21:33-61.
46. Linden W. *Stress Management. From Basic Science to Better Practice.* London: Sage; 2005.
47. Hescham S, Grace L, Kellaway LA, Bugarith K, Russell VA. Effect of exercise on synaptophysin and calcium/calmodulin-dependent protein kinase levels in prefrontal cortex and hippocampus of a rat model of developmental stress. *Metab Brain Dis.* 2009;24:701-709.
48. Gerber M, Puhse U. Review article: do exercise and fitness protect against stress-induced health complaints? A review of the literature. *Scand J Public Health.* 2009;37:801-819.
49. Hautanen A, Adlercreutz H. Altered adrenocorticotropin and cortisol secretion in abdominal obesity: implications for the insulin resistance syndrome. *J Intern Med.* 1993;234:461-469.
50. Rosmond R, Dallman MF, Bjorntorp P. Stress-related cortisol secretion in men: relationships with abdominal obesity and endocrine, metabolic and hemodynamic abnormalities. *J Clin Endocrinol Metab.* 1998;83:1853-1859.
51. Deuster PA, Petrides JS, Singh A, Lucci EB, Chrousos GP, Gold PW. High intensity exercise promotes escape of adrenocorticotropin and cortisol from suppression by dexamethasone: sexually dimorphic responses. *J Clin Endocrinol Metab.* 1998;83:3332-3338.
52. Kjaer M. Regulation of hormonal and metabolic responses during exercise in humans. *Exerc Sport Sci Rev.* 1992;20:161-184.
53. Luger A, Deuster PA, Kyle SB, et al. Acute hypothalamic–pituitary–adrenal responses to the stress of treadmill exercise. Physiologic adaptations to physical training. *N Engl J Med.* 1987;316:1309-1315.
54. Korkushko OV, Frolkis MV, Shatilo VB. Reaction of pituitary–adrenal and autonomic nervous systems to stress in trained and untrained elderly people. *J Auton Nerv Syst.* 1995;54:27-32.

55. Blaney J, Sothmann M, Raff H, Hart B, Horn T. Impact of exercise training on plasma adrenocorticotropin response to a well-learned vigilance task. *Psychoneuroendocrinology.* 1990;15:453-462.
56. Sinyor D, Schwartz SG, Peronnet F, Brisson G, Seraganian P. Aerobic fitness level and reactivity to psychosocial stress: physiological, biochemical, and subjective measures. *Psychosom Med.* 1983;45:205-217.
57. Sothmann MS, Gustafson AB, Garthwaite TL, Horn TS, Hart BA. Cardiovascular fitness and selected adrenal hormone responses to cognitive stress. *Endocr Res.* 1988;14:59-69.
58. Boutcher SH, Nurhayati Y, McLaren PF. Cardiovascular response of trained and untrained old men to mental challenge. *Med Sci Sports Exerc.* 2001;33:659-664.
59. de Geus EJ, van Doornen LJ, Orlebeke JF. Regular exercise and aerobic fitness in relation to psychological make-up and physiological stress reactivity. *Psychosom Med.* 1993;55: 347-363.
60. Summers H, Lustyk MK, Heitkemper M, Jarrett ME. Effect of aerobic fitness on the physiological stress response in women. *Biol Res Nurs.* 1999;1:48-56.
61. Blumenthal JA, Sherwood A, Babyak MA, et al. Effects of exercise and stress management training on markers of cardiovascular risk in patients with ischemic heart disease: a randomized controlled trial. *JAMA.* 2005;293:1626-1634.
62. Eriksen HR, Ihlebaek C, Mikkelsen A, Gronningsaeter H, Sandal GM, Ursin H. Improving subjective health at the worksite: a randomized controlled trial of stress management training, physical exercise and an integrated health programme. *Occup Med (Lond).* 2002;52:383-391.
63. Schonert-Hirz S. *Meine Stressbalance. Rezepte für Vielbeschäftigte von Dr. Stress.* Frankfurt: Campus Verlag; 2006.
64. Milani RV, Lavie CJ. Reducing psychosocial stress: a novel mechanism of improving survival from exercise training. *Am J Med.* 2009;122:931-938.
65. Rozanski A, Blumenthal J. Cardiac rehabilitation, exercise training, and psychosocial risk factors: REPLY. *J Am Coll Cardiol.* 2005;47:212-213.
66. Heather SL, Davidson J, Blumenthal JA. Nonpharmacologic treatments for depression in patients with coronary heart disease. *Psychosom Med.* 2005;67:58-62.
67. Blumenthal JA, Babyak MA, Doraiswamy PM, et al. Exercise and pharmacotherapy in the treatment of major depressive disorder. *Psychosom Med.* 2007;69:587-596.
68. Martens EJ, Hoen PW, Mittelhaeuser M, de Jonge P, Denollet J. Symptom dimensions of post-myocardial infarction depression, disease severity and cardiac prognosis. *Psychol Med.* 2010;40:1-8.
69. Milani RV, Lavie CJ. Impact of cardiac rehabilitation on depression and its associated mortality. *Am J Med.* 2007;120:799-806.
70. Milani RV, Lavie CJ, Cassidy MM. Effects of cardiac rehabilitation and exercise training programs on depression in patients after major coronary events. *Am Heart J.* 1996;132:726-732.
71. Lavie CJ, Milani RV. Effects of cardiac rehabilitation programs on exercise capacity, coronary risk factors, behavioral characteristics, and quality of life in a large elderly cohort. *Am J Cardiol.* 1995;76:177-179.
72. Lavie CJ, Milani RV. Prevalence of anxiety in coronary patients with improvement following cardiac rehabilitation and exercise training. *Am J Cardiol.* 2004;93:336-339.
73. Lavie CJ, Milani RV. Prevalence of hostility in young coronary artery disease patients and effects of cardiac rehabilitation and exercise training. *Mayo Clin Proc.* 2005;80:335-342.
74. Lucini D, Milani RV, Costantino G, et al. Effects of cardiac rehabilitation and exercise training on autonomic regulation in patients with coronary artery disease. *Am Heart J.* 2002;143: 977-983.
75. Milani RV, Lavie CJ, Mehra MR. Reduction in C-reactive protein through cardiac rehabilitation and exercise training. *J Am Coll Cardiol.* 2004;43:1056-1061.
76. Milani RV, Lavie CJ. Prevalence and profile of metabolic syndrome in patients following acute coronary events and effects of therapeutic lifestyle change with cardiac rehabilitation. *Am J Cardiol.* 2003;92:50-54.

77. Giannuzzi P, Saner H, Björnstad H, et al. Secondary prevention through cardiac rehabilitation: position paper of the working group on cardiac rehabilitation and exercise physiology of the European Society of Cardiology. *Eur Heart J.* 2003;24:1273-1278.

78. Balady GJ, Williams M, Ades PA, et al. Core components of cardiac rehabilitation/secondary prevention programs: 2007 update. A scientific statement from the American Heart Association Exercise, Cardiac Rehabilitation, and Prevention Committee, the Council on Clinical Cardiology; the Councils on Cardiovascular Nursing, Epidemiology and Prevention, and Nutrition, Physical Activity, and Metabolism; and the American Association of Cardiovascular and Pulmonary Rehabilitation. *Circulation.* 2007;115:2675-2682.

79. World Health Organization. Rehabilitation after Cardiovascular Diseases, with Special Emphasis on Developing Countries. Report of a WHO Expert Committee, WHO Technical Report Series, No. 831. 1993; Geneva: World Health Organization.

80. Piepoli MF, Corra U, Benzer W, et al. Review. Secondary prevention through cardiac rehabilitation: from knowledge to implementation. A position paper from the Cardiac Rehabilitation Section of the European Association of Cardiovascular Prevention and Rehabilitation. *EJCPR.* 2010;17:1-17.

81. Jordan J, Barde B, Zeiher AM. *Contributions Toward Evidence-Based Psychocardiology: A Systematic Review of the Literature.* Washington DC: American Psychological Association; 2007.

82. Linden W. Psychological treatments in cardiac rehabilitation: review of rationales and outcomes. *J Psychosom Res.* 2000;48:443-454.

83. American Association of Cardiovascular and Pulmonary Rehabilitation. *Guidelines for Cardiac Rehabilitation and Secondary Prevention Programs.* Champaign: Human Kinetics; 2004.

84. Oldridge NB, Guyatt GH, Fischer ME, Rimm AA. Cardiac rehabilitation after myocardial infarction: combined experience of randomized clinical trials. *JAMA.* 1988;260:945-950.

85. Linden W, Stossel C, Maurice J. Psychosocial interventions for patients with coronary artery disease: a meta-analysis. *Arch Intern Med.* 1996;156:745-752.

86. Dusseldorp E, van Elderen T, Maes S, Meulman J, Kraaij V. A meta-analysis of psychoeducational programs for coronary heart disease patients. *Health Psychol.* 1999;18:506-519.

87. Rees K, Bennett P, West R, Davey SG, Ebrahim S. Psychological interventions for coronary heart disease. *Cochrane Database Syst Rev.* 2004;2:CD002902002E.

88. van Dixhoorn J, White A. Relaxation therapy for rehabilitation and prevention in ischaemic heart disease: a systematic review and meta-analysis. *Eur J Cardiovasc Prev Rehabil.* 2005; 12:193-202.

89. Clark AM, Hartling L, Vandermeer B, McAlister FA. Meta-analysis: secondary prevention programs for patients with coronary artery disease. *Ann Intern Med.* 2005;143:659-672.

90. Linden W, Phillips MJ, Leclerc J. Psychological treatment of cardiac patients: a meta-analysis. *Eur Heart J.* 2007;28:2972-2984.

91. Frasure-Smith N, Lesperance F, Prince RH, et al. Randomised trial of home-based psychosocial nursing intervention for patients recovering from myocardial infarction. *Lancet.* 1997; 16(350):473-479.

92. Berkman LF, Blumenthal J, Burg M, et al. Effects of treating depression and low perceived social support on clinical events after myocardial infarction: the Enhancing Recovery in Coronary Heart Disease Patients (ENRICHD) randomized trial. *JAMA.* 2003;289:3106-3116.

93. Friedman M, Thoresen CE, Gill JJ, et al. Alteration of type A behavior and its effect on cardiac recurrences in post myocardial infarction patients: summary results of the recurrent coronary prevention project. *Am Heart J.* 1986;112:653-665.

94. Gulliksson, M. *Studies of Secondary Prevention after Coronary Heart Disease with Special Reference to Determinants of Recurrent Event Rate.* Digital Comprehensive Summaries of Uppsala Dissertations from the Faculty of Medicine, 472, 2009;ISSN 1651-6206.

95. Sirur R, Richardson J, Wishart L, Hanna S. The role of theory in increasing adherence to prescribed practice. *Physiother Can.* 2009;61:68-77.

96. Furze G, Lewin RJ, Murberg T, Bull P, Thompson DR. Does it matter what patients think? The relationship between changes in patients' beliefs about angina and their psychological and functional status. *J Psychosom Res.* 2005;59:323-329.
97. Maeland JG, Havik OE. Psychological predictors for return to work after a myocardial infarction. *J Psychosom Res.* 1987;31:471-481.
98. Maeland JG, Havik OE. Use of health services after a myocardial infarction. *Scand J Soc Med.* 1989;17:93-102.
99. Goulding L, Furze G, Birks Y. Randomized controlled trials of interventions to change maladaptive illness beliefs in people with coronary heart disease: systematic review. *J Adv Nurs.* 2010;66:946-961.
100. Bandura A. Health promotion by social cognitive means. *Health Educ Behav.* 2004;31: 143-164.
101. Fernandez RS, Davidson P, Griffiths R, Juergens C, Salamonson Y. Development of a health-related lifestyle self-management intervention for patients with coronary heart disease. *Heart Lung.* 2009;38:491-498.

Part V
Psychological Management

Chapter 19
The Psychological Treatment
of Cardiac Patients

Alena Talbot Ellis and Wolfgang Linden

Keywords Psychological treatment • Cardiac patients • INTERHEART study • Cardiac rehabilitation • Anxiety • Depression • Personality factors • Type-A personality • Type-D personality • Gender • Clinical practice

19.1 Chapter Objective

This chapter is meant to provide an overview of the existing research literature from the vantage point of how it can guide clinical practice in behavioral cardiac care. The authors are clinical psychologists who work as researchers and as clinicians. We have learned that psychologists and other mental health experts working in general health settings face a daily need to provide competent patient care even when research findings are not entirely consistent. In this vein, we urge researchers to work together with clinicians to enhance quality of care through research.[1] As research moves from the laboratory to the clinic, there are many threats to the internal validity of research protocols. Health professionals who bridge science and practice often experience a dilemma in the quest for clean methodologies in the face of clinical reality and its inherent constraints. For example, many treatment research questions are best answered in patients who have only one diagnosis and who are not taking medications, yet it is exceedingly difficult to find such patients. Comorbidity of psychological problems is highly prevalent, particularly among older patients. Even if a methodologically "pure" study was conducted, the results might then not generalize. We raise these issues in the introductory section in order to sensitize the reader to the views and values that guided our writing.

In order to provide the planned overview and build a bridge from science to practice, this chapter proceeds by reviewing the nature of the clinical problem at hand,

A. Talbot Ellis • W. Linden (✉)
Department of Psychology, University of British Columbia, Vancouver, BC, Canada
e-mail: wlinden@psych.ubc.ca

P. Hjemdahl et al. (eds.), *Stress and Cardiovascular Disease*,
DOI 10.1007/978-1-84882-419-5_19, © Springer-Verlag London Limited 2012

describing types of psychological interventions available, and summarizing research on what interventions are best for which patients. Three topics that have received limited attention in the past are given special consideration here: (a) gender differences in treatment needs and outcomes, (b) the use of routine screening and patient identification, and (c) the question of when and for whom psychological treatment is indicated. The goal is to provide clear practice guidelines as well as to highlight unresolved research questions.

19.2   The Nature of the Problem

Due to advances in medical interventions for coronary heart disease (CHD), cardiac patients are surviving longer. This also puts them at an increased risk for subsequent cardiac events, including myocardial infarction (MI), cardiac arrhythmias, or sudden cardiac death. The advances in cardiology increase the number of patients requiring long-term attention and costly health care services. We posit here that psychological interventions, in addition to traditional cardiology care and basic cardiac rehabilitation programs, can also aid in reducing the risk of secondary cardiac events.

There is overwhelming evidence that psychological and behavioral factors play a pivotal role in the etiology of heart disease and its recurrence, as detailed elsewhere in this book. Fortunately, these behavioral factors are open to change whereas other risk factors like age and genetics are not. Placing behavioral risk factors in their proper context is greatly aided by reviewing results from the INTERHEART study.[2] INTERHEART was an international case-control study conducted in 52 countries that examined the factors associated with MI in 15,152 individuals who had experienced an MI vs 14,820 controls. Outlined in Table 19.1 are the individual odds ratios for each risk factor along with a cumulative total. It is apparent that combined psychosocial factors (including depression, perceived stress, low locus of control, and major life events) independently increased the risk of MI 2.5-fold. It is also important to mention that many of these risk factors are interrelated and therefore may have a cumulative effect. For example, individuals who exercise less are more likely to have abdominal obesity. Similarly, individuals who suffer from depression are also less likely to exercise.[3] As INTERHEART revealed, the cumulative risk of suffering an MI faced by individuals with all of these risk factors present is 129 times greater than the risk in those without. These data outline the remarkable opportunities inherent in behavioral and emotional risk factor reduction.

Building sound rationales for treatment requires an understanding of the mechanisms by which risk factors lead to disease. Rozanski et al.[4] identified three pathways by which psychosocial factors can impact CHD and subsequent cardiac events:

1. They can contribute to the maintenance of health risk behaviors such as smoking or inactivity.
2. They can directly influence the development of atherosclerosis and result in cardiac events and

Table 19.1 Odds ratios (OR) for risk factors from the INTERHEART study

Rank	Risk factor	OR (and CI)
1	Lipids (top vs lowest quintile)	3.87 (3.4–4.4)
2	Diabetes	3.08 (2.8–3.4)
3	Current smoking	2.95 (2.7–3.2)
4	All psychosocial	2.51 (2.2–2.9)
5	Hypertension	2.48 (2.3–2.7)
6	Abdominal obesity	1.36 (1.2–1.5)
7	Diet (protective effect)	0.70 (0.64–0.77)
8	Exercise (protective effect)	0.72 (0.65–0.79)
9	Alcohol intake (higher intake, lower risk!)	0.79 (0.73–0.86)
	All risk factors together	*129.2 (90.2–185.0)*

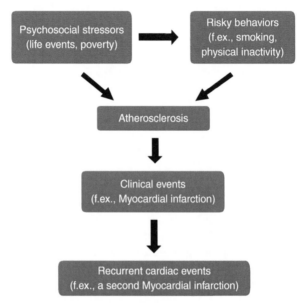

Fig. 19.1 Pathway to disease (Adapted from Rozanski et al.[4])

3. They can increase the risk of recurring cardiac events through acute or chronic pathophysiological means or by contributing to the maintenance of health risk behaviors which are imperative to target in cardiac rehabilitation (see Fig. 19.1).

The issue arises on how these complex pathways may be translated into efficacious treatment approaches.

19.3   Cardiac Rehabilitation

Cardiac risk factors are clearly open to primary prevention via public education campaigns about smoking, self-care, and lifestyle. However, the focus of this chapter is on secondary and tertiary prevention. Most tertiary prevention is embedded in cardiac rehabilitation efforts. Cardiac populations have been consistently found to display marked distress when entering inpatient care units or out-patient cardiac rehabilitation programs, including increased levels of depression and anxiety. Further, a significant portion of these individuals continue to experience elevated distress and impairments in social and vocational functioning years after hospitalization.[5] Psychosocial interventions aim to decrease these consequences and aid in stemming the course of disease progression.

19.3.1 Depression

Clinical depression and depressive mood are fairly prevalent in cardiac patients, and its inherent risk for event recurrence or mortality has been extensively studied. A separate chapter is therefore devoted to this topic alone (Chap. 12 by Hoen, Kupper and DeJonge). Suffice it to say here that recognition and treatment of depression is an integral part of multicomponent cardiac rehabilitation.

19.3.2 Anxiety

Estimates of the prevalence rates for anxiety disorders, including panic disorder and generalized anxiety disorder (GAD) in cardiac patients are approximately 18–26%.[6] A gradient with respect to anxiety symptoms and risk of CHD has also been shown.[7] While depression is primarily associated with increased risk of MI or secondary cardiac events, anxiety is also associated with increased risk of sudden cardiac death, possibly due to ventricular arrhythmia caused by decreased heart rate variability and impaired vagal control.[8] Mechanisms involved in the increased cardiac risk associated with depression and panic disorder are discussed by Esler elsewhere in this book (Chap. 3). However, research in this field is still scant.

19.3.3 Personality Factors

While Type-A personality may first come to mind when considering personality factors that contribute to cardiac events, it has been argued that the critical elements of Type-A personality that are associated with coronary heart disease are anger and hostility (which includes elements of cynicism, anger, and mistrust[9]). Inconsistent findings regarding Type-A behavior are likely due to the fact that some studies have used self-report tools to measure Type-A behavior whereas others are based on observation and rating of overt behavior. The studies treating Type-A as an "observed behavior" have produced more consistent results showing that Type-A is indeed a risk factor.[4] Prospective studies have found one component of Type behavior, namely, hostility, to predict the development of CHD[10] and it has been linked to increased incidences of MI and mortality.[4,11] Intervention trials have found that treatment focused on reducing Type-A behavior, including hostility, in conjunction with stress-management resulted in better health outcomes including a reduction in MI recurrence.[12]

While the concept of Type-A personality as coronary prone is no longer widely accepted, Type-D personality (or distressed personality) is coming into focus. Individuals with Type-D personality display two main traits, social inhibition and negative affect, and can present with depressive symptoms, chronic tension, anger, pessimism, lack of perceived social support, and a low level of subjective well-being. Prospective studies have found that Type-D personality style is associated with 4 to 8 times increased risk of mortality, recurrent MI, or sudden cardiac death.[13] Type-D personality features also include an increased vulnerability to vital exhaustion.[14] Vital exhaustion is characterized by feelings of excessive fatigue and lack of energy, increased irritability, and feelings of demoralization,[15] and has been shown to increase the risk of MI and other cardiac events, perhaps due to increased blood coagulability and impaired fibrinolysis.[16,17] Appels et al.[18,19] have provided preliminary evidence for the usefulness of an intervention for vital exhaustion. Breathing therapy was administered to 30 patients and found to decrease mean exhaustion scores.[18] An additional, small-scale pilot study assessed group therapy designed to reduce stressors leading to exhaustion, and to support recovery by promoting rest and making rest more efficient. The protocol included identification of stressors and help with stress coping, relaxation, and exercise to promote more efficient rest, and reduction of hostility. Results indicated a reduction in subsequent cardiac events for patients with no previous history of CHD; however, this did not translate to a decreased risk for those with a history of CHD.[19] While promising, both of these studies need large-scale replication.

19.3.4   Stress

Over time, chronic stress-induced elevations in heart rate and even more so in blood pressure are thought to create lasting detrimental changes in cardiovascular functioning, including elevation of the tonic blood pressure level, leading to development of cardiovascular disease.[20] Increased reactivity to and delayed recovery from stress has been shown to increase the progression of atherosclerosis,[21,22] and personality factors such as high trait levels of anger/hostility and worry have been shown to predict increased reactivity and delayed recovery.[23,24] Further, daily life stress, including increased levels of family and vocational stress has been found to accelerate disease progression in women[25] and acute life stressors, such as bereavement,[26] earthquakes, and terrorists attacks,[27,28] have been associated with increased rates of cardiac events. Therefore, most psychosocial interventions focus on stress reduction as a component of rehabilitation to reduce further cardiovascular "wear and tear," and secondary cardiac events.

Stress reduction techniques can take two forms. One approach is to emphasize physiological arousal reduction and autonomic balance through relaxation training, meditation, and/or biofeedback, all of which are designed to improve a person's autonomic, self-regulatory skills. Such methods can be taught in a standardized, manual-driven fashion, and two or more methods can be packaged together (e.g., relaxation and temperature biofeedback[29]).

A second approach is to view stress as a multistep process involving triggers, coping behaviors, cognitions, and physiological stress responses.[30] Thus, treatment or intervention may require the teaching of a broad array of problem-solving skills. Treatments using this second, less narrowly focused approach, target deficient cognitive and behavioral stress coping skills, and require more individually tailored, multicomponent interventions because the presumed stress coping deficits are not likely the same across all patients. Indeed, multicomponent, individualized psychological treatments lead to better health outcomes such as greater reduction in blood pressure than do single-component treatments like relaxation training.[31]

19.3.5   Social Support

Low social support has been associated with poor health outcomes; Berkman and colleagues[32] found that individuals with restricted social network were at three times greater risk for all-cause mortality. Conversely, higher levels of *perceived* social support have been found to buffer against the detrimental impact of depression on cardiac mortality rates.[33]

Research assessing the impact of social support has traditionally examined social network size or the number of social interactions and not perceived levels of support.[32] Similarly, many interventions focus on changes in network size and support-seeking behavior rather than in positive appraisals of existing social supports. Furthermore, evidence indicates that educating people in how to not only receive support but to also *offer* support (i.e., a reciprocity principle of support), offers the greatest benefits.[34,35]

19.3.6   Quality of Life

Although addressing the above targets in psychosocial intervention will certainly serve to increase quality of life, treatment goals may include other aspects as well, such as increasing marital support, addressing concerns and difficulties in sexual functioning, helping to adjust with returning to work, as well as addressing existential dilemmas that often arise with major illness.

19.4   The Nature of Psychological Interventions for Cardiac Patients

Previous sections of this chapter already touched on treatment techniques and approaches for various risk factors. As much as risk factors for CHD tend to aggregate and compound one another, the target areas for psychosocial intervention also cluster together. For example, anxiety and depression have a high rate of comorbidity, and Type-D personality features include lack of perceived social support and increased negative affect including depressive symptoms. Accordingly, multicomponent interventions are usually implemented. These interventions tend to involve behavioral targets including weight loss, smoking cessation, nutrition, improved exercise adherence, and efforts to reduce psychological distress such as relaxation strategies, more complex stress management approaches including behavioral change and cognitive retraining, reduction of Type-A behavior, treatment of depression, anxiety, and panic, or any combination of these various methods.[36]

Sotile[5] proposed a model of Effective Emotional Management for structuring psychosocial interventions in medical settings that entails five factors:

1. *Managing the physiological and psychological consequences of stress.* This component includes providing education about the impact of stress on the body, including explanation of the fight or flight response, vital exhaustion, and the General Adaptation Syndrome.
2. *Learning and using an effective method of relaxation.* Often in practice, a combination of strategies is taught including Diaphragmatic Breathing, Progressive Muscular Relaxation, Healing Imagery, and Biofeedback. As well, healthcare professionals can encourage the recall of previously learned or naturally occurring relaxation strategies. Education regarding the benefit of exercise for stress management and prevention of exhaustion is also encouraged.
3. *Controlling personality-based coping patterns.* Sotile[5] describes three reasons for this component. First, assessing coping styles can facilitate matching of delivery of information to an individual's psychological framework. Second, it allows for education regarding potential problems that may be associated with a particular coping style, and third, it aids in providing information regarding the interplay of different coping styles within the family unit and recognition of how this can impact the rehabilitation process. In particular, Type-A behavior patterns, hostility, and anger are targeted.
4. *Managing marital and family issues.* As mentioned above, an individual's social support system can have a huge impact on rehabilitative success. Sotile recommended involving the family in the rehabilitation process, normalizing their own emotional struggles and providing education about helpful versus unhelpful behaviors throughout the rehabilitation process.
5. *Controlling cognitive frames of reference.* This component follows a cognitive behavioral approach, and involves informing patients and families of how their thoughts affect their feelings and behaviors. This allows one to target maladaptive and distressing thinking patterns and replace them with more positive and realistic cognitive frameworks.

The American Association of Cardiovascular and Pulmonary Rehabilitation (AACPR)[37] also recognizes the necessity of adding psychosocial intervention and offers guidelines on what to address in both inpatient and outpatient settings. At an inpatient level, services should include support, education, and anticipatory guidance focused on helping patients and family members to cope with the stresses of hospitalization; help with relaxation including instruction in abdominal breathing and imagery; careful monitoring of clinical levels of distress and referral to specialized services if present; smoking cessation initiation; and discharge planning sessions with both patients and significant others including acknowledging the likelihood of experiencing depression and anxiety upon adjusting to the consequences of their illness, and proactively discussing sexual functioning concerns. The AACPR also acknowledges the need to encourage family participation and reinforcement of positive health behaviors.[37] After discharge, patients should be screened for post-traumatic stress symptoms related to their hospitalization or medical intervention (see also the Chap. 13 by von Känel and Gander). Topics that should be covered in outpatient interventions, regardless of whether in group or individual format, include sexual adjustment and the effect of illness and medication on mood and sexual response; strategies for modifying problem behaviors; hostility and depression and education regarding the impact of these variables on health; the importance of obtaining social support; and general stress management and relaxation training. The AACPR also recognizes the importance of follow-up and continued care once rehabilitation has ended.

19.5   Research on the Efficacy of Psychological Interventions

In order to ascertain the efficacy of psychological interventions for cardiac patients, and indeed the efficacy of any healthcare intervention, well-designed and executed randomized controlled trials (RCTs) are considered the gold standard. The choice of control group can be tricky in psychosocial cardiac rehabilitation because all patients already receive medical treatment and some also participate in exercise rehabilitation or nutrition counseling. All of these treatments are likely to activate perceived social support given that much of rehabilitation occurs in groups.

Guidelines are now available for the design of RCTs. The CONSORT statement, along with the explanation and elaboration document, gives specific guidelines on what information to collect and report.[38] Similarly, the Society for Behavioral Medicine has formed an Evidence-Based Behavioral Medicine committee that disseminates recommendations for designing and implementing behavioral medicine trials (http://www.sbm.org/ebbm/). Accordingly, in this chapter, when possible, RCTs have been provided as evidence for intervention efficacy.

19.5.1   How Well Do Psychological Interventions Work?

As noted above, individual RCTs of psychological interventions have often found support for their efficacy in reducing risk factors for disease progression and recurrence. However, differences between trials exist[36,37] in:

(a) Intervention protocols and targets
(b) Types of service providers involved in an intervention
(c) Whether treatment is individual or group based
(d) When treatment is initiated and
(e) Whether treatments are individualized
(f) Outcomes chosen, and how they were assessed

As such, psychological interventions for cardiac patients are rarely the same across settings, as currently no manualized treatment – a specific protocol for how to implement the intervention, ensuring consistency of treatment across settings and across therapists – has been agreed upon, making it challenging to assess overall efficacy. Indeed, while several small-scale studies have found evidence in favor of the addition of psychosocial interventions and indicate that distress and mortality rates can be reduced, some large clinical trials have failed to show the overall benefits of psychological treatments expected.[39] These seeming contradictions call for explanation and integration. Also, when examining a literature based on small trials, there may be publication bias.

In support of psychosocial components of cardiac rehabilitation are two large-scale studies. Friedman and colleagues[40] examined the impact of reduction of Type A behavior on cardiac recurrence in the Recurrent Coronary Prevention Project (RCPP). Note that the RCPP was not a full random assignment trial because the control group had not been randomized into this arm; therefore, only data from the randomized groups are described here. Eight hundred sixty-two post-MI patients were randomly assigned to either a low impact active treatment group ($n=270$) who received group cardiologic counseling (average of 20 sessions over 3 years) or a high impact active treatment group ($n=592$) who received both standard group cardiologic counseling and Type-A behavioral counseling (average of 29 sessions over 3 years), including instruction in progressive muscular relaxation and what was essentially cognitive behavioral therapy. A significant proportion of those patients receiving the Type-A behavior intervention showed reduction in this behavior (44%), as well as a reduction in nonfatal MI recurrences. The comparison of high versus low impact treatment revealed a distinct gradient effect because more treatment exposure also led to greater improvements. Important to note is that recruitment for the study was at least 6 months following an acute MI. Patients in the control condition did not improve.

Second, the Ischemic Heart Disease Life Stress Monitoring Program (IHDLSM[41,42]) found initial success in terms of mortality reduction. The IHDLSM was based on the notion that periods of stress often precede recurrent cardiac events. Stress levels in 453 male MI patients randomly assigned to an experimental group ($n = 229$) and a control group ($n = 224$) were monitored for 1 year via telephone using Goldberg's General Health Questionnaire (GHQ). When stress levels rose, individually tailored interventions, which included emotional support, education, and, when necessary, referral to other professionals (e.g., five participants were referred to psychiatrists) were implemented by project nurses to reduce stress. Results indicated that men in the experimental group had significantly lower GHQ scores than those in the control group. There were no differences in the degree of rehospitalization; however, individuals in the experimental group were approximately 50% less likely to suffer cardiac death ($n = 27$ vs $n = 48$). Important to note is that these benefits were not wholly apparent until the fourth month of treatment. Long-term follow-up of the study indicated that treatment benefits extended up to 6 months following treatment completion with regard to out-of-hospital (i.e., sudden) cardiac death.[42] Frasure-Smith[43] later reanalyzed the data from IHDLSM, taking into account in-hospital stress levels after the index MI. At 5-year follow-up, those in the control group initially identified as "high stress" showed a three-fold increase in cardiac death and a 1.5 fold increase in recurrent MI compared to those with initial low distress. Treatment did not benefit individuals classified as "low stress" indicating that intervention may only be beneficial for those in distress at the time of treatment initiation.

Intriguingly, the beneficial findings in IHDLSM did not hold when these researchers attempted to replicate and extend the intervention to both men and women (acronym M-HART). In fact, a trend was noted toward greater cardiac and all-cause mortality for women.[44] The authors suggest that the disappointing findings were due to improvements in overall post-MI medical management that translated into reductions in overall mortality rates, necessitating very large sample sizes to detect group differences. Further, they suggest that the M-HART program may have actually increased distress for women due to monthly telephone reminders of their MI and uncovered family or social strains with home visits. Later, these researchers reexamined the data with respect to reduction in distress,[45] and found that individuals who showed reductions in distress (operationalized by reductions in GHQ scores) after two nurse home-visits showed significantly lower cardiac mortality rates, remission rates, and anxiety and depression at 1-year follow-up than those who did not show this reduction. Therefore, the authors suggest that only interventions that are successful in changing physiological, behavioral, or psychological factors will have success in reducing mortality and improving prognosis.

Other larger-scale studies have not found evidence in support of psychosocial intervention. For example, Jones and West[46] conducted a multicentre RCT examining the impact of a 7-week intervention with 2,328 post-MI patients. The intervention consisted of education about MI, treatment and recovery, identification of stress and stress triggers, relaxation training, improvement in stress coping, group discussion, and individual counseling. At 6-month follow-up, there were no differences in rates of depression or anxiety between groups, and in fact the prevalence rates were unchanged from the time of discharge. Further, there were no differences in rates of secondary cardiac events. There was a nonsignificant difference in mortality rates at 6-month follow-up (34 for treatment group and 47 for controls), which was not apparent at 12-month follow-up. Important to note is that mortality was low in this trial (7% over 12 months) and the trial therefore lacked statistical power.[36] Further, the intervention period was relatively short and did not include a risk factor management component.

The Enhancing Recovery in Coronary Heart Disease Patients (ENRICHD) trial also showed disappointing findings,[39] as discussed in Chap. 12 by Hoen, Kupper and de Jonge. ENRICHD was a multicentre randomized trial of a cognitive-behavioral intervention conducted with post-MI patients who had elevated depression scores and low perceived social support on admission to hospital for an acute MI. Patients were randomly assigned to a usual care group ($n = 1,243$) or an intervention group ($n = 1,238$). The intervention consisted of CBT and individual sessions, which were tailored to meet each patient's needs and lasted for 6 months or until optimal treatment outcomes were met. Patients high on scores of depression were referred to psychiatrists for pharmacotherapy if needed and group therapy was also offered after three individual sessions. The study found no difference in mortality or recurrent MI rates within the 4-year follow-up period. Depression scores and levels of perceived social support were improved in the intervention group at 6-month follow-up but were no longer different from controls by 30 and 42 months, respectively.

Triggered by the lack of success in affecting mortality rates, Carney and colleagues[47] noted several limitations in their primary analysis. Therefore, they conducted a reanalysis that shed more light on the nonsignificant findings. They recognized that patients with as few as two depressive symptoms as recently as 1 week prior to recruitment were included in the study. This indicates that many of the subjects recruited may have had transient mood changes that may have resolved spontaneously, thus masking effects for those with more persistent depression. Further, these authors recognized that the primary analysis failed to address whether the intervention was successful for those who actually completed it. Patients who were too ill to participate for a length of time and those who died during the intervention phase of the study were included in the final survival analysis according to the intention-to-treat principle. The ENRICHD reanalysis therefore focused on the subgroup of patients who were more likely to have experienced persistent depression according to the Diagnostic and Statistical Manual IV (DSM – IV) criteria for major or minor depression, and who had a Beck Depression Inventory score of ≥ 10 at baseline – and who also completed the intervention phase. The final sample included 409 usual care patients and 449 intervention patients. Results indicate that those whose depression was unresponsive to treatment were at greater risk for mortality. Therefore, similar to Cossette and colleagues'[45] findings, the benefits of psychosocial intervention may only translate to individuals whose distress is actually reduced.[47]

The evidence for the success of psychosocial intervention in reducing distress and mortality or recurrence rates is somewhat mixed, although the reanalyses described above help shed light on the factors that may mask intervention effects.

Comprehensive meta-analyses have typically focused on the overall efficacy of treatment but have also considered patient characteristics and differences in treatment protocols that may have influenced the success of interventions.[48,49] Nunes et al.[50] conducted a meta-analysis examining psychological treatment for Type-A behavior. The authors found that intervention significantly reduced Type-A behavior, and that multiple modalities of treatment delivery translated to greater success. In particular, successful intervention included a psychoeducational component, a method to increase coping (either relaxation or cognitive therapy) and a behavioral intervention. While the 1-year follow-up for mortality and recurrence showed marginal success, the 3-year follow-up showed an approximately 50% reduction in recurrent MI. However, 3-year follow-up results were only available for two studies. The authors also noted several methodological flaws in the studies and emphasized the need for replication with longer follow-up periods. Also highlighting the need for cautious interpretation is the fact that only 7 of the 18 studies were conducted with individuals documented to have CHD; the remainder enrolled healthy individuals.

A meta-analysis of 23 studies examined the effects of psychosocial interventions when added to other rehabilitation efforts.[51] Results indicated that despite the diversity of psychosocial interventions with respect to length, target behavior, and type of service provider, they were associated with reductions in psychological distress, and positive effects on risk indicators including heart rate, cholesterol levels, and systolic blood pressure. Further, psychosocial intervention was associated with a 46% reduction in recurrence of cardiac events within 2 years and a 39% reduction for a longer follow-up period. There was also a significant 41% reduction in all-cause mortality for follow-up of 2 years or less; only 3 studies examined longer-term follow-up and long-term effects on mortality are uncertain.

Most meta-analyses aggregate psychological treatments into a single category, "active treatment," whereas van Dixhoorn and White[52] conducted a meta-analysis solely on the benefit of relaxation therapy for rehabilitation. Twenty-seven studies were identified that met the criteria. Physiological benefit was seen in the form of reduced resting heart rate, improved exercise tolerance even in the absence of exercise training, and increased heart rate variability. Psychological benefit was also noted with reduction in depression scores, however this effect was largely carried by two studies, and a reduction in state but not trait anxiety was also found. With respect to cardiac effects, there were significant reductions in angina pectoris at rest, and exercise-induced ischemia. The authors also found a significant reduction in composite cardiac events, $(OR = 0.29)$ and cardiac mortality $(OR = 0.29)$ in follow-ups up to 2 years posttreatment. Finally, three studies showed increased rates of return to work at 6 months with relaxation therapy. Important to note is that these benefits largely derived from relaxation taught in a full training format rather than brief instruction. Additionally, the authors note several limitations to their analyses, including inclusion of studies with small sample sizes and few RCTs; there is also a possibility of publication bias in meta-analyses such as this one, and the results need to be interpreted with caution.

Consistent with the reanalyses of major clinical trials discussed above, Dusseldorp and colleagues[48] found that psychological treatment of cardiac patients reduces subsequent mortality if the treatment actually reduces psychological distress. This finding is of great importance in understanding results of treatment studies in the area. It also has major implications for clinical practice: it would seem reasonable to treat until improvement is seen rather than stop at a fixed number of sessions because that was the mandated treatment length of the trial. Of course, such treatment cannot be infinite in length and continuing to treat patients who show no signs of improvement is not well advised. Analysis of 37 studies indicated that interventions including stress management and health education components were associated with a 34% reduction in cardiac mortality and a 29% reduction in MI recurrence at 2–10 years of follow-up. However, this was largely dependent on psychological distress and behavioral risk factors being successfully reduced. For example, studies showing success in this respect demonstrated a 36% reduction in recurrent MIs versus 2% for studies that did not show this success; and 31% versus 14% reductions in mortality, respectively.

Additionally, the most recently published meta-analysis by Linden et al.[49] found that psychosocial interventions when added to other active rehabilitation efforts reduced the odds of mortality by 27% in follow-up periods of 2 years or less, and reduced the recurrence of nonfatal cardiac events up to 43% for follow-up longer than 2 years, but this applied only to male participants. Those patients with little emotional distress did not benefit, and patients who received treatment soon after their cardiac event also did not derive a lot of benefit. On the other hand, patients recruited many months after their surgery or hospitalization who were still in distress showed the greatest mortality reduction (72% in the first 2 years) when distress was treated. Curiously, some clinical trials have offered psychological treatments to all patients even though some were not distressed to begin with; such studies predictably suffer from "floor effects," that is, inability to show further improvement, and failed to find treatment effective.[53]

Reviews have also indicated that beneficial effects of rehabilitation may weaken over time irrespective of whether there is a psychological intervention component.[54] Therefore, it is essential that researchers conduct long-term follow-up studies to assess treatment efficacy.

19.6   The Issue of Gender in Cardiac Rehabilitation

There is growing evidence that careful consideration of the patient's gender may be pivotal in assuring equal quality services for men and women alike. In order to enact efficacious rehabilitation, patients need to actively participate but participation rates in rehabilitation programs are often low despite the overwhelming evidence for benefits.[55,56] Participation is typically around 25–31% for men and a paltry 11–20% for women.[57-59] Furthermore, persistence is poor as 40–50% of patients fail to remain in the program after 6 months.[59,60]

A review of possible predictors of participation and adherence to program attendance reported that the physicians' endorsement and attitude toward the effectiveness of a cardiac rehabilitation predicted ongoing participation, as did ease of physical access and transportation.[59] Individual variables such as high self-efficacy and social support, along with high levels of socioeconomic status and education also predicted increased participation. Predictors of lack of participation included lack of insurance coverage and gender – women were less likely to participate. The lower rate of participation in women was hypothesized to be due to lower referral rates, old age, obesity, disease severity, family obligations, and role resumptions. Other studies have supported these findings and indicate that the variables found to be critical for adherence are specific to the disease, the treatments themselves, the cost and efforts of prevention, and characteristics of the health care environment ([61]; see also Chap. 20 by Rozanski et al.).

Not surprisingly, emotional states can also impact participation and adherence. Lane and colleagues[62] found that higher ratings of anxiety and depression prior to an MI event predicted nonattendance. Further, Caulin-Glaser and colleagues[63] found that depressed women were more likely to not complete cardiac rehabilitation than nondepressed women. Given that female cardiac patients are at greater risk for depression than male patients, this may in part explain why participation is lower in women than in men. However, it also highlights the need to be proactive in the detection and treatment of depression in all patients (see also the Chap. 12 by Hoen et al.).

The meta-analysis conducted by Linden et al. highlights that psychosocial interventions have not shown improvements in mortality and morbidity for women. This observation is critical because mortality rates are positively associated with the higher age of the average female cardiac patient, with increased illness severity at time of diagnosis and higher rates of comorbid disease such as diabetes.[64] Research has also found specific psychosocial factors that contribute to the poorer prognosis in women than men, such as feelings of guilt and inadequacy due to the inability to care for others including their often older spouses,[65] and increased ratings of depression.[66,67] As mentioned above, women are less likely to be referred for cardiac rehabilitation, and even if referred, they adhere less and show less improvement when participating than do men.[68] Therefore, the current challenge for the field is to develop interventions that meet the unique needs of female cardiac patients.[69]

Preliminary research focused on developing strategies specifically for women have shown promising results. For example, a recent RCT by Orth-Gomér et al.[70] examined a women only, group-based psychosocial intervention for CHD, and showed a two thirds decrease in mortality rates (25 vs 8 in the intervention group; $p < 0.007$) across a 9-year follow-up period. The ambitious intervention was based on cognitive-behavior therapy principles and focused on stress reduction and coping surrounding marriage or vocation, along with education surrounding CHD, recognizing cognitive distortions, combating depression and anxiety, and improving social relations and support. Further research in sex-specific interventions is needed in order to develop successful and comprehensive programs.

19.7   Conclusions and Recommendations for Clinical Practice

Emotional distress is prevalent in cardiac patients and evidence supports the addition of a psychosocial treatment component for those patients with elevated distress. The studies reviewed above suggest that multicomponent, long-term psychological interventions lead to better outcomes than brief, single-technique interventions. There is a distinct gradient effect in that more treatment exposure leads to better outcomes via greater patient behavior change.[40] To maximize the benefit achievable for all cardiac patients, clinicians need to focus on removing barriers to participation in cardiac rehabilitation and to facilitate adherence to behavioral prescriptions. Practitioners need to recognize the pivotal role of their endorsement of cardiac rehabilitation, and there is a need for addressing transportation barriers, and increasing self-efficacy and social support.[59] There is also a strong case for the need to address gender issues in referral, treatment, and retention. Traditional approaches to cardiac rehabilitation seem to have been tailored for men and do not appeal to women who feel that their needs are not fully met.[69]

Another issue of concern is our limited knowledge about the natural trajectory of change in distress over time. The analysis by Linden and colleagues[49] highlights the need for distress tracking, not only right after diagnosis and initial treatment but continually throughout rehabilitation and follow-up. Some initially distressed patients get better on their own, some do not change, and others continue to get worse.[71] Schrader and colleagues[71] found that of individuals with signs of mild depression upon admission to hospital, 16% were still moderately to severely depressed 3 months later, and of those with moderate to severe depression at time of admission, 60% remained moderately to severely depressed. If distress screening was implemented only at the stage of referral to cardiac rehabilitation, then those who continue to show distress or get worse later on would not receive adequate care. Consistent with this observation is that when distressed patients are treated very early after an MI, they do not benefit in terms of mortality reduction; on the other hand, identifying and treating patients who are still distressed many months after an MI has been shown to lead to significantly longer survival.[49] Two meta-analyses[48,49] suggest that the psychological treatment of cardiac patients needs to continue until distress is measurably reduced. What actually should happen in clinical practice, namely, to treat until success, is not adequately tested in clinical trials of psychological therapy where treatment length is usually fixed.

Despite the existence of a large population of patients who experience significant psychosocial distress, routine distress screening is not common practice and many patients who could benefit from psychological treatment never receive it. The goal of screening is to assure equitable resource allocation and best patient care, that is, to proactively identify patients in need of professional help. However, these laudable goals can be achieved only when distress screening has become routine.

Grissom and Phillips[72] suggest that the most significant barriers to consistent screening by physicians are: (1) lack of training in detecting and treating depression; (2) skepticism that treating depression will improve medical outcomes; and (3) limitations of depression assessment tools, including lengthy administration and scoring procedures. While providing every patient with an extensive psychological battery to assess distress is certainly not feasible in terms of cost and resources, screening tools with relatively few items have now been developed to identify those who may require more extensive assessment or referral to psychological services. For example, the Hospital Anxiety and Depression Scale[73] or the Screening Tool for Psychological Distress (STOP-D[74];) are such measures. The STOP-D taps into the most common psychosocial problems in cardiac patents, namely, depression, anxiety, stress, hostility/anger, and inadequate social support, has only five items and takes only 1–2 min to complete. It has shown similar success in identifying those in distress as longer validated scales.[74] In summary, we posit that screening for psychological distress need not be cumbersome or expensive.

19.8   Conclusion

Given the high prevalence of psychosocial distress in cardiac patients and its impact on morbidity, mortality, and quality of life, it follows that psychosocial interventions should be key components of rehabilitative care. While the implementation of various elements of psychological intervention in a cardiac rehabilitation program is dependent on the institutions' philosophy of care and resources, the reader should be heartened by the fact that relatively inexpensive psychosocial interventions have the potential for substantial improvements in function and quality of life, and may reduce mortality and cardiac events. Last but not least, clinical practice is sensitive to cost-benefit considerations. Numerous studies have found evidence that multicomponent rehabilitation programs are cost-effective because they reduce subsequent hospitalizations and surgeries (e.g., [75]).

Urgently needed are the following:

1. Studies of natural trajectories of distress and determination of the best time for offering treatment
2. Efficacy evaluations of routine use of women-centered rehabilitation programs
3. Studies on the implementation of simple routine screening protocols and assessment of their outcomes
4. Identification of the minimal set of elements needed for effective psychological treatment of cardiac patients.

References

1. Linden W, Wen FK. Therapy outcome research, social policy and the continuing lack of accumulating knowledge. *Prof Psychol Res Pract.* 1990;21:482-488.
2. Yusuf S, Hawken S, Ounpuu S, et al. For the INTERHEART study investigators. Effect of modifiable risk factors associated with myocardial infarction in 52 countries (the INTERHEART study): case control study. *Lancet.* 2004;364:937-952.

3. Strawbridge WJ, Deleger S, Roberts RE, Kaplan GA. Physical activity reduces the risk of subsequent depression for older adults. *Am J Epidemiol.* 2002;156:328-334.
4. Rozanski A, Blumenthal JA, Kaplan J. Impact of psychological factors on the pathogenesis of cardiovascular disease and implications for therapy. *Circulation.* 1999;99:2192-2217.
5. Sotile WM. *Psychosocial Interventions for Cardiopulmonary Patients.* Champaign: Human Kinetics; 1996.
6. Haworth JE, Moniz-Cook E, Clark AL, Wang M, Waddington R, Cleland JGF. Prevalence and predictors of anxiety and depression in a sample of chronic heart failure patients with left ventricular systolic dysfunction. *Eur J Heart Fail.* 2005;7:803-808.
7. Kubzansky LD, Kawachi I, Weiss ST, Sparrow D. Anxiety and coronary heart disease: a synthesis of epidemiological, psychological, and experimental evidence. *Ann Behav Med.* 1998;20:47-58.
8. Kawachi I, Sparrow D, Vokonas PS, Weiss ST. Symptoms of anxiety and risk of coronary heart disease: the Normative Aging study. *Circulation.* 1994;90:2225-2229.
9. Donker FJS. Cardiac rehabilitation: a review of current developments. *Clin Psychol Rev.* 2000;20:923-943.
10. Koskenvuo M, Kaprio J, Rose RJ, et al. Hostility as a risk factor for mortality and ischaemic heart disease in men. *Psychosom Med.* 1998;50:330-340.
11. Chaput LA, Adams SH, Simon JA, et al. Hostility predicts recurrent events among postmenopausal women with coronary heart disease. *Am J Epidemiol.* 2002;156(12):1092-1099.
12. Burell G, Ohman A, Sundin O, et al. Modification of the type A behavior pattern in postmyocardial infarction patients: a route to cardiac rehabilitation. *Int J Behav Med.* 1994;1:32-54.
13. Denollet J, Sys SU, Stroobant N, Rombouts H, Gillebert TC, Brutsaert DL. Personality as independent predictor of long term mortality in patients with coronary heart disease. *Lancet.* 1996;347:417-421.
14. Pedersen SS, Denollet J. Type D personality, cardiac events, and impaired quality of life: a review. *Eur J Cardiovasc Prev Rehabil.* 2003;10:241-248.
15. Appels A. Mental precursors of myocardial infarction. *Br J Psychiatry.* 1990;156:465-471.
16. Appels A, Mulder P. Fatigue and heart disease. The association between 'vital exhaustion' and past, present and future coronary heart disease. *J Psychosom Res.* 1989;33:727-738.
17. Kop WJ, Hamulyak K, Pernot C, Appels A. Relationship of blood coagulation and fibrinolysis to vital exhaustion. *Psychosom Med.* 1997;60:352-358.
18. Appels A, Bar F, Lasker J, Flamm U, Kop W. The effect of a psychological intervention program on the risk of a new coronary event after angioplasty: a feasibility study. *J Psychosom Res.* 1997;43(2):209-217.
19. Appels A, Bär F, van der Pol G. Effects of treating exhaustion in angioplasty patients on new coronary events: results of the randomized exhaustion intervention trial (EXIT). *Psychosom Med.* 2005;67:217-223.
20. Schwartz AR, Gerin W, Davidson KW, et al. Toward a causal model of cardiovascular responses to stress and the development of cardiovascular disease. *Psychosom Med.* 2003;65:22-35.
21. Barnett PA, Spence JD, Manuck SB, Jennings JR. Psychological stress and the progression of carotid artery disease. *J Hypertens.* 1997;15:49-55.
22. Chida Y, Steptoe A. Greater cardiovascular responses to laboratory mental stress are associated with poor subsequent cardiovascular risk status: a meta-analysis of prospective evidence. *Hypertension.* 2010;55:1026-1032.
23. Anderson JC, Linden W, Habra ME. The importance of examining blood pressure reactivity and recovery in anger provocation research. *Int J Psychophysiol.* 2005;57:159-163.
24. Lai JY, Linden W. Gender, anger expression style, and opportunity for anger release determine cardiovascular reaction to and recovery from anger provocation. *Psychosom Med.* 1992; 54:297-310.
25. Wang HX, Leineweber C, Kirkeeide R. Psychosocial stress and atherosclerosis: family and work stress accelerate progression of coronary disease in women. The Stockholm Female Coronary Angiography Study. *J Intern Med.* 2007;261:245-254.

26. Kaprio J, Koskenvuo M, Rita H. Mortality after bereavement: a prospective study of 95,647 persons. *Am J Public Health*. 1987;77:283-287.
27. Leor J, Poole WK, Kloner RA. Sudden cardiac death triggered by an earthquake. *N Engl J Med*. 1996;334:413-419.
28. Meisel SR, Kutz I, Dayan KI, et al. Effects of the Iraqi missile war on incidence of acute myocardial infarction and sudden death in Israeli civilians. *Lancet*. 1991;338:660-661.
29. Jacob RG, Chesney MA, Williams DM, et al. Relaxation therapy for hypertension: design effects and treatment effects. *Ann Behav Med*. 1991;13:5-17.
30. Linden W. *Stress Management: From Basic Science to Better Practice*. Thousand Oaks: Sage; 2005.
31. Linden W, Moseley JV. The efficacy of behavioral treatments for hypertension. *Appl Psychophysiol Biofeedback*. 2006;31:51-63.
32. Berkman LF, Leo-Summers L, Horwitz RI. Emotional support and survival after myocardial infarction: a prospective, population-based study of the elderly. *Ann Intern Med*. 1992;117:1003-1009.
33. Frasure-Smith N, Lesperance F, Gravel G, et al. Social support, depression, and mortality during the first year after myocardial infarction. *Circulation*. 2000;101(16):1919-1924.
34. Ahern MM, Hendryx MS. Social capital and risk for chronic illnesses. *Chronic Illn*. 2005;1:183-190.
35. Hogan B, Linden W, Najarian B. Social support interventions: do they work? *Clin Psychol Rev*. 2002;22:381-440.
36. Linden W. Psychological treatments in cardiac rehabilitation: review of rationales and outcomes. *J Psychosom Res*. 2000;48:443-454.
37. Balady GJ, Williams MA, Ades PA, et al. Core components of cardiac rehabilitation/secondary prevention programs: 2007 update: a scientific statement from the American Heart Association Exercise, Cardiac Rehabilitation, and Prevention Committee, the Council on Clinical Cardiology; the Councils on Cardiovascular Nursing, Epidemiology and Prevention, and Nutrition, Physical Activity, and Metabolism; and the American Association of Cardiovascular and Pulmonary Rehabilitation. *Circulation*. 2007;115:2675-2682.
38. Moher D, Schulz KF, Altman DG. The CONSORT statement: revised recommendations for improving the quality of reports of parallel-group randomised trials. *Lancet*. 2001;357(9263):1191-1194.
39. Writing committee for the ENRICHD investigators. Effects of treating depression and low perceived social support on clinical events after myocardial infarction: the enhancing recovery in coronary heart disease patients (ENRICHD) randomized trial. *JAMA*. 2003;289:3106-3116.
40. Friedman M, Thoreson C, Gill J, et al. Alteration of type a behavior and reduction in cardiac recurrences in post-myocardial infarction patients. *Am Heart J*. 1984;108:237-248.
41. Frasure-Smith N, Prince R. The ischemic heart disease life stress monitoring program: impact on mortality. *Psychosom Med*. 1985;47:431-445.
42. Frasure-Smith N, Prince R. Long-term follow-up of the ischemic heart disease life stress monitoring program. *Psychosom Med*. 1989;51:485-513.
43. Frasure-Smith N. In-hospital symptoms of psychological stress as predictors of long-term outcome after acute myocardial infarction in men. *Am J Cardiol*. 1991;67:121-127.
44. Frasure-Smith N, Lesperance F, Prince R, et al. Randomised trial of home-based psychosocial nursing intervention for patients recovering from myocardial infarction. *Lancet*. 1997;350(9076):473-479.
45. Cossette S, Frasure-Smith N, Lesperance F. Clinical implications of a reduction in psychological distress on cardiac prognosis in patients participating in a psychosocial intervention program. *Psychosom Med*. 2001;63(2):257-266.
46. Jones DA, West RR. Psychological rehabilitation after myocardial infarction: multicentre randomized controlled trial. *BMJ*. 1996;313(7071):1517-1521.
47. Carney RM, Blumenthal JA, Freedland KE, et al. Depression and late mortality after myocardial infarction in the Enhancing Recovery in Coronary Heart Disease (ENRICHD) study. *Psychosom Med*. 2004;66(4):466-474.

48. Dusseldorp E, Van Elderen T, Maes S, Meulman J, Kraail V. A meta-analysis of psycho-educational programs for coronary heart disease patients. *Health Psychol.* 1999;18:506-519.
49. Linden W, Phillips MJ, Leclerc J. Psychological treatment of cardiac patients: a meta analysis. *Eur Heart J.* 2007;28:2972-2984.
50. Nunes EV, Frank KA, Kornfeld DS. Psychological treatment for the type a behavior pattern and for coronary heart disease: a meta-analysis of the literature. *Psychosom Med.* 1987;48: 159-173.
51. Linden W, Stossel C, Maurice J. Psychosocial interventions for patients with coronary artery disease: a meta-analysis. *Arch Intern Med.* 1996;156(7):745-752.
52. van Dixhoorn J, White A. Relaxation therapy for rehabilitation and prevention in ischaemic heart disease: a systematic review and meta-analysis. *Eur J Cardiovasc Prev Rehabil.* 2005; 12(3):193-202.
53. Linden W, Satin JR. Avoidable pitfalls in behavioral medicine outcome research. *Ann Behav Med.* 2007;33:143-147.
54. Clark AM, Hartling L, Vandermeer B, McAlister FA. Meta-analysis: secondary prevention programs for patients with coronary artery disease. *Ann Intern Med.* 2005;143:659-672.
55. Lau J, Antman E, Jimenez-Silva J, et al. Cumulative meta-analysis of therapeutic trials for myocardial infarction. *N Engl J Med.* 1992;327:248-254.
56. Osevala NM, Malani PN. Cardiac rehabilitation in older adults: benefits and barriers. *Clin Geriatr Med.* 2008;16:22-24.
57. Ades PA, Waldmann ML, McCann WJ, Weaver SO. Predictors of cardiac rehabilitation participation in older coronary patients. *Arch Intern Med.* 1992;152(5):1033-1035.
58. Barber K, Stommel M, Kroll J, et al. Cardiac rehabilitation for community-based patients with myocardial infarction: factors predicting discharge recommendation and participation. *J Clin Epidemiol.* 2001;54:1025-1030.
59. Jackson L, Leclerc J, Erskine Y, Linden W. Getting the most out of cardiac rehabilitation: a review of referral and adherence predictors. *Heart.* 2005;91:10-14.
60. Oldridge NB, Guyatt GH, Fischer ME, Rimm AA. Cardiac rehabilitation after myocardial infarction: combined experience of randomized clinical trials. *JAMA.* 1988;260:945-950.
61. Poole G, Hunt Matheson D, Cox DN. *The Psychology of Health and Health Care: A Canadian Perspective.* 3rd ed. Toronto: Pearson Prentice-Hall; 2008.
62. Lane D, Carroll D, Ring C, Beevers DG, Lip GYH. Predictors of attendance at cardiac rehabilitation after myocardial infarction. *J Psychosom Res.* 2001;51:497-501.
63. Caulin-Glaser T, Maciejewski PK, Snow R, LaLonde M, Mazure C. Depressive symptoms and sex affect completion rates and clinical outcomes in cardiac rehabilitation. *Prev Cardiol.* 2007;10:15-21.
64. Mosca L, Manson JE, Sutherland SE, et al. Cardiovascular disease in women. A statement for healthcare professionals from the American Heart Association. *Circulation.* 1997;96: 2468-2482.
65. MacKenzie G. Role patterns and emotional responses of women with ischemic heart disease 4 to 6 weeks after discharge form hospital. *Can J Cardiovasc Nurs.* 1993;4:9-15.
66. Katz C, Martin RD, Landa B, Chadda KD. Relationship of psychological factors to frequent symptomatic ventricular arrhythmia. *Am J Med.* 1985;78:589-594.
67. Frasure-Smith N, Lesperance F, Talajic M. Depression and 18-month prognosis after myocardial infarction. *Circulation.* 1995;91(4):999-1005.
68. Shuster PM, Waldron J. Gender differences in cardiac rehabilitation patients. *Rehabil Nurs.* 1991;16:248-253.
69. Abbey SE, Stewart DE. Gender and psychosomatic aspects of ischemic heart disease. *J Psychosom Res.* 2000;48:417-423.
70. Orth-Gomér K, Schneiderman N, Wang HX, Walldin C, Blom M, Jernberg T. Stress reduction prolongs life in women with coronary disease: the Stockholm Women's Intervention Trial for Coronary Heart Disease (SWITCHD). *Circ Cardiovasc Qual Outcomes.* 2009;2:25-32.
71. Schrader G, Check F, Hordacre AL, Guiver N. Predictors of depression three months after cardiac hospitalization. *Psychosom Med.* 2004;66:514-520.

72. Grissom GR, Phillips RA. Screening for depression: this is the heart of the matter. *Arch Intern Med.* 2005;165:1214-1215.
73. Bjelland I, Dahl AA, Haug TT, Neckelmann D. The validity of the hospital anxiety and depression scale: an updated literature review. *J Psychosom Res.* 2002;52:69-77.
74. Young QR, Ignaszewski A, Fofonoff D, Kaan A. Brief screen to identify 5 of the most common forms of psychosocial distress in cardiac patients: validation of the screening tool for psychological distress. *J Cardiovasc Nurs.* 2007;22:525-534.
75. Ades PA, Pashkow FJ, Nestor JR. Cost-effectiveness of cardiac rehabilitation after myocardial infarction. *J Cardiopulm Rehabil.* 1997;17:222-231.

Chapter 20
Integrating the Management of Psychosocial and Behavior Risk Factors into Clinical Medical Practice

Alan Rozanski

Keywords Psychosocial risk factors • Behavioral risk factor • Chronic stress • Negative emotions • Stress management • Coronary artery disease

Coronary heart disease (CHD) constitutes the leading cause of death in Western societies and is increasingly prevalent in developing nations. Advances in modern medical treatment for CHD has helped to tame the clinical consequences of heart disease, but the overall prevalence of CHD risk factors remains very high in society and is increasing in epidemic proportion for obesity and diabetes, both among adults and children. Hence, a high prevalence of CHD is predicted for well into the twenty-first century. It is apparent, therefore, that the development of better strategies for reducing the overall risk burden for CHD has become necessary.

Strategies for reducing CHD risk have focused on the promotion of better nutritional choices and avoidance of overeating and overweight, increasing physical activity, smoking cessation, and improving medication adherence. In addition, psychosocial risk factors directly contribute to the development and/or progression of CHD, and importantly, these factors can substantially impair patients' ability to maintain healthy lifestyle habits and adhere to recommended behavioral changes.[1] To date, however, the management of psychosocial risk factors has been poorly integrated into the clinical management of patients with suspected CHD. There a number of reasons for this. First, whereas there is a general awareness that certain psychological factors such as depression are causative of CHD, the magnitude of these relationships is generally underestimated by physicians. Secondly, although

A. Rozanski
Cardiology Fellowship Training Program, Department of Medicine,
St. Luke's Roosevelt Hospital Center, Columbia University College of Physicians and Surgeons,
New York, NY, USA
e-mail: ar77@columbia.edu

P. Hjemdahl et al. (eds.), *Stress and Cardiovascular Disease*,
DOI 10.1007/978-1-84882-419-5_20, © Springer-Verlag London Limited 2012

there are Guidelines on cardiac rehabilitation and secondary prevention which include lifestyle interventions (e.g., the AACVPR/ACC/AHA guidelines) and several Guidelines on the primary prevention of CHD, there are no existing practical guidelines that instruct physicians as to how to integrate the management of psychological risk factors into ordinary clinical care. Third, the evidence base concerning the effectiveness of behavioral interventions that incorporate psychological practices is limited, with conflicting results among the few large behavioral interventions trials that have been conducted among cardiac patients.[2-8] However, in recent years, an increasing number of evidence-based psychological approaches that can help improve patients' health behaviors have emerged. If these approaches could be integrated into clinical medicine, they may offer means for improving clinical care and reducing CHD risk factors.

Accordingly, in this chapter, I will provide a broad perspective as to psychological factors that are causative risk factors for CHD, pointing out pertinent epidemiological and pathophysiological associations. Second, I will provide an overview of various means by which psychosocial interventions can be used in ordinary clinics to help patients better manage "conventional" behavioral risk factors, such as smoking and poor diet, as well as adverse psychological factors, such as chronic stress. Finally, I will discuss practical means for developing a health delivery approach that could incorporate psychological principles into the management of patients with suspected or known CHD.

20.1 The Spectrum of Psychosocial Risk Factors That Cause Disease

Epidemiological study has established a wide spectrum of psychosocial risk factors that may contribute to the pathogenesis of CHD and/or may increase the risk for adverse coronary events. These factors can be divided into (1) chronic stress; (2) negative thought and emotions; (3) the inability to fulfill basic psychological needs; and (4) inadequate rest and relaxation ("R&R") (Table 20.1). Each of these domains is discussed below:

20.1.1 Chronic Stress

Stress is "good" when it challenges us in a meaningful way and we can cope with it. Coping with such stress engages our innate need for purpose and helps us to develop a sense of mastery and self-esteem. By contrast, when stress is uncontrollable or cannot be mastered, and persists for long periods of time, such unpleasantness may lead to widespread pathophysiological damage. Chronic stress is unique among psychosocial risk factors because it can be produced and quantified in animals and then studied for its adverse pathophysiological effects in a controlled environmental

Table 20.1 Spectrum of psychosocial risk factors

A. *Negative thought patterns and emotions*
  1. Depressive syndromes
  2. Anxiety syndromes
  3. Worry
  4. Hostility and anger
  5. Rumination
  6. Resentment
  7. Pessimism
B. *Chronic stress*
  1. Work stress
  2. Marital stress and dissatisfaction
  3. Social isolation and lack of social support
  4. Low socioeconomic status
  5. Caregiver strain
  6. Trauma or abuse in childhood
  7. Perceived injustice
C. *Unsatisfied basic psychological needs*
  1. Sense of purpose
  2. Social connectedness
  3. Sense of security
  4. Autonomy
D. *Lack of rest and relaxation*
  1. Sleep loss
  2. Difficulty in unwinding
  3. Lack of vacations
  4. Time pressure

setting (see Chap. 2 by Shively). For example, when male cynomolgus monkeys are placed into new groups, they initially fight with each other to establish a social hierarchy of most dominant to most subordinate monkeys. If the monkeys are placed into new groups every few months, a chronic socially adverse environment is thus established, with the male dominant monkeys in such unstable groups developing significantly more atherosclerosis than dominant monkeys in stable social groups.[9] This effect of chronic stress stems from continual stimulation of the hypothalamic-pituitary-adrenocortical (HPA) axis and the sympathetic nervous system (SNS) system.[10] Studies demonstrate that such continual stimulation is associated with elevated inflammatory proteins, such as C-reactive protein,[11,12] a heightened frequency of metabolic syndrome and central obesity,[11,12] signs of hypercoagulability,[10,13] hypertension,[14,15] autonomic impairment,[16] evidence of accelerated aging,[17] and accentuated heart rate and blood pressure responsiveness, with prolonged recovery, when chronically stressed individuals or animals are exposed to acute stress.[10] This heightened cardiovascular reactivity has been linked to accelerated atherosclerosis.[1] In addition, as demonstrated by McEwen et al.,[18] the brain itself appears to be a target organ for chronic stress, as manifested by functional enlargement of the amygdala and diminution in the size of the hippocampus and prefrontal cortex. These issues are addressed in greater detail in other chapters in this book.

The epidemiological evidence that links chronic stress to adverse outcomes is extensive. For example, the INTERHEART case–control study examined predictors of myocardial infarction among 12,461 acute post-MI patients who were matched to comparable control subjects. A crude index of chronic stress was strongly predictive of myocardial infarction, with a risk ratio that was comparable to other measured CHD risk factors in this large study.[19] Increasing epidemiological data has identified relationships between CHD and specific forms of chronic stress (Table 20.1). Among these stressors, chronic work stress has been particularly studied. For instance, the presence of high job demand but low job latitude, or high demand and low "reward" in terms of pay, job security, satisfaction, or recognition, has both been shown to increase CHD risk.[10,20,21] In addition, an increasing literature has linked chronic marital stress to adverse cardiac outcomes, including its progression during serial carotid ultrasound and CAC scan studies.[22-25] Among other forms of stress, caregiver strain is also quite common today, but its direct effect on cardiac outcomes has received little study to date.

20.1.2   Chronically Negative Thought Patterns and Emotions

An increasing number of negative cognitive and emotional patterns have been linked to adverse clinical outcomes (Table 20.1; see also Chap. 19 by Talbot Ellis and Linden). Chronic negative thoughts and emotions are appropriately grouped together because of their bi-directional relationship. Negative thoughts lead to negative emotions, but the converse is also true. That is, negative emotional states tend to produce a general cognitive restrictiveness, characterized by less flexible and less creative thinking, a narrowed scope of attention, and decreased problem-solving skills, as shown by Fredrickson et al.[26] Substantial pathophysiology may ensue when people experience chronically negative thoughts or emotions. These effects have best been illustrated for depression (Fig. 20.1). As with chronic stress, major depression leads to chronic HPA and SNS activation which may result in adverse effects such as insulin resistance and increased risk for diabetes, abdominal obesity, osteoporosis, platelet dysfunction, elevation in inflammatory proteins, and endothelial dysfunction[27-34] (see also Chap. 12 by Hoen et al. and other chapters in this book). These changes combine to produce a pro-atherosclerotic environment. Epidemiological study has demonstrated a strong relationship between the presence of major depression and CHD events, with a potency that is comparable to other major CHD risk factors, such as hypertension, diabetes, or smoking.[1] Notably, a gradient relationship has been noted between the measured magnitude of depressive feelings and adverse clinical outcomes, with even mild depressive symptoms causing increase in clinical events.[35] Anxiety syndromes are also strongly linked to adverse cardiac events, as shown for general anxiety disorder,[36,37] phobic anxiety,[38,39] panic disorder,[40,41] and posttraumatic stress disorder.[42] Such data illustrate the degree to which people are physiologically intolerant of chronic negative emotions.

Fig. 20.1 Prolonged depressed feelings lead to chronic activation of the hypothalamic-pituitary-adrenocortical (*HPA*) axis and the sympathetic nervous system (*SNS*), with resultant widespread peripheral effects that combine in synergistic fashion to promote atherosclerosis and other morbidities

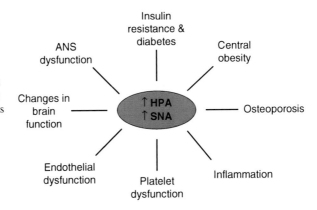

In addition, various negative cognitive states have been linked to CHD. For instance, within the Normative Aging Study, a dose–response relationship was noted between *chronic worry*, a cognitive component or precursor state of anxiety, and CHD.[43] A second negative cognitive state is *rumination*, the tendency to repetitively think about negative events. Experimental laboratory study has demonstrated that ruminators show heightened heart and blood pressure reactivity to acute stress and delayed recovery of these responses.[44] A third negative cognitive state is *resentment*. While resentment, per se, has not yet been well studied for its cardiovascular effects, data indicate that its flip side, the state and trait of being forgiving, tends to favorably diminish cardiovascular reactivity (i.e., the magnitude of heart rate and blood pressure responses) to acute stress stimuli.[45] A new area of study is *perfectionism*. Perfectionism is a negative cognitive state that is characterized by a tendency to set excessively high standards for personal performance. Perfectionists typically tend to be highly self-critical. In one study, individuals manifesting perfectionism manifested higher cortisol secretion than others during an experimental psychological stress (Fig. 20.2).[46,47] A second study has linked perfectionism to higher mortality.[47] While much more study is needed with respect to each of these cognitive states, combined, these data provide supportive evidence that negative cognitions, like negative emotions, are associated with adverse pathophysiological sequelae.

An emotional/thought complex that has been commonly studied for its cardiac effects is *anger and hostility*. Overall, the clinical effects of anger and hostility appear less profound than that of depression and anxiety, but a recent meta-analysis of 25 studies involving community samples and 19 studies involving patients with known heart disease found that in both groups, there was an approximately 20–25% increase in cardiac events among patients manifesting anger and hostility compared to those who did not.[48] In addition, a number of studies have also demonstrated that anger and hostility are associated with accelerated atherosclerosis among patients studied by serial carotid ultrasound measurements.[1]

Recently, there has been increasing interest in whether the flip side of negative emotions, *positive emotions*, provides health buffering effects. From a cognitive perspective, there is a general tendency for people to act friendlier and feel more optimistic when in positive emotional states, and Fredrickson et al. have demonstrated

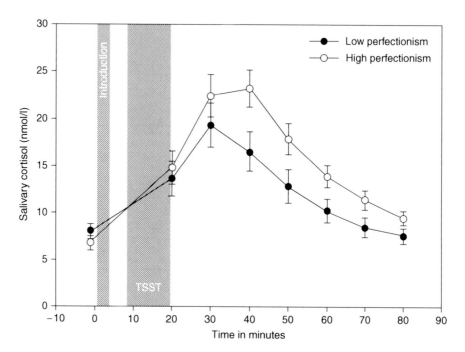

Fig. 20.2 Assessment of cortisol reactivity to psychological stress among subjects with high versus low levels of perfectionism. Salivary cortisol secretion was measured before and after subjects underwent the Trier Social Stress Test (*TSST*). Cortisol reactivity was greater among subjects with high levels of perfectionism[46]

that positive emotions tend to help build individuals' personal resources and provide them with increased resilience for coping with adversity.[49] The physiological effects of positive emotions are now an increasing focus of study. In laboratory studies which have compared exposure to humorous versus sad or stressful video stimuli, exposure to positive emotion–evoking film clips was shown to produce favorable changes in arterial wall stiffness,[50] improved endothelial function,[51] and shortened hemodynamic recovery following acute mental stress.[52] Pre-exposure to negative films has been shown to have the opposite effects on each of these parameters. Epidemiological studies concerning the effects of positive emotions have rapidly accumulated and a meta-analysis of 70 such studies has found the presence of positive well-being to be associated with reduced mortality.[53]

A cognitive pattern that has been extensively studied for both its positive and negative aspects has been the study of *optimism versus pessimism*. A consistent gradient relationship has been demonstrated in this regard: Optimists tend to have better health outcomes compared to those who are neutral in their thought tendencies, while pessimists have worse outcomes.[54-56] The largest study to date of the effects of optimism versus pessimism has been the follow-up of 97,253 women in the Women's Health Initiative.[57] Compared to pessimistic women, optimistic women had a sub-stantially reduced risk ratio for cardiac mortality (0.70, 95% CI 0.55–0.90).

20.1.3   Satisfaction of Psychological Needs

Human beings have basic psychological needs that produce a sense of vitality when fulfilled, and a sense of tension when unfulfilled. Clinical studies have demonstrated that long-term lack of fulfillment of basic psychological needs can be health damaging, while fulfillment promotes health. Theorists have differed regarding the scope of basic psychological needs but there is widespread agreement that social connection is one of these basic needs. Epidemiological data has consistently demonstrated a powerful gradient relationship between social connectedness and a wide variety of health outcomes.[10] Both long-term mortality and the risk for cardiac events increase progressively with decreasing sizes of individual social networks and with the quality of social connections[1,10,58] (Fig. 20.3). Numerous studies have delineated pathophysiological mechanisms by which lack of social integration and social isolation exert their negative health effects.[1,10]

Another potent basic psychological need is the need for a sense of meaning and purpose in life. While this need was popularized by Victor Frankl,[59] only in recent years has it received epidemiological evaluation.[60-62] For example, within the MacArthur Study of Successful Aging, older adults who reported being more useful to friends and family enjoyed greater longevity during a subsequent 7-year follow-up than did elderly individuals who reported never or rarely feeling useful at the time of baseline interview.[60] Similar findings were noted by Boyle et al. in their 5-year follow-up of 1,238 elderly individuals assessed at baseline for their sense of life purpose.[62] More study is indicated, however, in non-elderly populations. In addition, epidemiological and physiological study is needed to examine the potential health benefits of fulfilling other basic psychological needs, such as the need for feeling secure and the need for autonomy.

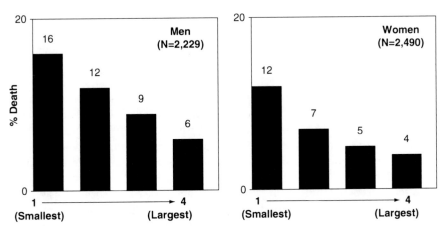

Fig. 20.3 Mortality results among individuals who were characterized at baseline according to the size of their social network size in the Alameda county study. Both for men and for women, mortality rates were highest in those with small social networks and lowest in those with high social networks[58]

20.1.4 Rest and Relaxation

Rest and relaxation ("R&R") is another important domain of health that has received increasing attention relative to medical outcomes. The most central aspect of this domain is *sleep* (see also Chap. 14 by Åkerstedt and Perski). Sleep may be impaired because of the presence of a sleep-disordered breathing problem, such as sleep apnea, insomnia, or the voluntary decision to reduce one's sleep. Both sleep apnea and insomnia have been linked to adverse clinical outcomes, and increasing data link voluntary sleep loss to important pathophysiological and clinical sequelae. An early seminal study in this regard subjected healthy young men to six nights of 4-h sleep periods.[63] This sleep debt was sufficient to induce alterations in glucose metabolism, a trend toward diminished insulin sensitivity, and an increase in evening cortisol levels. Subsequent study has demonstrated that even mild sleep loss is sufficient to induce low-grade inflammation.[64] In addition, chronic sleep loss can exert significant effects on the neuroendocrine control of appetite, leading to excessive food intake[65] and to increase in body mass index.[66] In addition, there is increasing epidemiological data that links short sleep to adverse clinical events.[67,68]

Unwinding after work is also a potentially important determinant of health. Unwinding can be accomplished through engagement in mental, social, or physical activities that are enjoyable or by employing direct relaxation techniques. Since opportunities to unwind during daily work is limited for most workers, most unwinding is generally limited to after work hours and weekends. Unwinding can be impaired due to continued involvement in job-related activities or other demanding (e.g., domestic) activities after work or due to excessive worry regarding work after hours. After-work pre-occupation with job-related issues can lead to prolonged physiological activation during evening hours.[69,70] There is increasing epidemiological evidence that lack of unwinding leads to reduced longevity.[71-73] For example, van Amelsvoort et al. observed a stepwise increase in mortality according to the perceived need for recovery from work.[72]

A third form of "R&R" includes the taking of *vacations* which afford time for extended rest and relaxation, re-connection with others, investment in personal interests, and a reduction of tension. In a study of 1,500 women, those who took more frequent vacations (≥2 per year) reported less tension, depression and fatigue, and more marital satisfaction compared to those women who took infrequent vacations (only once in 2 years).[74] An association between infrequent vacations and adverse outcomes has also been observed in a 20-year follow-up of women from the Framingham Heart Study[75] and a 9-year follow-up from the Multiple Risk Factor Intervention Trial.[76]

A fourth form of "R&R" is the ability to maintain a *sense of leisure*. This sense is highly related to how time pressed one feels. The greater the sense of time pressure, the less leisure one is capable of feeling. Due to technology, modern life is inherently more fast-paced and potentially time pressed,[77] but despite the apparent ubiquity of this issue, it has been poorly studied for its health effects. In one case–control study, a dose–response relationship was noted between having a sense of time urgency and sustaining a nonfatal myocardial infarction,[78] but clearly, prospective study is needed.

20.2 Integrating Psychological Principles into the Management of Behavioral and Psychosocial Risk Factors

Despite the epidemiological and pathophysiological evidence linking psychosocial risk factors to CAD, the treatment of these risk factors is not currently well integrated into clinical medicine. Within clinical practice, there is a persistent separation between the management of "behavioral" CAD risk factors – smoking, poor diet, overeating, and sedentary behavior – and the psychosocial risk factors reviewed in this chapter. Fostering a more unified integration of these factors would be desirable for two reasons. First, psychosocial risk factors such as depression, anxiety, social isolation, chronic stress, time pressure, and lack of sleep are important determinants of poor health habits and their presence represents a significant barrier to modifying adverse behaviors, such as overeating and smoking. Secondly, as reviewed, psychosocial risk factors are causative CAD risk factors and thus deserve treatment in their own right. Among psychosocial risk factors, those of a psychiatric nature generally deserve referral to health care professionals that are skilled in treating such illnesses. However, issues such as motivating patients and providing behavioral suggestions and instructions that support patients to make health habit change can be managed within the context of medical practice, either directly by physicians or by adjunctive staff, such as nurses, dieticians, and other office personnel. In recent years, several behavioral management techniques have been developed and tested for their ability to help patients modify health behaviors, such as overeating, smoking and lack of exercise, and psychosocial problems, such as chronic stress, difficulty unwinding, poor sleep hygiene, and time pressure.

The induction of behavioral change involves three critical components: enhancing motivation, providing assistance in the execution of health goals, and providing help in long-term behavioral maintenance (Fig. 20.4). Examples of behavioral management approaches that can be used to enhance these three components of behavioral change are listed in Table 20.2 and discussed below. While various techniques may be assigned to one category of behavioral change, these techniques frequently overlap in terms of their ability to provide assistance in motivation, goal execution, or behavioral maintenance.

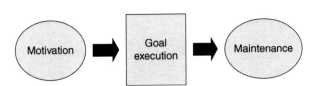

Fig. 20.4 Behavioral interventions can be targeted to address the three major determinants of successful behavior change: (1) motivation, (2) goal execution, or (3) long-term maintenance of behavioral change

Table 20.2 Examples
of behavioral interventions
to help patients in health
habit change

A. *Promotion of motivation*
    Autonomy
    Self-efficacy
    Time management
B. *Execution of goals*
    Implementation intentions
    Self-monitoring
    Energy management
    Stress management
C. *Promotion of long-term maintenance*
    Social support
    Feedback
    Contingency plans

20.2.1 Methods to Improve Motivation

20.2.1.1 Fostering of Autonomy

People are more motivated when they choose goals based on their own volition rather than being told what to do. This principle is commonly referred to as "autonomy."[79] This principle is highly relevant to medical practice, as it is common to use external forms of motivation, such as attempting to instill fear as to the health consequences if patients do not comply with recommended behavioral change. The practical difference involved in coaching patients from the principle of autonomy can sometimes be subtle but yet important. For instance, a physician dealing with a sedentary patient with heightened cardiovascular risk can and should provide patients with an explanation of the benefits that can be accrued from regular physical activity. To promote autonomy, however, the physician should then pause and ask the patient: *"Based on what I have told you, do you see a reason(s) as to why you might want to exercise"*? The goal of this type of question is to foster within patients a sense of purpose and ownership over their health goals. Secondly, it is helpful to foster patients' ownership as to *how* they personally prefer to accomplish their health goals rather than simply telling patients how to exercise, lose weight, etc. In support of this approach, greater reductions in hemoglobin A_{1c} have been observed among diabetics who perceived more autonomy support from their health providers compared to those who did not,[80] and similar data has been noted for smoking and weight loss interventions.[81,82]

20.2.1.2 Self-Efficacy

People are more likely to make efforts toward goals they believe they can achieve. This concept concerning the importance of self-belief has been termed "self-efficacy", as proposed by Bandura.[83] Its implication relative to cardiac practice is that prescriptions regarding health habit change should be tailored to the individual patient's belief regarding what he/she can actually achieve. For example, recommendations for adequate exercise in adults call for at least 30 min of moderate exercise or 20 min of vigorous exercise at least three times per week, with additional resistance exercises at least twice per week.[84] However, these recommendations are frequently too difficult for sedentary patients. Coaching such patients for "small win" means asking patients to identify the smallest physical activity program to which they can commit, even as little as a few minutes of extra walking per day. A program of follow-up is then necessary to ensure that targeted increases in activity, according to patient ability, occur over time.

20.2.1.3 Time Management

Time management is an important but often overlooked aspect of behavioral health management. A full discussion of time management approaches that can support behavioral change is beyond the scope of this chapter. However, one foundational principal is that when people weigh competing goals, there is a tendency to *overvalue* goals that are present-centered and *undervalue* goals which are future-oriented.[85] This principle suggests a role for discussing time management in clinical medical practice. When physicians discuss health goals with patients, these discussions are frequently held in the abstract, without consideration of the competing priorities in patients' lives. However, after patients leave the confines of their doctors' offices and return to their daily routines, health goals commonly are not perceived as pressing as various daily life obligations, such as work deadlines or important family obligations. For example, an overweight male with evidence of heart disease may be strongly advised by his physician to lose weight. The patient may sincerely want to embrace his physician's injunction and advice regarding weight loss, and, at the time of actually being counseled, the patient may prioritize his health over his work. The next day, however, pressing work may receive a higher valued priority and the patient may thus decide to put off the start of his health goal, in this case the start of a new diet, *"until tomorrow"*. Commonly, this dynamic gets repeated on subsequent days until discouragement sets in. Physicians can help counter this problem by pointing out this dynamic to patients and helping them to form behavioral anchors, such as those described below, before patients leave their offices.

20.2.2 Methods to Improve the Execution of Health Goals

20.2.2.1 Implementation Intentions

New health goals involve the adoption of "practices." As opposed to habits which are ingrained, automatic, and do not require much effort, new practices are vulnerable since they require effort and mindful intention and are subject to impediment by common barriers, such as feeling fatigued or unmotivated. Gollwitzer et al. developed an approach called "implementation intentions" that has the capacity to help new practices function as if they were habits.[86] Simply, intentional intentions call for the identification of some anchor, either in time or place, which cues an individual to perform their intended new practice. Gollwitzer proposes a specific conditional formulation for implementation intentions: "When it is X, I will do Y." For instance, someone may declare the following intention: "When I finish work at 6 p.m. at night, I will drive to the gym before coming home." In the absence of this implementation intention, each night this individual may negotiate in his or her mind, while driving home, whether he or she is too tired, too stressed, or time pressured by other priorities to exercise that evening. Implementation intentions are designed to take such inner conflict out of the equation. To work, however, individuals have to be well motivated toward their new intended health practice before formulating an implementation intention. Implementation intentions have been experimentally applied to various health practices.[87] A meta-analysis of 94 studies confirmed the ability of implementation intentions to assist in the execution of various health and life goals.[88]

20.2.2.2 Self-Monitoring

Self-monitoring may be used as a means of setting concrete goals, increasing self-awareness, improving motivation, and providing personal feedback. For instance, self-weighing is a ubiquitous objective means of charting one's course toward weight loss. Studies indicate that regular self-weighing is associated with more weight loss and/or less weight gain in weight loss trials.[89-91] Similarly, the use of pedometers can be used to self-monitor one's daily steps. A target of 10,000 steps per day has been recently promulgated as a rough general mean target for active physical activity, but as aforementioned, recommendations around step progression should preferably be adjusted to the individuals' baseline physical activity and sense of what constitutes an appropriate pedometer step progression for oneself. A recent meta-analysis of 26 studies found that pedometer use was associated with a 27% increase in physical activity compared to baseline.[92] A goal of 10,000 steps per day was a predictor of increased physical activity, and pedometer use was associated with significant decreases in body mass index and systolic blood pressure.

20.2.2.3 Stress and Energy Management

Common barriers to health goal execution include feelings of stress, low moods, and fatigue. Thayer et al. studied the relationship between these parameters by requesting volunteers to simultaneously monitor their activities, mood, and energy and tension levels at frequent intervals during daily activity.[93] They found a relatively low frequency of negative moods when individuals reported low tension (regardless of energy) and a high frequency of negative moods when people reported being both tense and tired. Interestingly, however, when subjects reported high tension but concomitantly high-energy, positive moods prevailed. While tense-tired, individuals were found to be highly prone to "quick fix" behaviors designed to increase energy (e.g., sweet foods) or reduce tension (e.g., smoking, watching television).

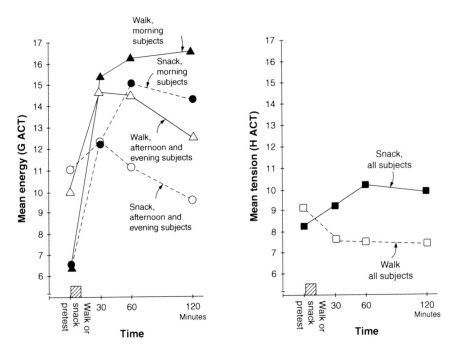

Fig. 20.5 On left, comparison of change in mean self-rated energy level in subjects at baseline and after brisk walking for 10 min or after ingesting a candy bar in the morning and in the afternoon. Mean energy increased after both exercise and the sugar snack. On right, change in mean self-rated tension levels after exercise and the snack. Mean tension levels at 1–2 h within the morning and afternoon subjects were increased after the snack and decreased after the exercise[94]

An important paradox concerning periods of tense-tiredness is that while people tend to be more cognitively restricted and less capable at such times, that is when people often feel the greatest urgency to solve chronic problems. Instead, people can often be better served by ignoring perceived sources of tension during periods of tense-tiredness and focusing on increasing energy instead. As one's energy increases, mood and cognition may improve, and problems can then be viewed from a broader perspective and solved more effectively. Importantly, since periods of tense-tiredness may precede the formation of negative moods,[93] teaching patients how to monitor their energy and learning how to increase it prophylactically may be beneficial. For instance, if a patient notes that he or she tends to get tired around 4 p.m. each day, a short rest or performance of progressive relaxation exercises may restore energy and reduce the likelihood of low moods at that time. Examples of other approaches to increasing energy include doing side work that is innately interesting, use of music or other entertainment, and brief periods of exercise. Thayer et al. demonstrated that short bursts of physical energy were as effective as sweet calorie dense foods for increasing energy, but exercise resulted in decreased tension in the following 1–2 h while sweet food ingestion served to increase tension (Fig. 20.5).[94]

The management of tense-tiredness can also be assisted by approaches designed to reduce tension without trying to actively manage the *source* of tension. These approaches can range from simple breathing exercises to specific techniques designed to produce physical and emotional unwinding, including mindful meditation, biofeedback exercises, yoga, and tai-chi.

20.2.3 Methods for Promoting Long-Term Behavioral Maintenance

Many patients succeed in the initial institution of new heath behaviors, including substantial weight loss, but then commonly suffer relapse over the long term. Providing patients with assistance toward long-term maintenance of new behavioral practices is thus a central component of behavioral interventions. Important in this regard is helping patients to garner *social support*. Social support can take many forms, such as physician-office support, referral to community-based programs, establishing buddy systems or more spousal and family support, and more recently, making use of internet-based programs. Studies consistently demonstrate that lack of social support is an important predictor of patient non-adherence.[95]

Provision for *on-going feedback* is another central component for enhancing long-term behavioral maintenance. Feedback from physicians and their staff ensures that barriers to maintaining health practices can be identified and discussed, and it serves to build patient awareness and cue them that their health providers are engaged and consider their health practices to be important.

Not uncommonly, relapse occurs because patients get thrown by an unanticipated breakdown, such as that caused by stressful life events, problems in balancing competing life priorities, or development of an inter-current illness. As such events commonly occur over time, it is useful to develop *prophylactic contingency plans* for dealing with breakdowns. Contingency planning can vary in complexity and can be tailored to suit a patient's inherent coping style. Some patients, for example, tend to be perfectionists, and tend to view any breakdown as a sign of failure. A general conceptual approach to contingency planning is to have patients maintain a minimum floor for their health practices, so that they always are on the "playing field." For example, a patient who has successfully instituted a plan to exercise at a gym for 30–60 min for most days of the week may prophylactically agree to a "backup" plan to do neighborhood walking for 15 min per day in the event that life events or obligations prohibit the patient from going to the gym for a period of time.

20.3 Integrating Behavioral Interventions into Clinical Management

The behavioral management techniques discussed herein represent examples of a larger number of techniques that can be used to support behavioral change in patients. Currently, however, there is no paradigm to inform and instruct physicians

Table 20.3 Suggested open-ended questions to screen for psychosocial risk factors

1. "How has your mood been recently?" or "Do you ever feel down?"
2. "Do you feel anxious or unduly worried?"
3. "Are you under undue pressure at work or at home?"
4. "If need be, do you have someone to turn to for support?"
5. "How is your sleeping?"
6. "Do you have difficulty unwinding after work or at the end of the day?"
7. "How would you describe your energy level?"
8. "Do you feel unduly time pressed?"

on how to incorporate the behavioral interventions discussed in this chapter. Future work is needed to design and test programs that could assist physicians. The success of any approach would depend on simple and effective screening for psychosocial issues that might impinge on behavior or health. Physicians are already accustomed to conducting an extensive review of systems in a matter of minutes and with experience, psychosocial screening can similarly be conducted by a series of short questions, such as those suggested in Table 20.3. Alternatively, such questions could be addressed by experienced office personnel when feasible. Some interventions among those noted above can be easily incorporated into clinical practice without significantly increasing the time for physician–patient interactions. Examples would include asking patients to form one specific implementation intention before leaving the office, and advising patients to self-monitor their weight each week or their daily physical activity using pedometers. In subsequent visits, patients could be provided feedback on their self-monitored behaviors. To help with social support, physician offices might create a local catalog of relevant support groups and community programs that are available for patient use.

Dealing with such issues as time pressure, poor life balance, fatigue, stress, and negative emotions can be more challenging and time consuming. The development of a stepped-model approach could be tested for assisting physicians in this regard, the lowest level being advice dispensed at the physician–patient level, the middle level being aid provided by adjunctive office personnel, and the highest level being referral to mental healthcare professionals. An example of interventions that can be handled at the physician–patient level might include advice in the realm of "R&R" (e.g., advice regarding napping or avoiding undue sleep restriction). Examples of services that can be offered by office personnel include providing patients with coaching assistance aligned to principles that increase motivation (e.g., autonomy and self-efficacy), practical help to assist patients in their execution of health goals (e.g., more detailed review of implementation intentions) or to teach patients how to better monitor and preserve their energy or reduce stress (e.g., breathing exercises), assistance in identifying and instituting social support, and more structured and frequent feedback. The third level of intervention, referral to mental healthcare professionals, should be considered when significant psychological distress is uncovered during routine psychosocial screening, including evidence of major depression or anxiety syndromes. In addition, issues such as poorly managed chronic stress and insomnia may be deserving of referral for specialized counseling.

20.4 Summary

A wide variety of psychosocial problems are causative of CHD including the presence of chronic negative emotions, such as depression and anxiety; negative thought patterns, such as pessimism; chronic stress; the lack of satisfaction of basic psychological needs, such as the needs for social relationships and for meaningful purpose; and inadequate "R&R." The pathophysiological effects of negative psychological factors serve to increase the risk of atherosclerosis, hypertension, diabetes, metabolic syndrome and increase the risk for premature aging, reduced longevity, and the development of premature cardiac events. Psychosocial risk factors and conventional "behavioral" risk factors, such as overeating and sedentary behavior, are highly linked. In recent years, evidence-based behavior approaches have been developed that can improve health behaviors and/or reduce psychosocial distress. A number of these approaches have been reviewed in this chapter but methods for widespread delivery of these behavioral management techniques in a practical and cost-effective manner await further prospective development.

References

1. Rozanski A, Blumenthal JA, Davidson KW, et al. The epidemiology, pathophysiology, and management of psychosocial risk factors in cardiac practice: the emerging field of behavioral cardiology. *J Am Coll Cardiol*. 2005;45:637-651.
2. Thomas RJ, King M, Lui K, et al. AACVPR/ACC/AHA 2007 performance of measures of cardiac rehabilitation for referral to and delivery of cardiac rehabilitation/secondary prevention services. *J Cardiopulm Rehabil Prev*. 2007;27:260-290.
3. Graham I, Atar D, Borch-Johnsen K, et al. European guidelines on cardiovascular disease prevention in clinical practice: executive summary. Fourth Joint Task Force of the European Society of Cardiology and Other Societies on Cardiovascular Disease Prevention in Clinical Practice. *Eur Heart J*. 2007;28:2375-2414.
4. Friedman M, Thoresen CE, Gill JJ, et al. Alteration of type A behavior and its effect on cardiac recurrences in post-myocardial infract patients: summary results of the Recurrent Coronary Prevention Project. *Am Heart J*. 1986;112:653-665.
5. Frasure-Smith N, Prince R. The ischemic heart disease life stress monitoring program: impact on mortality. *Psychosom Med*. 1985;47:431-445.
6. Jones DA, West RR. Psychological rehabilitation after myocardial infarction: multicenter randomized control trial. *Br Med J*. 1996;313:1517-1521.
7. Frasure-Smith N, Lesperance F, Prince RH, et al. Randomized trial of home-based psychosocial nursing intervention for patients recovering from myocardial infarction. *Lancet*. 1997;350: 473-479.
8. The ENRICHD Investigators. Effects on treating depression and low perceived social support on clinical events after a myocardial infarction: the Enhancing Recovery in Coronary Heart Disease Patients (ENRICHD) randomized trial. *JAMA*. 2003;289:3106-3116.
9. Kaplan JR, Manuck SB, Clarkson TB, et al. Social status, environment and atherosclerosis in cynomolgus monkeys. *Arteriosclerosis*. 1982;2:359-368.
10. Rozanski A, Blumenthal JA, Kaplan J. Impact of psychological factors on the pathogenesis of cardiovascular disease and implications for therapy. *Circulation*. 1999;99:2192-2217.
11. Jain S, Mills PH, Kanel RV. Effects of perceived stress and uplifts on inflammation and coagulability. *Psychophysiology*. 2007;44:154-160.

12. Brunner EJ, Hemmingway H, Walker BR. Adrenocortical, autonomic, and inflammatory causes of the metabolic syndrome: nested case-control study. *Circulation*. 2002;106:2659-2665.

13. Brydon L, Magid K, Steptoe A, et al. Platelets, coronary heart disease, and stress. *Brain Behav Immun*. 2006;20:113-119.

14. Schnall PL, Schwartz JE, Landsbergis PA, et al. A longitudinal study of job strain and ambulatory blood pressure: results from a three-year follow-up. *Psychosom Med*. 1998;60: 697-706.

15. Vrijkotte TGM, van Doornen LJP, de Geus EJC. Effects of work stress on ambulatory blood pressure, heart rate, and heart rate variability. *Hypertension*. 2000;35:880-886.

16. Lucini D, Di Fede G, Parati G, et al. Impact of chronic psychological stress on autonomic cardiovascular regulation in otherwise healthy subjects. *Hypertension*. 2005;46:1201-1206.

17. Epel ES, Blackburn EH, Lin J, et al. Accelerated telomere shortening in response to life stress. *Proc Natl Acad Sci USA*. 2004;101:17312-17315.

18. McEwen BS. Physiology and neurobiology of stress and adaptation: central role of the brain. *Physiol Rev*. 2007;87:873-904.

19. Yusuf S, Hawkin S, Ounpuu S, et al. Effect of potentially modifiable risk factors associated with myocardial infarction in 52 countries (the INTERHEART study): case-control study. *Lancet*. 2004;364:937-952.

20. Karasek R, Baker D, Marxer F, et al. Job decision latitude, job demands, and cardiovascular disease: a prospective study of Swedish men. *Am J Public Health*. 1981;71:694-705.

21. Siegrist J. Adverse health effects of high-effort/low-reward conditions. *J Occup Health Psychol*. 1996;71:694-705.

22. Orth-Gomer K, Wamala SP, Horsten M, et al. Marital stress worsens prognosis in women with coronary heart disease: the Stockholm Female Coronary Risk Study. *JAMA*. 2000;248: 3008-3014.

23. Coyne JC, Rohrbaugh MJ, Shoham V, et al. Prognostic importance of marital quality for survival of congestive heart failure. *Am J Cardiol*. 2001;88:526-529.

24. Eaker ED, Sullivan LM, Kelly-Hayes M, et al. Marital status, marital strain, and risk of coronary heart disease or total mortality: the Framingham Offspring Study. *Psychosom Med*. 2007;69:509-513.

25. Gallo LC, Troxel WM, Kuller LH, et al. Marital status, marital quality, and atherosclerotic burden in postmenopausal women. *Psychosom Med*. 2003;65:952-962.

26. Fredrickson BL. The role of positive emotions in positive psychology: the broaden-and-build theory of positive emotions. *Am Psychol*. 2001;56:218-226.

27. Koschke M, Boettger MK, Schulz S, et al. Autonomy of autonomic dysfunction in major depression. *Psychosom Med*. 2009;71:852-860.

28. Timonen M, Salmenkaita I, Jokelainen J, et al. Insulin resistance and depressive symptoms in young adult males: findings from Finnish Military Conscripts. *Psychosom Med*. 2007;69: 723-728.

29. Vaccarino V, McClure C, Johnson D, et al. Depression, the metabolic syndrome and cardiovascular risk. *Psychosom Med*. 2008;70:40-48.

30. Everson-Rose SA, Lewis TT, Karavolus K, et al. Depressive symptoms and increased visceral fat in middle-aged women. *Psychosom Med*. 2009;71:410-416.

31. De Groot M, Anderson R, Freedland KE, et al. Association of depression and diabetes complications: a meta-analysis. *Psychosom Med*. 2001;63:619-630.

32. Michelson D, Stratakis C, Hill L, et al. Bone mineral density in women with depression. *N Engl J Med*. 1996;335:1176-1181.

33. Howren MB, Lamkin DM, Suls J. Associations of depression with C-reactive protein, IL-1, and IL-6: a meta-analysis. *Psychosom Med*. 2009;71:171-186.

34. Broadley AJM, Jones CJH, Frenneaux MP. Arterial endothelial function is impaired in treated depression. *Heart*. 2002;88:521-524.

35. Lesperance F, Frasure-Smith N, Talajiv M, et al. Five-year risk of cardiac mortality in relation to initial severity and one-year changes in depression symptoms after myocardial infarction. *Circulation*. 2002;105:1049-1053.

36. Martens EJ, Dejong P, Na B, et al. Scared to death? Generalized anxiety disorder and cardiovascular events in patients with stable coronary heart disease. *Arch Gen Psychiat.* 2010;67:750-758.

37. Frasure-Smith N, Lesperance F. Depression and anxiety as predictors of 2-year cardiac events in patients with stable coronary artery disease. *Arch Gen Psychiat.* 2008;65:62-71.

38. Kawachi I, Colditz GA, Ascherio A, et al. Prospective study of phobic anxiety and risk of coronary heart disease in men. *Circulation.* 1994;89:1992-1997.

39. Albert CM, Chae CU, Rexrode KM, et al. Phobic anxiety and risk of coronary heart disease and sudden cardiac death among women. *Circulation.* 2005;111:480-487.

40. Smoller JW, Pollack MG, Wassertheil-Smoller S, et al. Panic attacks and risk of incident cardiovascular events among postmenopausal women in the Women's Health Initiative Observational Study. *Arch Gen Psychiat.* 2007;64:1153-1160.

41. Walters K, Rait G, Petersen I, et al. Panic disorder and risk of new onset coronary heart disease, acute myocardial infarction, and cardiac mortality: cohort study using the general practice research database. *Eur Heart J.* 2008;29:2981-2988.

42. Kubzansky LD, Koenen KC, Spiro A, et al. Prospective study of posttraumatic stress disorder symptoms and coronary heart disease in the normative aging study. *Arch Gen Psychiat.* 2007;64:109-116.

43. Kubzansky LD, Kawachi I, Spiro A III, et al. Is worrying bad for your heart? A prospective study of worry and coronary heart disease in the Normative Aging Study. *Circulation.* 1997;95:818-824.

44. Glynn LM, Christenfeld N, Gerin W. The role of rumination in recovery from reactivity: cardiovascular consequences of emotional states. *Psychosom Med.* 2002;64:714-726.

45. Lawler KA, Younger JW, Piferi RL, et al. A change of heart: cardiovascular correlates of forgiveness in response to interpersonal conflict. *J Behav Med.* 2003;26:373-393.

46. Wirtz PH, Elsenbruch S, Emini L, et al. Perfectionism and the cortisol response to psychosocial stress in men. *Psychosom Med.* 2007;69:249-255.

47. Fry PS, Debats DL. Perfectionism and the five-factor personality traits as predictors of mortality in older adults. *J Health Psychol.* 2009;14:513-524.

48. Chida Y, Steptoe A. The association of anger and hostility with future coronary heart disease. *J Am Coll Cardiol.* 2009;59:936-946.

49. Fredrickson BL. What good are positive emotions? *Rev Gen Psychol.* 1998;3:300-319.

50. Vlachopoulos C, Xaplanteris P, Alexopoulos N, et al. Divergent effects of laughter and mental stress on arterial stiffness and central hemodynamic. *Psychosom Med.* 2009;71:1-8.

51. Miller M, Mangano C, Park Y, Goel R, Plotnick GD, Vogel RA. Impact on cinematic viewing on endothelial function. *Heart.* 2006;92:261-262.

52. Frederickson BL, Levenson RW. Positive emotions speed recovery from the cardiovascular sequelae of negative emotions. *Cognition Emotion.* 1998;12:191-220.

53. Chida Y, Steptoe A. Positive psychological well-being and mortality: a quantitative review of prospective observational studies. *Psychosom Med.* 2008;70:741-756.

54. Kubzansky LD, Sparrow D, Vokonas P, et al. Is the glass half empty of half full? A prospective study of optimism and coronary heart disease in the normative aging study. *Psychosom Med.* 2001;63:910-916.

55. Giltay EJ, Geleijnse JM, Zitman FG, et al. Dispositional optimism and all-cause and cardiovascular mortality in a prospective cohort of elderly Dutch men and women. *Arch Gen Psychiat.* 2004;61:1126-1135.

56. Giltay EJ, Kamphuis MH, Kalmijn S, et al. Dispositional optimism and the risk of cardiovascular death. *Arch Intern Med.* 2006;166:431-436.

57. Tindle HA, Chang YF, Kuller LH, et al. Optimism, cynical hostility, and incident coronary heart disease and mortality in the women's health initiative. *Circulation.* 2009;120:656-662.

58. Berkman LF, Syme SL. Social networks, host resistance, and mortality: a nine-year follow-up study of Alameda county residents. *Am J Epidemiol.* 1979;109:186-204.

59. Frankl VE. *Man's Search for Meaning: An Introduction to Logotherapy.* New York: Simon & Schuster; 1959.

60. Gruenewald TL, Karlamangla AS, Greendale GA, et al. Feelings of usefulness to others, disability, and mortality in older adults: the MacArthur study of successful aging. *J Gerontol.* 2007;62B:P28-P37.
61. Okamoto K, Tanaka Y. Subjective usefulness and 6-year mortality risks among elderly persons in Japan. *Psychol Sci.* 2004;59B:P246-P249.
62. Boyle PA, Barnes LL, Buchman AS, et al. Purpose in life is associated with mortality among community-dwelling older persons. *Psychosom Med.* 2009;71:575-579.
63. Speigel K, Leproult R, Van Cauter E. Impact of sleep debt on metabolic and endocrine function. *Lancet.* 1999;354:1435-1439.
64. Irwin MR, Wang M, Compomayor CO, et al. Sleep deprivation and activation of morning levels of cellular and genomic markers of inflammation. *Arch Intern Med.* 2006;166:1756-1762.
65. Speigel K, Talasi E, Penev P, et al. Sleep curtailment in healthy young men is associated with decreased leptin levels, elevated ghrelin levels and increased hunger and appetite. *Ann Intern Med.* 2004;141:846-850.
66. Kuntson KL, Speigel K, Penev P, et al. The metabolic consequences of sleep deprivation. *Sleep Med Rev.* 2007;11:163-178.
67. Gallicchio L, Kalesan B, et al. Sleep duration and mortality: a systematic review and meta-analysis. *J Sleep Res.* 2009;18:145-147.
68. Cappuccio FP, D'Elia L, Strazzullo P, et al. Sleep duration and all-cause mortality: a systematic review and meta-analysis of prospective studies. *Sleep.* 2010;33:585-592.
69. Brosschut JF, Peiper S, Thayer JF. Expanding stress theory: prolonged activation and preservative cognition. *Psychoneuroendocrinology.* 2005;30:1043-1049.
70. Frankenhauser M. Coping with stress at work. *Int J Health Serv.* 1981;11:491-510.
71. Suadicani P, Hein HO, Gyntelberg F. Are social inequalities associated with the risk of ischemic heart disease as a result of psychosocial working conditions? *Atherosclerosis.* 1993;101:165-175.
72. Van Amselvoort LGPM, Bultmann IJK, Swaen GMH, et al. Need for recovery after work and the subsequent risk of cardiovascular disease in a working population. *Occup Environ Med.* 2003;60:i83-i87.
73. Kivimaki M, Leino-Arjas P, Kaila-Kangas L, et al. Is incomplete recovery from work a risk marker of cardiovascular death? Prospective evidence from industrial employees. *Psychosom Med.* 2006;68:402-407.
74. Chikani V, Reding D, Gunderson P, et al. Vacations improve mental health among rural women: the Wisconsin Rural Womens's Health Study. *Wisconsin Med J.* 2005;104:20-23.
75. Eaker ED, Pinsky J, Castelli WP, et al. Myocardial Infarction and coronary death among women: psychosocial predictors from a 20-year follow-up of women in the Framingham study. *Am J Epidemiol.* 1992;135:854-864.
76. Gump B, Mattews K, et al. Are vaccinations good for your health? The 9-year mortality experience after the multiple risk factor intervention trial. *Psychosom Med.* 2000;62:608-612.
77. Gleick J. *Faster: The Acceleration of Just About Everything.* New York: Pantheon Press; 1999.
78. Cole S, Kawachi I, Liu S, et al. Time urgency and risk of non-fatal myocardial infarction. *Int J Epidemiol.* 2001;30:363-369.
79. Ryan RM, Deci EL. Self-determination theory and the development, and well-being. *Am Psychol.* 2000;55:68-78.
80. Williams GC, Freeman ZR, Deci EL. Supporting autonomy to motivate patients with diabetes for glucose control. *Diabetes Care.* 1998;21:1644-1651.
81. Williams G, Cox E, Kouides R. Presenting the facts about smoking to adolescents. *Arch Pediat Adol Med.* 1999;153:959-964.
82. Williams GC, Grow VM, Freeman ZR, et al. Motivational predictors of weight loss and weight-loss maintenance. *J Pers Soc Psychol.* 1996;70:115-126.
83. Bandura A. *Social Learning Theory.* Englewood Cliffs: Prentice Hall; 1977.
84. Haskell W, Lee IM, Pate R, et al. Physical activity and public health. Updated recommendation for adults from the American College of Sports Medicine and the American Heart Association. *Circulation.* 2007;116:1081-1093.

85. Loewenstein G, Thaler RH. Anomolies: intertemporal choice. *J Econ Perspect.* 1989;3:181-193.
86. Gollwitzer PM. Implementation intentions: strong effects of simple plans. *Am Psychol.* 1999;54:493-503.
87. Orbeil S, Hodgldns S, Sheeran P. Implementation intentions and the theory of planned behavior. *Pers Soc Psychol B.* 1997;23:945-954.
88. Gollwitzer PM, Sheeran P. Implementation intentions and goal achievement: a meta-analysis of effects of processes. *Adv Exp Soc Psychol.* 2006;38:69-119.
89. O'Neil PM, Brown JD, et al. Weighing the evidence: benefits of regular weight monitoring for weight control. *J Nutr Educ Behav.* 2005;37:319-322.
90. Linde JA, Jeffrey RW, French S, et al. Self-weighing in weight gain prevention and weight loss trials. *Ann Behav Med.* 2005;30:210-216.
91. Wing RR, Tate DF, Gorin AA, et al. A self-regulation program for maintenance of weight loss. *N Engl J Med.* 2006;355:1563-1571.
92. Bravata DM, Smith-Spangler C, Sundaram V, et al. Using pedometers to increase physical activity and improve health. *JAMA.* 2007;298:2296-2304.
93. Thayer RE, Newman R, McClain TM. Self regulation of mood: strategies for changing a bad mood, raising energy and reducing tension. *J Pers Soc Psychol.* 1994;67:910-925.
94. Thayer RE. Energy, tiredness, and tension effects of a sugar snack vs moderate exercise. *J Pers Soc Psychol.* 1987;52:119-125.
95. DiMatteo MR. Social support and patient adherence to medical treatment: a meta-analysis. *Health Psychol.* 2004;23:207-218.

Part VI
Conclusions

Chapter 21
Concluding Remarks

Paul Hjemdahl, Annika Rosengren, and Andrew Steptoe

Keywords Acute stress • Cardiovascular disease • Cardiovascular outcomes •
Coronary heart disease (CHD) • Psychosocial factors • Stress

This book illustrates the importance of stress and psychosocial factors in the etiology, development, and management of atherosclerotic cardiovascular disease, especially coronary heart disease (CHD). Studies in animals show that stress can cause atherosclerotic disease and have provided some plausible mechanisms. Experimental studies in humans have demonstrated that acute stress can engage neuro-humoral and other mechanisms designed to provide survival benefits but which, when engaged too intensively or too frequently, may initiate disease processes and cause cardiovascular complications in susceptible individuals. Observational studies have provided evidence that various factors related to the multifaceted and sometimes illusive concept of "stress" can both fuel atherosclerotic disease processes and precipitate acute cardiovascular events; measurements of mechanistic markers have helped to translate laboratory findings into "real life." Several chapters in this book have thus described the mechanistic background to stress-related cardiovascular disease. Several chapters then address clinical situations in which "stress" is of

P. Hjemdahl (✉)
Department of Medicine, Solna, Clinical Pharmacology Unit, Karolinska Institute,
Karolinska University Hospital/Solna, Stockholm, Sweden
e-mail: paul.hjemdahl@ki.se

A. Rosengren
Institute of Medicine, Sahlgrenska Academy, Sahlgrenska University Hospital,
Ostra, Gothenburg, Sweden
e-mail: annika.rosengren@hjlgu.se

A. Steptoe
Department of Epidemiology and Public Health, University College London, London, UK
e-mail: a.steptoe@ucl.ac.uk

P. Hjemdahl et al. (eds.), *Stress and Cardiovascular Disease*,
DOI 10.1007/978-1-84882-419-5_21, © Springer-Verlag London Limited 2012

importance. The different authors describe their conceptual frameworks, and provide slightly varying definitions of "what is stress." These accounts and interpretations will give the reader food for thought, and we felt no need to synchronize different statements on definitions into any unifying concept of stress.

Acute stress may precipitate serious cardiovascular events and sudden death in predisposed individuals as discussed by Tofler et al. in Chap. 9. Stress may also cause stress cardiomyopathy, often referred to as the Takotsubo syndrome, which appears to be related to sympathetic overactivity and is important to recognize since it is reversible and associated with a good prognosis, as discussed by Wittstein in Chap. 10. Most authors in this book have focused on stress and cardiac disease since this is the field mostly studied. However, stress may also have cerebrovascular consequences and precipitate stroke.

Depression has been much discussed in the context of myocardial infarction (MI) and has been rather extensively studied in cardiac patients. However, many questions remain unsolved, as discussed by Hoen et al. in Chap. 12. Depression no doubt worsens the prognosis of MI patients, but "how close the relationship is" and "the direction of causality" are still somewhat uncertain. Depression can activate relevant disease mechanisms, but disease can also cause depression and there is overlap with other psychosocial and personality factors. It may be important if the depression is a premorbid condition or triggered by the MI, whether it is an episode of severe major depression or only minor depressive symptoms, and what other comorbidities are present. Furthermore, depressed patients are less likely to adhere to treatments and lifestyle advice which will worsen their prognosis in general and confound mechanistic interpretations of findings in depressed cardiac patients. Finally, how to treat depressed cardiac patients is not yet satisfactorily solved. Antidepressant drug trials are small and short lasting, i.e., underpowered for evaluations of cardiovascular outcomes, and the effects of drug treatment on depression ratings over and above those of placebo are relatively modest in both cardiac and other patients. Studies of psychotherapy alone or in combination with drug therapy have yielded equivocal results, as discussed also by Talbot-Ellis and Linden (Chap. 19). The overview by Hoen et al. (Chap. 12) covers many important yet illusive issues surrounding depression and cardiovascular disease in a balanced manner.

The ability of individuals to recuperate following stress is important, and disturbed sleep is increasingly acknowledged as both a consequence of chronic stress and a contributor to it. Chronically disturbed sleep is associated with an increased risk of developing obesity and the metabolic syndrome, and carries a worsened cardiovascular prognosis, as discussed by Åkerstedt and Perski in Chap. 14. Identifying and helping patients to manage significant sleep problems is an important aspect in the care of stressed cardiac patients.

Physical fitness is an important issue in cardiovascular prevention, and exercise programs are generally employed in cardiac rehabilitation as discussed by Saner and Burell in Chap. 18. Increasing physical activity will counteract weight gain and metabolic derangements including HPA-axis activation that may lead to diabetes and atherosclerotic disease manifestations (Chaps. 5 and 16). Increased physical fitness is also associated with an increase in vagal activity, which may reduce the risk of sudden cardiac death (Chap. 3), and attenuation of several haemostatic mechanisms which are related to arterial thrombosis (Chap. 6). Exercise may also have beneficial psychological effects and can aid in the management of anxiety and depressive symptoms in cardiac patients. However, exercise programs are difficult to implement in depressed patients, and lack of exercise is a factor contributing to the worsened prognosis of depressed cardiac patients (Chaps. 12 and 19). A very important issue is how to actually make sedentary and distressed individuals want to change their lifestyle – most patients know what to do but few do it without the proper motivation, counseling, and support. This is dealt with in several chapters.

Stress management programs have shown mixed results, as discussed in particular in Chaps. 12, 18 and 19. Psychological interventions can improve both the quality of life and the prognosis of cardiac patients. However, as discussed by Talbot-Ellis and Linden in Chap. 19, it is important – in studies and in the clinic – to focus on the right patients, i.e., not patients who are only mildly or temporarily distressed after a cardiac disease episode, and to implement multi-component and long-term treatment programs among patients with significant distress. In their extensive review and analysis of the literature on psychological treatment, they point out that studies of psychological treatment that fail to demonstrate medical benefits tend to suffer from "floor effects" (inclusion of patients who are only mildly distressed with little room for improvement), and have employed too simple and/or short-lasting interventions, and had too short follow-ups. Psychological treatment studies have also tended to be underpowered, and meta-analyses of many small studies to deal with this problem have resulted in "lumping" studies together in ways that may dilute findings because of differences in study design and interventions. Success in changing behavior is not achieved by all participants. This also dilutes the findings of trials when they are analyzed at the group level, and illustrates the problems associated with intention-to-treat vs. per protocol and subgroup analyses of clinical trials. Additionally, meta-analyses, as well as re-analyses of some large studies, suggest that success is related to the level of distress of the patient and perseverance of the program. Thus, the message in the Chapter on psychological treatment is that it works, but that the right patients should be targeted and that the interventions should be based on multidisciplinary, multi-component, and long-term efforts.

Women seem to do less well in stress management programs, and Talbot-Ellis and Linden remind us that this appears to be related to fewer referrals, lower participation rates, and poorer retention of women compared to men in these programs. Some studies show that women may not benefit at all from interventions designed to help men. However, there are also examples of successful interventions among women. Better attention to the special needs of women and more positive attitudes among physicians toward stress management are advocated in order to improve accrual and treatment results.

As noted above, increasing physical fitness is an important issue in cardiovascular prevention and rehabilitation. Saner and Burell argue in Chap. 18 that the best results are achieved with programs that integrate exercise and psychological stress management. All behavioral interventions face the barriers of non-participation and poor adherence, especially in the long term. Multidisciplinary efforts to deal with both physical and psychological aspects in the management of stress and to achieve lifestyle change are recommended. However, as discussed by Rozanski in Chap. 20, much can be achieved also in the doctor's office by identifying barriers to lifestyle change, discussing them with the patient, and supporting the patient in his/her efforts, at the same time recognizing when more intense management and involvement of other professionals in the care of the patient is needed.

Much of the evidence accrued in the field is based on observational studies, both smaller mechanistic studies and large epidemiological studies, which link various environments and phenotypes to manifestations of cardiovascular disease and its risk factors. As described in the Introduction, the possibility of confounding should always be considered in observational studies. In retrospective case–control studies, the baseline measurements may be inadequate for the control of confounding factors, whereas prospective cohort studies can include measurements needed for this reason. However, confounding by unmeasured or unknown factors cannot be adjusted for. Several authors point out that more longitudinal studies are needed to establish the sequence of events and direction of causality. Also, we feel there is a need for more high-quality clinical trials of sufficient magnitude and duration to further document the utility of psychosocial and behavioral interventions.

Publications should be complete and transparent, i.e., based on prespecified criteria which should be made available to the public in a similar manner as for clinical drug trials (in publications and/or databases such as ClinicalTrials.gov), since the awareness of problems with publication bias and selective reporting is increasing due to commercial actors and interests (see Introduction). Bias and interests in "marketing" ways to deal with medical problems are not confined to drug companies, but may also influence academic researchers since fame and funding are at stake. This does not mean that subgroup analyses and post-hoc analyses should be avoided. If clearly stated how and why they were performed, they contribute to the advancement of research by modifying hypotheses, as shown by Talbot-Ellis and Linden in the Chapter on psychological treatment.

Clearly, psychosocial factors and stress need to be addressed more seriously in patient care than is often the case today. The present knowledge, albeit not complete and not fully proven in some respects, should be better incorporated into everyday patient care and into Guidelines. Health professionals need to be informed about simple ways of identifying stress and dealing with it in everyday patient care (Chapters by Rozanski, and by Talbot-Ellis and Linden) and at workplaces (Chapters by Kivimäki et al., and by Lucini and Pagani). Clinics need to be organized so that psychosocial needs can be attended to in a multidisciplinary manner with staff of their own and/or collaborations with health care professionals who can help patients change their lifestyle and/or cope better with their stressful situations.

As pointed out by Rozanski in Chap. 20, implementation of behavioral change is a task which involves not only telling the patient what to do (stop smoking, eat better, exercise more, etc.) but also influencing the attitudes and priorities of the patient, setting realistic goals which the patient can incorporate as being his/her own goals, and following up that the goals set are gradually achieved. Factors that may adversely affect compliance need to be identified and dealt with. Simple tools to use are suggested by Talbot-Linden and by Rozanski. A key issue for success in achieving behavioral change is motivation based on autonomy, self-efficacy, and time management. A long-term perspective is needed, and persistence is enhanced by social support and feedback. Saner and Burell argue that group interventions are more efficient than individual sessions, that efforts must be focused on behavioral skills training, and that staff engaged in behavioral intervention programs need appropriate training. Differences between men and women need to be taken into account. An important factor to consider is attitudes among doctors who fail to recognize the importance of psychosocial factors or take the opportunity to attend to them. Advances in medical therapies have reduced cardiovascular morbidity and mortality in recent years, but skills in the management of psychosocial problems can further improve prevention and treatment results. We hope this book will provide some inspiration to increase both further study of the importance of stress for cardiovascular disease and better implementation of the knowledge that exists.

Index

A

Acute cardiovascular disease
  air pollution, 154
  cocaine, 154
  heavy physical exertion, 153–154
  marijuana, 154
  respiratory infection, 154
Acute coronary syndrome (ACS), 113,
    155, 173
Acute stress
  adrenaline, 48–49
  cardiac responses, 44–46
  coagulation and fibrinolysis, 99
  cortisol secretion, 41
  defense reaction, 41
  limb blood flow, 46–47
  platelet activation, 97–99
  pro-coagulant responses, 100–101
  renal blood flow, 47–48
Adenosine triphosphate (ATP), 261
Adrenaline, 34
Adrenocorticotropin hormone (ACTH), 73
Aerobic physical activity.
    See Physical activity
Allostatic systems, 290
American Association of Cardiovascular and
    Pulmonary Rehabilitation (AACPR),
    344
Angiotensin-converting enzyme (ACE), 181
ANS. *See* Autonomic nervous system (ANS)
Anti-thrombotic mechanisms
  blood coagulation and fibrinolysis, 92–93
  platelets, 90–92
Anxiety syndromes, 362

Arrythmogenic mechanisms
  ECG-derived proarrhythmic
    changes, 143
  electrical recovery, 142
  electroencephalographic study, 143
  myocardial ischaemia, 141
  stress-induced cardiac response, 143
Atherosclerosis
  activated platelets, 112
  acute coronary disease, 114–115
  CHD, 113–114
  endothelial dysfunction, 112
  fatty streak, 113
  immune function and hypertension, 115
  LDL-cholesterol, 112
  macrophages, 112
  plaque rupture, 113
Autonomic nervous system (ANS), 218, 302
Autonomic responses
  acute stress, 41–44
  adrenaline, 48–49
  cardiovascular homeostasis, 32–34
  catecholamine measurements, 36–38
  CGRP, 34
  cholinergic mechanisms, 40
  defence reaction, 31, 41
  endothelial function, 41
  limb blood flow, 46–47
  NPY, 34
  pathophysiological considerations, 49–50
  recurrent/chronic mental stress, 38–40
  renal blood flow, 47–48
  renin–angiotensin system, 40
  sympatho-adrenal system, 35–36

P. Hjemdahl et al. (eds.), *Stress and Cardiovascular Disease*,
DOI 10.1007/ 978-1-84882-419-5, © Springer-Verlag London Limited 2012

B

Baroreflex sensitiviy, 304
Beck depression inventory
    (BDI), 216
Behavioral risk factor, 384, 385
    autonomy, principle of, 368
    clinical management, 372–373
    goal execution, 367, 368
    implementation intentions, 369–370
    long-term behavioral maintenance, 372
    motivation, 367, 368
    self-efficacy, 368–369
    self-monitoring, 370
    stress and energy management,
        370–372
    time management, 369
Behavior, stress
    negative and positive responses, 306
    psychosocial coping, 307–308
    unhealthy lifestyle, 307
Blood coagulation
    methodology and biomarkers, 95
    pro-and anti-thrombotic mechanisms,
        92–93
    sympatho-adrenal activation, 97
Brain imaging
    acute stress challenges, 131
    amygdala activity, 136
    autonomic activity, 131
    baroreceptor reflex activity, 137
    blood pressure manipulations, 136
    brainstem sites, 132
    cardiovascular control, 131
    dorsal anterior cingulate cortex, 136
    ECG-derived proarrhythmic
        changes, 143
    electrical recovery, 142
    electroencephalographic
        study, 143
    fMRI, 137
    functional abnormalities, 141
    HRV measures, 135
    humoral stress responses, 143
    myocardial ischaemia, 141
    neuroimaging techniques, 130
    stress-induced cardiac response, 143
    subgenual cingulate and autonomic
        nuclei, 137
    valsalva manoeuvre, 132
Brain metabolism, 261
Brain natriuretic peptide (BNP), 179
Broken heart syndrome. See Stress
    cardiomyopathy (SCM)

C

Calcitonin gene-related peptide (CGRP), 34
Cardiac randomized evaluation
    of antidepressant and psychotherapy
        efficacy trial (CREATE), 224
Cardiac rehabilitation
    anxiety, 340
    depression, 340
    patient's gender issue, 349–350
    personality factors, 340–341
    physical fitness, 382
    quality of life, 342
    social support, 342
    stress, 341–342
Cardiovascular homeostasis
    autoregulatory mechanisms, 34
    baroreflexes, 34
    blood pressure, 33
    neuro-hormonal activity, 32
    pressor response, 33
Catecholamines, 183
Central nervous system (CNS), 72
Chronic negative thoughts, 362–364
Chronic stress
    anxiety, 103–104
    caregiving, 102
    continual stimulation, 361
    depression, 102–103
    INTERHEART case–control
        study, 362
    job stress, 101–102
    low socio-economic status, 101
    pathophysiological effects, 360
    vital exhaustion, 104
Clinician-Administered PTSD Scale
    (CAPS), 238
Cold pressor testing (CPT), 187
Comprehensive rehabilitation programs,
    321, 322
Coronary artery atherosclerosis (CAA)
    ovarian function, 20–21
    sex differences, 21–22
    social isolation, females, 22
    social reorganization, males, 19–20
    social subordination and depression,
        females, 22–24
Coronary artery bypass graft (CABG), 221
Coronary artery risk development in young
    adults (CARDIA) study, 120
Corticotropin releasing hormone, 72
C-reactive protein (CRP), 206
Cushing's syndrome (CS), 82
Cynomolgus monkeys, 17

D

Depression and coronary heart disease
  cardiac rehabilitation, 340
  cardiovascular disease, 214
  chronic psychosocial stress, 102–103
  collaborative care, 228
  confounding, 216
  diagnostic criteria DSM-IV, 214
  haemostatic effects, 102–103
  health care–related behavior, 227
  heart rate variability (HRV), 218–219
  hypothalamus-pituitary-adrenal axis, 220
  inflammation, 219
  lifestyle modification, 222
  LVEF, 216
  MDD, 214
  mechanistic pathways, 227
  mediation testing, 222
  medication adherence, 221
  meta-analyses, 215
  myocardial infarction, 382
  physical exercise, 227
  platelet function, 220
  post-MI patients, 217
  psychological treatment, 223–224
  psychosocial risk factors, 217
  screening, 226–227
  serotonin metabolism, 220–221
  social isolation, 218
  subtypes of depression, 225–226
  Type D personality, 218
  vital exhaustion, 218
Depressive disorder
  cardiac risk mechanism, 66
  coronary heart disease, 62
  sympathetic nervous and adrenaline
      secretion, 63
  sympathetic pathophysiology, 63–64
  therapy, 67
Diabetes
  metabolic syndrome (*see* Metabolic
      syndrome)
  sleep, 267

E

Electrocardiographic (ECG), 177
Energy management, 370–372
Enhancing recovery in coronary heart
      disease (ENRICHD),
      225, 347
Essential hypertension. *See* Hypertension
Estrogen therapy, 21

F

F–18 fluorodeoxyglucose (FDG), 180
Fibrinolysis
  methodology and biomarkers, 95
  pro-and anti-thrombotic mechanisms,
      92–93
  sympatho-adrenal activation, 97
Follicle-stimulating hormone (FSH), 81
Functional syndromes, 303

G

GH-releasing hormone (GHRH), 266
Glucocorticoid Receptor (GR), 75–78
Glucocorticoids
  biological effects, 78–79
  body composition, 83
  circulation and metabolism, 75
  emotional dysregulation, 84
  endocrine effects, 81–82
  endothelial function and oxidative
      stress, 83
  immune system, 82
  inflammation and tissue repair, 83–84
  intermediary metabolism
      and cardiovascular system,
      79–81
  plasma lipoprotein and carbohydrate
      metabolism, 83
  transcriptional regulation
      and activation, 78
Gonadotropin releasing hormone
      (GnRH), 81
G protein–coupled receptor kinase 5
      (GRK5), 187

H

Haemostatic effects
  acute stress, 97–101
  anxiety, 103–104
  arterial thrombosis, 89
  caregiving, 102
  depression, 102–103
  job stress, 101–102
  low socio-economic status, 101
  methodology and biomarkers, 93–95
  pathways and (patho)physiological
      process, 90
  pro-and anti-thrombotic
      mechanisms, 90–93
  sympatho-adrenal activation, 96–97
  vital exhaustion, 104

Health belief model, 328
Heart rate variability, 36, 302
High-quality studies
    Kuopio ischemic heart disease risk factor
        study, 204
    long-term exposure, 204–206
    Malmö diet and cancer (MDC) study, 203
    work, lipids, fibrinogen (WOLF) Stock-
        holm study, 203
Hypertension
    aversive stressors, 278–279
    epidemiological studies, 277
    experimental models, 276
    neurogenic hypertension, 283
    personality characteristics, patients, 277
    public policy implementation, 278
    renin-angiotensin system, 280–281
    sleep, 265–266
    stress biological markers, 280
    stress-induced hypertension, 276
    sympathetic nervous system, 281–282
Hypothalamic-pituitary-adrenal (HPA) axis
    biological effects, 78–79
    body composition, 83
    circulation and metabolism, 75
    CV risk factors, 82
    emotional dysregulation, 84
    endocrine effects, 81–82
    endothelial function and oxidative
        stress, 83
    immune system, 82
    inflammation and tissue repair, 83–84
    intermediary metabolism and cardiovascular
        system, 79–81
    plasma lipoprotein and carbohydrate me-
        tabolism, 83
    stress response, 73–74
    stress system, 72–73
    transcriptional regulation and activation, 78

I
I-metaiodobenzyl-guanidine (I-MIBG), 181
Immune system, 267–268
Inflammation
    activated platelets, 112
    acute coronary disease, 114–115
    ambulatory blood pressure monitoring, 117
    aspirin, 117
    cardiovascular disease, 122–123
    CHD, 113–114
    endothelial dysfunction, 112
    fatty streak, 113
    hostility, 117

IL–6 and fibrinogen, 118
IL–1β gene expression, 116
immune function and hypertension, 115
LDL-cholesterol, 112
macrophages, 112
plaque rupture, 113
population studies, 120–122
psychophysiological/mental stress
    testing, 116
Insomnia, 264–265
INTERHEART study, 199–200
Ischemic heart disease life stress monitoring
    (IHDLSM) program, 345, 346

L
Left ventricular ejection fraction (LVEF), 216
Lifestyle hypertension, 283
Light transmittance aggregometry (LTA), 93
Locus ceruleus (LC), 72
Low density lipoprotein (LDL), 112

M
Major depressive disorder (MDD), 213
Metabolic syndrome
    caloric imbalance, 289
    characteristics, 288
    cross-sectional studies, 291–292
    definition, 288, 289
    drug treatment studies, 289
    obesity (see Obesity)
    prospective studies, 293–294
    psychosocial factors, 292
    risk factors, 288
    Whitehall II study, 291–292
M-HART program, 346
MIND-IT study, 224
Multicenter investigation of limitation of
        infarct size (MILIS), 152
Multi-ethnic study of atherosclerosis
        (MESA), 121
Muscle sympathetic nerve activity
        (MSNA), 137
Myocardial infarction (MI)
    depression, 382
    psychological treatment, 338
    risk factors, 240–241

N
Negative emotions, 362–364
Neural systems
    amygdala activity, 136

autonomic activity, 131
baroreceptor reflex activity, 137
blood pressure manipulations, 136
brainstem sites, 132
cardiovascular control, 131
dorsal anterior cingulate cortex, 136
fMRI, 137
HRV measures, 135
valsalva manoeuvre, 132
Neurogenic hypertension, 283
Neuropeptide Y (NPY), 34
Noradrenaline transporter (NET), 61
Nucleus of the solitary tract (NTS), 136

O
Obesity
allostatic systems, 290
animal studies, 291
mechanism and experimental studies, 291
methodological problems, 290
risk factors, 290
sleep, 267
Obstructive sleep apnea, 265

P
Panic disorder
adrenaline co-transmission, 60–61
cardiac risk mechanism, 65–66
epinephrine, 62
myocardial infarction and sudden death, 59
neuronal noradrenaline re-uptake, 61–62
single-fibre firings, 60
sympathetic nervous and adrenaline
secretion, 59
sympathetic pathophysiology, 63–64
therapy, 67
Paraventricular nucleus (PVN), 72
Periaqueductal grey matter (PAG), 132
Phenylethanolamine methytransferase
(PNMT), 61
Phospholamban (PLN), 186
Physical activity
all-cause mortality, 320
blood pressure, 321
clinical indications, 323
comprehensive rehabilitation programs,
321, 322
ENRICHD trial, 327
health belief model, 328
hemostatic mechanisms, 320
lifestyle factors, 320
meta analysis, 322

myocardial ischemia, 320
nonfatal myocardial infarction, 322
psychological and social conditions, 322
psychological problems, 325–326
psychophysiological responses, 324–325
psychosocial risk factors, 323–324
RCPP trial, 327
self-monitoring techniques, 329
stress management programs, 326
SUPRIM program, 327
transtheoretical model, 328
Platelets
function, 93–95
pro-and anti-thrombotic mechanisms, 90–92
sympatho-adrenal activation, 96
Positive emotions, 363
Positron emission tomography (PET), 130
Post-traumatic stress disorder (PTSD)
antipsychotics, 252
atherothrombotic risk, 247–250
benzodiazepines, 253
beta blockers, 253
CAPS, 238
cardiac patients, 251
cardiovascular endpoints, 242–244
CHD, 251
definition, 238
diagnostic criteria, 239
inflammatory markers, 246
interventions, 252
pathways and mechanisms, 245–246
prevalence, 239–240
preventive strategies, 252
primary care PTSD screen instrument, 252
randomized controlled trials, 253
risk factors, MI, 240–241
smoking, 251
SSRIs, 252
sympathetic nervous system activation, 246
symptoms, 245
trauma-focused cognitive behavioral
therapy, 252
venlafaxine, 253
Proinflammatory cytokines, 267
Pro-thrombotic mechanisms
blood coagulation and fibrinolysis, 92–93
platelets, 90–92
Psychological stress
allostatic load, 3
animal research, 5–6
behavioural methods, 5
biological stress response, 4
cardiovascular disease, 2
clinical research, 10–11

Psychological stress (*cont.*)
  cortisol, 7
  epidemiological studies, 8–9
  experimental designs, 6
  glucocorticoids, 3
  homeostasis, 3
  laboratory stress testing, 7
  naturalistic and ambulatory monitoring, 8
  prevention and treatment, 11
  psychosocial stimuli, 6
  stressful stimuli, 3
Psychological treatment
  American Association of Cardiovascular
    and Pulmonary Rehabilitation, 344
  behavioral factors, 338
  cardiac rehabilitation (*see* Cardiac reha-
    bilitation)
  complex pathways, 338–339
  comprehensive meta-analyses, 348
  cumulative effects, 338
  effective emotional management, 343
  ENRICHD, 347
  Goldberg's General Health Questionnaire, 346
  individual odds ratios, 339
  INTERHEART study, 338
  Ischemic Heart Disease Life Stress
    Monitoring Program, 345
  M-HART program, 346
  myocardial infarction, 338
  recommendations, 351–352
  Type-A behavior, 345
Psychological triggers
  absolute risk, 162
  acute cardiovascular disease, 152
  acute depression, 155
  anger, 154–155, 161
  anxiety, 155, 161
  bereavement, 155, 161
  MILIS, 152
  pathophysiology, 157–158
  plaque vulnerability, 158–159
  population stressors, 156–157, 161–162
  possible triggers, 153
  terminology, 152
  triggered acute risk protection, 159
  work-related stress, 155–156
Psychoneurocardiology
  methods, 56
  sympathetic nerve biology, 56–57
Psychosocial risk factors, 384, 385
  behavioral risk factor (*see* Behavioral risk
    factor)

behavioral risk factor (*see* Behavioral risk
    factor)(continued)
  chronic negative thoughts and emotions,
    362–364
  chronic stress, 360–362
  psychological needs, 365
  reduction strategies, 359
  rest and relaxation, 366
Psychosocial work factors
  confounding, 206–207
  coronary heart disease, 208
  high-quality papers, 202–204
  INTERHEART study, 199–200
  meta-analysis, 201–202
  risk factors, 206
  theoretical models, 198–199

Q
Quality of life, 342

R
Randomized controlled trials (RCT), 11, 380
Rapid eye movement (REM), 260
Recurrent coronary prevention project, 345
Renin–angiotensin–aldosterone (RAAS), 34
Rest and relaxation (R&R), 366
Restless legs syndrome, 265

S
Selective serotonin reuptake inhibitors
  (SSRIs), 252
Sertraline heart attack randomized trial
  (SADHART), 224
Single photon emission tomography
  (SPET), 130
Sleep
  brain metabolism, 261
  CHD morbidity and mortality, 268–269
  circadian influences, 261–262
  definition, 260
  development, 260
  diabetes, 267
  endocrine effects, 266
  homeostatic regulation, 261
  hypertension, 265–266
  immune system, 267–268
  implications, physicians, 269
  insomnia, 264–265
  obesity, 267

obstructive sleep apnea, 265
periodic limb movements, 265
polysomnography, 260
rapid eye movement, 260
restless legs syndrome, 265
sleep disturbances, 259
stress, 262–264
Slow wave sleep (SWS), 260
Social stress
atherogenesis and CHD, 24–25
CAA and CHD risk, 17–18
low social status, 18–19
ovarian function, 20–21
sex differences, 21–22
social isolation, females, 22
social reorganization, males, 19–20
social strangers, 18
social subordination and depression,
females, 22–24
visceral fat deposition, 25–26
Socio economic status (SES), 117
Stress biological markers, 280
Stress cardiomyopathy (SCM)
acute emotional/physical trigger, 175, 177
cardiac MRI, 180
catecholamines, 172
clinical characteristics, 176
coronary thrombosis/acute plaque
rupture, 179
diagnostic criteria, 177
ECG, 177–179
endothelial dysfunction, 187
epicardial spasm, 184–185
genetic determinants, 187–188
hormonal influence, 186
I-MIBG imaging, 181
intraventricular obstruction, 185
microvascular dysfunction, 185
mood disorders and antidepressant use,
187
myocyte effects, 185–186
patient demographics and clinical
presentation, 175
PET, 180
plaque rupture, 183–184
prevalence, 173–174
prognosis and recurrence, 182
treatment, 181–182
ventricular ballooning, 179–180
ventricular systolic function,
recovery of, 180
Stress management

autoregressive spectral analysis,
304–306
behavior (see Behavior, stress)
behavioral risk factor, 370–372
chronic negative consequences, 302
clinical and social attention, 303
definition, 302
functional syndromes, 303
models, 302
multidimensional approach, 303
physical symptoms, 303
regulatory systems, 302
somatic symptom, 303
therapeutic approaches, 303
worksite intervention (see Worksite
intervention)
Stress management programs, 383
Subcutaneous abdominal tissue
(SAT), 26
Suprachiasmatic nuclei (SCN), 261
Sympathetic neural and adrenal medullary
mechanisms
cardiac risk mechanism, 64–67
depressive illness, 62–63
panic disorder, 57–62
pathophysiology, 63–64
psychoneurocardiology, 55–57
Sympatho-adrenal activation
β-blockade, 36
blood coagulation and fibrinolysis, 97
catecholamines, 35
HRV, 36
noradrenaline, 35
platelets, 96
radiotracer infusion technique, 36

T

Takotsubo cardiomyopathy. See Stress
cardiomyopathy (SCM)
Thrombolysis in myocardial infarction
(TIMI), 185
Thyroid stimulating hormone (TSH), 81
Transient left ventricular apical ballooning
syndrome. See Stress
cardiomyopathy (SCM)
Triggered acute risk protection therapy
beta-adrenergic blocking drugs, 160
medications, 160
Triggers and mechanisms of myocardial
infarction (TRIMM), 153
Triglyceride (TG), 83

V
Valsalva manoeuvre, 132
Vasoconstriction, 158
Visceral adipose tissue (VAT), 26
Von Willebrand factor (VWF), 91

W
Women's Ischemia Syndrome Evaluation
    (WISE) study, 122
Worksite intervention
    components, 313
    economic and social
        consequences, 309

lifestyle intervention and
    modification, 314
mental health problems, 308
multidimensional approach, 310
organizational structures, 308
psychological and physiological
    parameters, 311
relaxation technique, 312, 314
somatic symptoms, 308
stress assessment, 309–310